Navigating Black Maternal Mental Health and Well-Being

Rahmatu Kassimu
Dr. K.'s Health Minute, USA

Elizabeth Wachira
East Texas A&M University, Commerce, USA

IGI Global
Scientific Publishing
Publishing Tomorrow's Research Today

Vice President of Editorial Melissa Wagner
Director of Acquisitions Mikaela Felty
Director of Book Development Jocelynn Hessler
Production Manager Mike Brehm
Cover Design Jose Rosado

Published in the United States of America by
IGI Global Scientific Publishing
701 East Chocolate Avenue
Hershey, PA, 17033, USA
Tel: 717-533-8845 | Fax: 717-533-7115
Website: https://www.igi-global.com E-mail: cust@igi-global.com

Library of Congress Cataloging-in-Publication Data

Names: Kassimu, Rahmatu, 1987- editor. | Wachira, Elizabeth, 1986- editor.
Title: Navigating Black maternal mental health and well-being / edited by Rahmatu Kassimu, Elizabeth Wachira.
Description: Hershey, PA : Medical Information Science Reference, [2026] | Includes bibliographical references and index. | Summary: "This groundbreaking textbook aims to explore and address the multifaceted landscape of Black Maternal Mental Health, delving into critical topics such as cultural competence, trauma-informed care, and the intersectionality of race, gender, and socioeconomic factors"-- Provided by publisher.
Identifiers: LCCN 2024038901 (print) | LCCN 2024038902 (ebook) | ISBN 9798369342725 (h/c) | ISBN 9798369376508 (s/c) | ISBN 9798369342732 (eISBN)
Subjects: LCSH: African American mothers--Mental health--Textbooks. | African American mothers--Mental health services--Textbooks. | African American women--Mental health--Textbooks. | African American women--Mental health services--Textbooks.
Classification: LCC RC451.4.M58 N38 2024 (print) | LCC RC451.4.M58 (ebook) | DDC 616.890082--dc23/eng/20241114
LC record available at https://lccn.loc.gov/2024038901
LC ebook record available at https://lccn.loc.gov/2024038902
British Cataloguing in Publication Data
A Cataloguing in Publication record for this book is available from the British Library.

Table of Contents

Detailed Table of Contents

to address racism and bias, culturally competent care, and tailored interventions for improved outcomes. This serves as a valuable resource for healthcare professionals, policymakers, researchers, and advocates seeking to understand, address, and ultimately empower Black mothers in their maternal mental health journey.

This chapter examines the critical issue of improving maternal mental health for Black birthing parents through postpartum caregiver services. The purpose of this chapter is to highlight the significance of maternal mental health, particularly among Black birthing parents who face unique challenges and disparities in healthcare. The chapter explores the impact of postpartum care and caregiver services on mitigating mental health disparities and improving maternal health outcomes. Key topics include postpartum depression, health equity, cultural competence, and the importance of community and social support networks. Additionally, the chapter discusses mental health interventions and the role of Black maternal health organizations in advocating for better healthcare access and outcomes for Black birthing parents. Through an analysis of current practices and recommendations, this chapter aims to provide a comprehensive understanding of the strategies needed to enhance maternal mental health and ensure equitable and culturally competent postpartum care.

Perinatal loss is a profoundly emotional and life-altering experience for families. Black women face this loss disproportionately due to systemic inequities, racism, and socioeconomic challenges. This chapter seeks to honor and understand the unique experiences of Black women navigating perinatal bereavement, exploring how race, class, and gender intersect to create disparities in healthcare access and quality. It also highlights the additional layers of trauma many Black women endure. The author advocates for trauma-informed, culturally sensitive care that centers on safety, trust, and collaboration. Key strategies include empowering women in decision-making, embracing culturally affirming practices, and fostering supportive community connections. Guided by Womanist theory, this chapter offers practical tools to address inequities and create holistic and healing care. It encourages healthcare providers to adopt policies and practices that prioritize equity and compassion, creating a pathway to healing, resilience, and hope for Black women and their families.

"Echoes of Black Birth: Trauma Family Dynamics and the Path to Policy Solutions" looks at the experiences of Black people who have given birth, considering historical and modern factors. Jennifer Rutledge Pettie shows how systemic healthcare inequities harm Black families.Within the context of modern healthcare, this study examines the effects of medical racism and segregation. Medical racism is a critical issue since it prevents individuals from accessing healthcare. This chapter advocates for widespread changes to current systems after examining their detrimental impact on Black pregnant individuals. The prevalence of birth trauma is extensive, and it can have lasting consequences for one's psychological well-being and familial connections. Empirical evidence and anecdotal accounts substantiate this claim. This chapter presents several policy reforms aimed at improving maternal health, via establishment of robust social support systems, implementation of reproductive justice initiatives, and provision of culturally appropriate healthcare services.

Preface

Black maternal mental health is an urgent public health, cultural, and human rights issue that demands our focused attention. As editors of this volume, *Navigating Black Maternal Mental Health and Well-Being*, we are honored to bring together a collective of scholars, health professionals, and community advocates who explore the deep-rooted, multi-layered challenges facing Black mothers across diverse contexts. The impetus for this book stems from a shared recognition that current systems, medical, social, and policy, continue to fail Black birthing people, not by chance, but by design. These failures are the legacies of slavery, reproductive coercion, institutionalized racism, and decades of silencing and exclusion. Our goal is not only to examine these patterns but to amplify the work of those carving out new spaces for healing, justice, and systemic transformation.

Across the United States and beyond, Black women endure disproportionate rates of maternal morbidity and mortality, and equally distressing mental health challenges during the perinatal period. These disparities are neither isolated nor accidental. They are the result of chronic stress, inadequate care, systemic neglect, and cultural erasure. This book brings these dynamics to the forefront through contributions that span historical analysis, clinical research, community engagement, and personal advocacy. We center voices that are too often marginalized in academic literature—voices that speak to the lived realities of Black women navigating pregnancy, parenting, mental health, grief, trauma, and resilience in a world shaped by racialized healthcare structures.

As editors, one a scholar-practitioner in health promotion and the other a maternal health advocate and public health expert, we approached this project with deep care, urgency, and intentionality. We sought authors whose work is grounded in cultural competence, bioethics, intersectionality, and justice. Each chapter explores a facet of Black maternal mental health that deserves greater visibility: from perinatal anxiety and depression, to bereavement care, policy failures, coping strategies, and the powerful role of male partners and community networks. The book is designed not only as an academic resource but also as a call to action, for healthcare providers, policymakers, researchers, educators, doulas, and, most importantly, Black mothers and families themselves.

Chapter 1: Unraveling the Social Determinants of Black Maternal Health: A Comprehensive Exploration

This chapter explores how historical injustices and entrenched systemic racism continue to shape the maternal health outcomes of Black women in the United States. Arika Wiggins outlines how intersecting social determinants, including socioeconomic status, racial discrimination, healthcare inequities, and chronic stress, contribute to disparities in Black maternal health. The chapter calls for a multidimensional response that centers racial equity and supports culturally grounded, community-based care initiatives as a path toward sustainable systemic change.

Chapter 2: Navigating Black Maternal Mental Health and Wellbeing: Perinatal Anxiety and Depression in Black Mothers

Mercedes Moore delves into the roots of Black maternal mental health disparities, linking reproductive oppression under slavery to ongoing medical racism today. The chapter focuses on perinatal mood and anxiety disorders (PMADs) among Black mothers, emphasizing how these conditions are worsened by socioeconomic disadvantage, stigma, and lack of culturally competent care. It argues for an urgent overhaul of healthcare systems to better support Black mothers through tailored mental health resources and equitable birth practices.

Chapter 3: Prevalent Forms of Mental Health Issues and Coping Strategies Amongst Black Women

This chapter reviews the most common mental health challenges faced by Black women during the peripartum and postpartum periods, such as depression and anxiety. Najla Abdalla highlights the culturally relevant coping strategies employed by Black women to maintain their mental well-being and evaluates the effectiveness of current interventions. The chapter offers recommendations for healthcare professionals to adopt more responsive and culturally informed approaches to improve outcomes.

Chapter 4: Perinatal Anxiety and Depression in Black Mothers

In this follow-up exploration, Mercedes Moore expands on how historical trauma, especially reproductive exploitation during slavery, continues to reverberate in the modern treatment of Black mothers. The chapter underscores alarming statistics, such as a 40% rate of postpartum depression among Black women, and critiques the myth that privilege or access shields Black women from adverse outcomes. Moore advocates for radically reimagined healthcare systems that are explicitly designed with Black maternal well-being at the center.

Chapter 5: You Good, Sis? Analyzing the Role of Individual and Interpersonal Factors on Mental Health in Former Teenage Mothers of Color

This chapter examines how former teenage mothers of color navigate mental health challenges through the lens of Life Course Theory. The authors analyze how factors like maternal self-efficacy, emotional support, coping mechanisms, and racism-related stress impact long-term mental health. Their findings suggest that while individual resilience is vital, addressing systemic inequities and enhancing interpersonal support is equally crucial to improving outcomes for women of color who experienced early motherhood.

Chapter 6: The Maternal Mental Health of Black Women Working

Jennifer Edwards sheds light on the unique mental health burdens faced by Black women in the workforce who are pregnant or parenting. The chapter argues that the professional success of Black mothers is inseparable from their maternal mental health and urges workplaces to adopt diversity, equity, inclusion, and belonging (DEIB) strategies that address this intersection. Recommendations include redesigning benefits packages, offering flexible schedules, and fostering environments that actively support maternal well-being.

Chapter 7: Addressing Maternal Mental Health Trauma in Black and Brown Communities: A Culturally Competent and Bioethical Approach

This chapter integrates bioethical principles with culturally competent care to examine how systemic racism and structural inequities affect the mental health of Black and Brown birthing people. The authors analyze the ethical implications of disparities in diagnosis, treatment, and policy while focusing on tools such as the Edinburgh Postnatal Depression Scale. By emphasizing autonomy, justice, and beneficence, the chapter calls for healthcare reforms that uphold ethical responsibility and promote equitable maternal mental health care.

Chapter 8: Community-Based Approaches to Black Maternal Mental Health

Aliyu Tijani Jibril advocates for a shift from institutional to community-centered solutions in addressing Black maternal mental health disparities. Highlighting the failures of universal screening, structural racism, and inadequate treatment access, the chapter proposes culturally responsive interventions rooted in local knowledge and support systems. It offers practical policy recommendations to empower Black communities and healthcare workers alike in fostering a more equitable and inclusive maternal care environment.

Chapter 9: Improving Maternal Mental Health for Black Birthing Parents Through Postpartum Caregiver Services

This chapter discusses the transformative potential of postpartum caregiver services in mitigating the mental health disparities experienced by Black birthing parents. Chinonye Egbulem emphasizes the importance of community-based support, culturally competent care, and mental health interventions tailored to the unique needs of Black parents. The chapter also spotlights the role of maternal health organizations in advocating for equitable access and concludes with strategies to integrate postpartum support into mainstream healthcare systems.

Chapter 10: Transforming Perinatal Bereavement Care: Centering Trauma-Informed and Culturally Competent Practices for Black Women

Solimar Santiago-Warner addresses the often-overlooked experience of perinatal loss among Black women, emphasizing how intersecting oppressions intensify grief and trauma. Guided by Womanist theory, the chapter advocates for trauma-informed, culturally affirming care practices that prioritize trust, autonomy, and emotional safety. It offers practical recommendations for providers and systems to create supportive, healing environments that recognize the profound and unique impact of perinatal bereavement in Black communities.

Chapter 11: Echoes of Black Birth: Trauma Family Dynamics and the Path to Policy Solutions

This closing chapter takes a policy-focused lens to examine how medical racism, family trauma, and systemic neglect intersect to shape the experiences of Black birthing people. Jennifer Rutledge Pettie combines empirical evidence with personal narratives to advocate for reproductive justice, robust support systems, and culturally appropriate care. The chapter offers a roadmap for policy reforms that can address trauma at both the individual and structural levels, with the goal of transforming maternal health outcomes for Black families.

We are proud that this collection spans a range of perspectives and geographic contexts. Some authors write from inside the academy, while others come from community practice or advocacy spaces. Together, they illustrate that the crisis of Black maternal mental health cannot be solved in isolation, it requires a sustained, multi-sectoral, and justice-centered approach. From systemic inequities in healthcare access to the impacts of perinatal mood disorders, the chapters probe the question: What does it mean to birth and mother while Black in today's world? And how can we move from survival to thriving, from fragmented care to holistic well-being?

Crucially, the chapters also highlight resilience, innovation, and the cultural strengths of Black motherhood. Whether exploring trauma-informed bereavement care or the role of family dynamics, the contributors emphasize that change is possible, and is already happening, in the hands of those who dare to reimagine care. The solutions shared in this book range from policy reform and institutional accountability to grassroots, community-based interventions and culturally tailored mental health services. We believe these approaches hold immense promise for healing and transformation when grounded in cultural humility, compassion, and equity.

In closing, we dedicate this volume to the Black mothers, birthing people, and families who continue to resist, rebuild, and rise in the face of historical and ongoing injustice. We hope that *Navigating Black Maternal Mental Health and Well-Being* serves as a resource, a mirror, and a movement-builder. May it empower readers to advocate, listen, and lead. May it challenge institutions to do better—and be better. And may it inspire each of us to create systems of care where Black lives, births, and mental health are fully valued, protected, and celebrated.

Chapter 1

Unraveling the Social Determinants of Black Maternal Health:
A Comprehensive Exploration

Arika Y. Wiggins
https://orcid.org/0009-0007-3907-5332
Southeast Missouri State University, USA

ABSTRACT

Black women in the United States continue to face persistent inequities in maternal health outcomes, which are influenced by a myriad of social variables. Starting with a historical context of slavery and systemic racism, this chapter examines the socioeconomic factors, racial discrimination, healthcare access and quality, and the role of chronic stress in shaping the lived experiences and health outcomes of Black mothers. It emphasizes the need for a comprehensive approach that addresses the intersectionality of race, socioeconomic status, and gender in order to improve Black maternal health. The concluding section of the chapter underscores the significance of collective endeavors by community leaders, policymakers, and healthcare providers. To work towards eliminating systemic obstacles, the recommendation is to advance racial equity and allocate resources towards community-based initiatives that offer Black mothers culturally appropriate support and care.

DOI: 10.4018/979-8-3693-4272-5.ch001

THE PERSISTENT ISSUE: RACIAL DISPARITIES IN MATERNAL HEALTH OUTCOMES

The concept of social determinants of health recognizes that an individual's health outcomes are influenced by a complex interplay of factors beyond medical care including socioeconomic status, education, housing, and access to resources (Marmot & Allen, 2014). For Black women, the social determinants of health are deeply rooted in the legacy of slavery, systemic racism, and ongoing discrimination (Bailey et al., 2017). Understanding and addressing these social determinants is crucial for improving Black maternal health outcomes and achieving health equity.

Black women in the United States face a disproportionate burden of adverse maternal health outcomes as compared to their white counterparts. Racial disparities in maternal morbidity and death continue to exist, despite advancements in medical technology and overall enhancements in maternal health (Petersen et al., 2019). The reasons for these discrepancies are diverse and multifaceted, covering a wide range of social, economic, and environmental factors that impact the health and well-being of Black women (Crear-Perry et al., 2021). This chapter provides an exploration of the social determinants of Black maternal health, examining the historical context, current challenges, and potential interventions to address this critical public health issue.

A HISTORICAL CONTEXT

Before understanding the disparities in Black maternal health, it is essential to recognize the historical context of slavery and its ongoing effects on Black women's health and wellbeing. Black women endured inhumane treatment during the era of slavery, which included forced labor, sexual exploitation, and medical experimentation (Washington, 2006). Generations of health disparities were caused by the denial of fundamental human rights and the absence of bodily autonomy. (Owens & Fett, 2019).

Black women's experiences were nonetheless shaped by discriminatory laws and practices even after slavery was abolished. The marginalization of Black communities was sustained by Jim Crow Laws, redlining, and other institutionalized racism practices, which also restricted their access to high-quality healthcare, education, and employment prospects (Bailey et al., 2017). These historical injustices have significantly influenced the social factors affecting the health of Black women, leading to persistent inequities in maternal health outcomes.

In the early 20th century, the eugenics movement further exacerbated the mistreatment of Black women in healthcare settings. Eugenicists, who promoted the notion that some racial and ethnic groups were genetically inferior, subjected Black women to forced sterilizations and other forms of reproductive injustice (Roberts, 1997). The enduring impact of these past traumas continues to influence Black women' experiences and health outcomes in the present, as they navigate a healthcare system historically characterized by racism and prejudice (Prather et al., 2018).

ACCESS TO QUALITY HEALTHCARE

One of the primary social determinants of Black maternal health is access to quality healthcare. Receiving prompt and proper prenatal care is crucial for diagnosing and managing potential issues during pregnancy. However, Black women frequently encounter considerable hurdles accessing this care (Gadson et al., 2017). Challenges related to healthcare access are exacerbated in underserved communities due to factors such as shortage of healthcare providers, transportation constraints, and lack of insurance coverage (Howell, 2018).

Furthermore, Black women frequently experience prejudice and discrimination from healthcare professionals when they do receive medical care. Studies have shown that healthcare professionals are more likely to dismiss or underestimate the pain and symptoms reported by African American and Black patients, leading to delayed diagnoses and inadequate treatment (Hoffman et al., 2016). Scenarios such as these are known as implicit bias. This type of bias can lead to severe consequences for the health of Black mothers, as it may impede the detection and treatment of critical conditions such as preeclampsia and hemorrhage (Howell et al., 2018).

To address these disparities, it is crucial to implement policies and interventions that improve access to quality healthcare for Black women. This includes expanding insurance coverage, increasing the diversity of healthcare providers, and providing cultural competency training to reduce implicit bias (Howell et al., 2018). Additionally, community-based programs that offer maternal education, support, and resources for women of color can help bridge the gap in access to care and promote better health results (Tandon et al., 2013).

Case Study One: Tamara's Challenges With Finding Quality Maternal Healthcare

Tamara, a 28-year-old Black woman, lives in a rural area and works part-time as a home health aide. She is pregnant with her third child, she is concerned about symptoms she is having that she did not experience during her other pregnancies, and she is concerned about receiving quality prenatal care to ensure a healthy pregnancy and birth. Tamara has faced the following challenges related to accessing quality maternal healthcare:

1. Limited Healthcare Providers: In Tamara's rural town, there is a shortage of healthcare providers, particularly those who specialize in obstetrics and gynecology. The nearest obstetrics care is 50 miles away, and public transportation is not readily available if needed.
2. Inadequate Health Insurance Coverage: The company that Tamara works for does not provide health insurance benefits for part-time employees, and her part-time employment status prevents her from qualifying for Medicaid. She is having difficulty with locating reasonably priced healthcare providers that offer the necessary prenatal care.
3. Discrimination and Implicit Bias: When Tamara does secure an appointment with a healthcare provider, she experiences discriminatory treatment. The provider demonstrates a lack of interest in addressing her inquiries and appears to disregard her concerns. Tamara perceives that her pain and symptoms are not taken seriously, which is a regular occurrence for Black female patients in medical environments.
4. Lack of Cultural Competency: The healthcare providers that Tamara has encountered do not have knowledge of cultural and social diversity and fail to consider her unique cultural background and experiences as a Black woman living in a rural community. The absence of the provider's cultural competency hinders effective communication and trust between Tamara and her medical providers.
5. Limited Access to Specialty Care: Tamara ends up developing gestational diabetes during her pregnancy. She encounters difficulties in obtaining the required specialized medical care and treatment for her condition due to the scarcity of healthcare resources in her area and inadequate insurance coverage. Additionally, the diversity-related communication issues that Tamara experienced with her primary prenatal provider further compounds her challenges in accessing appropriate care.

The Outcome

Tamara's prenatal treatment ends up being inconsistent due to the hurdles she experienced with attempting to receive adequate healthcare. She misses important visits and does not obtain timely treatment for her gestational diabetes. As a result, Tamara experiences difficulties during her pregnancy, including pre-eclampsia, which remains undiscovered until she develops severe symptoms and is taken to the emergency room. She has an emergency cesarean section and delivers a premature baby who requires extensive care in the Neonatal Intensive Care Unit (NICU).

Reflective Overview

Tamara's experience highlights the critical role that access to quality healthcare plays in maternal health outcomes for Black women. The absence of accessible, affordable, and culturally competent healthcare services in Tamara's rural area caused significant obstacles to receiving sufficient prenatal care. The difficulties she experienced were heightened by the unconscious bias that she encountered from her healthcare providers, which resulted in the delay of diagnosis and treatment of severe conditions.

Tamara's story emphasizes the necessity of structural adjustments to increase Black women's access to high-quality healthcare, especially for those living in underserved areas. Addressing these disparities requires a multifaceted approach that includes increasing the number of available healthcare providers, extending insurance coverage, and offering cultural competency training. Furthermore, supporting patient-centered care models that give special consideration to the needs and experiences of Black women is crucial to improving maternal health outcomes.

SOCIOECONOMIC FACTORS

Socioeconomic status is another significant social determinant of Black maternal health, as it influences access to resources, education, and opportunities that shape health outcomes. Poverty is associated with a range of health risks including inadequate nutrition, chronic stress, and limited access to preventive care (Mehra et al., 2019). Poverty disproportionately affects Black women, who comprise nearly one-fourth of the population residing below the poverty line (National Partnership for Women & Families, 2023).

The intersection of race and socioeconomic status creates unique challenges for Black mothers. Black women continue to have greater rates of maternal morbidity and mortality than White women, even after adjusting for income and education (Petersen et al., 2019). This implies that the combined effects of racism and discrimination, in conjunction with socioeconomic disadvantage, elevate the vulnerability of Black mothers to unfavorable health consequences (Gavin et al., 2005).

Addressing socioeconomic disparities necessitates a comprehensive approach that includes policies to alleviate poverty, enhance access to education and career opportunities, and offer assistance for Black families (Mehra et al., 2019). Furthermore, healthcare professionals must acknowledge the influence of socioeconomic factors on health outcomes and deliver culturally sensitive care that is tailored to the specific needs of Black mothers (Howell et al., 2018).

Case Study Two: The Impact of Socioeconomic Status on Maya's Maternal Health

Maya is a 24-year-old African American single mother who lives in an urban, low-income neighborhood. To make ends meet and support her 2-year-old son, she works two part-time jobs as a cashier and a waitress. Maya recently found out that she is pregnant with her second child, and endures the following challenges that are related to socioeconomic factors:

1. Low Income and Financial Strain: Maya struggles to earn a living wage despite working two jobs. Her limited income makes it difficult to afford basic necessities such as nutritious food, secure housing, and quality childcare. Ultimately, the constant financial strain takes a toll on her physical health and mental well-being.
2. Food Insecurity: Since Maya lives in a food desert, she has limited access to fresh and nutritious foods. She primarily relies on convenience stores and fast-food restaurants for her meals, which are typically excessive in calories and lacking key nutrients. The inadequate quality of her diet puts her at risk of obesity and related complications during her pregnancy.
3. Inadequate Housing: Maya and her son live in a small, crowded apartment that is in a poorly maintained building. The apartment has issues with mold, pests, and inadequate ventilation, which can cause respiratory problems and increase the risk of allergies and infections.
4. Limited Access to Transportation: Maya does not own a car and relies on public transportation to commute to her jobs and access healthcare services. The unreliable and time-consuming nature of public transportation makes it difficult for her to attend prenatal check-ups and other important appointments on a regular basis.
5. Lack of Paid Family Leave: Now pregnant with her second child, Maya realizes that neither of her part-time jobs offers paid family leave. She is forced to continue working long hours throughout her pregnancy to maintain a stable income, which increases her risk of stress-related complications and limits her ability to attend prenatal care visits.

The Outcome

Due to the cumulative impact of these socioeconomic factors, Maya experiences numerous challenges throughout her pregnancy. She develops anemia due to poor nutrition and is diagnosed with gestational hypertension during her third trimester. Maya's demanding work schedule and lack of paid leave prevent her from attending all of her recommended prenatal check-ups, leading to delayed interventions for her conditions. Consequently, Maya goes into preterm labor at 35 weeks, and gives birth to a baby with low birth weight who has a short stay in the neonatal intensive care unit.

Reflective Overview

Maya's story illustrates how socioeconomic status can significantly influence maternal health outcomes for Black women. The combination of low income, food insecurity, inadequate housing, limited transportation, and lack of paid family leave creates a complex puzzle of barriers that hinder access to quality prenatal care and increases the risk of adverse pregnancy outcomes. A comprehensive strategy is required to address these socioeconomic disparities. Policies that promote affordable housing, living wages, access to nutritious food, dependable transportation, and paid family leave are all components. By improving the socioeconomic conditions for Black women, communities can work towards reducing maternal health inequities and promoting better outcomes for Black mothers and their children.

CHRONIC STRESS AND RACISM

Chronic stress and exposure to racism are significant social determinants of Black maternal health. Due to the combined effects of socioeconomic hardship, marginalization, and discrimination, Black women experience a disproportionate amount of stress (Geronimus et al., 2006). This prolonged stress can significantly affect both mental and physical health, raising the risk of illnesses such as depression, diabetes, and hypertension. (Black et al., 2009).

Research has shown that experiences of racism and discrimination, both interpersonal and institutional, contribute greatly to the chronic stress experienced by Black women (Nuru-Jeter et al., 2009). The "weathering hypothesis" suggests that the cumulative impact of racism and stress leads to accelerated aging and an increased risk for chronic diseases among Black women (Geronimus et al., 2006). This weathering effect has been linked to adverse birth outcomes, such as preterm birth and low birth weight (Braveman et al., 2017).

To address the effects of chronic stress and racism on Black maternal health, a thorough strategy is needed that involves treatments at the individual level as well as systemic reforms. The role of healthcare providers can involve screening for and addressing stress and mental health concerns that are voiced by Black mothers (Howell et al., 2018). Additionally, policies and interventions that aim to reduce racism and discrimination in service delivery, such as implicit bias training as part of diversity initiatives, can help create a more equitable and supportive environment for Black mothers (Bailey et al., 2017).

Case Study Three: The Toll of Chronic Stress and Racism on Jasmine's Pregnancy

Jasmine, a 34-year-old African American woman, is a successful attorney living with her fiancé in a predominantly white, affluent suburb. Despite her professional achievements, Jasmine constantly faces racial discrimination and microaggressions in her workplace and community. Jasemine is nine weeks pregnant with her first baby, and is experiencing chronic stress due to several types of racism in her neighborhood and place of employment:

1. Workplace Discrimination: As the only Black woman in her law firm, Jasmine experiences subtle albeit persistent forms of discrimination. Her colleagues often question her competence, ignore her input during meetings, and assign her less prestigious cases. This constant undermining of her abilities creates a stressful and hostile work environment for Jasemine.
2. Racial Microaggressions: Jasmine encounters frequent racial microaggressions in her daily life. She often experiences people in her community making insensitive comments and asking inappropriate questions about her appearance, and it is common for people in the community to express surprise at her articulate manner of speaking. These seemingly minor incidents accumulate over time, contributing to Jasemine feeling frustrated, angry, and alienated.
3. Imposter Syndrome: As a result of the pervasive racial stereotypes and discrimination, Jasmine begins to internalize feelings of self-doubt and imposter syndrome. She feels pressure to work twice as hard to prove her worth and constantly worries about making mistakes that could confirm negative stereotypes about Black women. She also becomes hyper-focused on always looking presentable when she is in public, especially in the community where she lives.
4. Racial Battle Fatigue: The cumulative impact of chronic stress and racism takes a toll on Jasmine's mental and physical health. She experiences symptoms of racial battle fatigue including anxiety, depression, and insomnia. These psychological stressors can have adverse effects on her pregnancy, increasing the risk of complications such as preterm labor and low birth weight.
5. Inadequate Support Systems: Jasmine's experiences with racism and discrimination make it difficult for her to find support systems besides her fiancé that thoroughly understand her struggles. She feels isolated and disconnected from her predominantly white social circle and lacks access to culturally sensitive mental health resources.

The Outcome

During her pregnancy, Jasmine's chronic stress levels remain high due to the ongoing racial discrimination and microaggressions that she faces daily. Despite receiving regular prenatal care, she develops pregnancy-induced hypertension and experiences symptoms of antenatal depression. Jasmine's doctor, who lacks cultural competency training, fails to fully acknowledge the impact of racism on her health and does not provide adequate mental health support or resources. As a result, Jasmine's condition worsens, and she is hospitalized for pre-eclampsia at 36 weeks, leading to an emergency cesarean section, a prolonged recovery period, and her prematurely born baby spending 6 weeks in the hospital.

Reflective Overview

Jasmine's story demonstrates the profound impact that chronic stress and racism can have on the maternal health of Black women, even those with a higher socioeconomic status, access to quality healthcare and insurance. The cumulative effects of racial discrimination, microaggressions, and the resulting psychological distress can lead to adverse pregnancy outcomes and exacerbate existing health disparities. Addressing these issues requires a multi-level approach that includes promoting diversity and inclusion in the workplace, providing cultural competency training for healthcare providers, and increasing access to culturally sensitive mental health resources. By acknowledging and addressing the role of racism as a chronic stressor, communities can work towards improving maternal health outcomes and promoting health equity for Black women.

ENVIRONMENTAL FACTORS

Environmental factors, such as housing conditions, neighborhood safety, and access to healthy food, also contribute to Black maternal health disparities. Black women have higher rates of living in neighborhoods with increased levels of poverty, crime, and environmental toxins, which can have a negative impact on health outcomes for pregnant women and their unborn babies (Mendez et al., 2016). Poor housing conditions such as overcrowding and exposure to lead and other toxins have been linked to adverse birth outcomes and developmental delays in children (Bashir, 2002).

Black communities are frequently disproportionately impacted by environmental factors such as limited access to nutritious dietary options (Walker et al., 2010). Lack of access to affordable and nutritious food can lead to poor maternal nutrition.

This substandard nutrition during pregnancy is associated with an increased risk of complications during pregnancy and adverse birth outcomes.

As with other social determinants of maternal health, a multi-sectoral approach that involves collaboration between healthcare providers, community organizations, and policymakers is required for addressing environmental disparities. Interventions such as improving access to safe and affordable housing, increasing the availability of healthy food options in underserved communities, and reducing exposure to environmental toxins can help promote better health outcomes for Black mothers and their families (Mendez et al., 2016).

Case Study Four: The Influence of the Neighborhood Environment on Brenda's Maternal Health

Brenda is a 26-year-old Black woman. She lives in an urban, low-income neighborhood with her partner, their five-year-old son, and their three-year-old daughter. Brenda is pregnant with her third child and works as a receptionist at a local community center.

Neighborhood Environmental Factors:

1. Limited Access to Healthy Food Options: Brenda's neighborhood lacks grocery stores that provide fresh, nutritious foods. Brenda struggles to maintain a healthy diet during her pregnancy because the neighborhood primarily consists of convenience stores and fast-food restaurants. Her risk of obesity during pregnancy, gestational diabetes, and other nutrition-related issues is increased by her restricted access to healthful dietary options.
2. Inadequate Green Spaces and Recreational Facilities: The neighborhood lacks safe, well-maintained parks and recreational facilities, which discourages Brenda from engaging in regular physical activity with her children. Additionally, abandoned lots and the lack of green spaces contribute to a sense of social isolation and detachment from nature, both of which can have damaging effects on mental health.
3. Environmental Pollution: Brenda's neighborhood is located near a busy highway and an industrial area, which exposes residents to elevated levels of air pollution, noise pollution, and toxic chemicals. Low birth weight, preterm birth, and congenital anomalies are among the adverse birth outcomes that may be exacerbated by exposure to these environmental pollutants.
4. Poor Housing Conditions: Brenda lives in a neighborhood where most of the homes are dilapidated, plagued by pest infestations, contain mold, and are covered

with lead paint. These substandard living conditions can aggravate respiratory problems, allergies, and other health concerns, including during pregnancy.

5. Community Violence and Safety Concerns: Brenda's neighborhood has a high prevalence of crime and community violence, which creates an ongoing sense of stress and worry. Brenda's inaccessibility to community resources, including prenatal education classes and support groups, is intensified by the absence of secure outdoor areas and her apprehension regarding potential violence.

The Outcome

The cumulative impact of these neighborhood environmental factors takes a toll on Brenda's health during her pregnancy. She develops gestational hypertension, which is aggravated by the chronic stress of living in an unsafe neighborhood. Additionally, the limited access to healthy food options contributes to excessive gestational weight gain and increases her risk of gestational diabetes. Despite receiving prenatal care, Brenda encounters problems in her third trimester and goes into preterm delivery at 36 weeks. She delivers a baby with a low birth weight who requires an extended stay in the NICU.

Reflective Overview

Brenda's story demonstrates how local environmental factors can have a substantial impact on the maternal health of Black mothers. Adverse pregnancy outcomes are caused by a complex combination of factors, including poor living conditions, community violence, pollution, a lack of access to healthy food options, and inadequate green areas. Addressing these neighborhood-level disparities requires a comprehensive, multi-sectoral approach that includes urban planning initiatives to increase access to healthy food and green spaces, policies to improve housing quality and safety, and community-based interventions to reduce violence and promote social cohesion. Improving maternal health outcomes and eliminating inequities for Black women and their families can be achieved in communities across the United States by promoting healthier and more equitable neighborhood environments.

SOCIAL SUPPORT AND COMMUNITY RESOURCES

Community resources and social support are essential for advancing the health and wellbeing of Black mothers. Strong social networks, which include friends, family, and neighbors, can provide practical, emotional, and educational support to expectant and new mothers (Giurgescu et al., 2015). Studies indicate that social support is linked to enhanced maternal mental well-being, decreased stress levels, and improved delivery outcomes (Dunkel Schetter et al., 2013).

However, Black women may encounter specific barriers to accessing and maintaining social support networks. Socioeconomic disadvantage, prejudice, and discrimination can strain interpersonal relationships and restrict opportunities for social interaction (Giurgescu et al., 2015). Additionally, the lack of culturally responsive support services and the stigma surrounding mental health concerns that continues to be common amongst many Black families and communities, may prevent Black women from seeking help when needed (Watson et al., 2019).

When providing prenatal and postpartum care, healthcare professionals can have a positive impact on the social support for Black women by evaluating social support networks and directing their patients to local resources and support services. (Howell et al., 2018). Community-based interventions, such as peer support groups and mentorship programs, can provide Black mothers with opportunities to connect with others who share similar experiences and challenges (Giurgescu et al., 2015). Additionally, policies that promote family-friendly workplace environments and increase access to affordable childcare can help reduce the strain on social support networks.

Case Study Five: The Role of Social Support and Community Resources in Simone's Maternal Health Journey

Simone is a 32-year-old Black woman who lives in a predominantly Black, urban neighborhood. She is a single mother of two children and is currently pregnant with her third child. Simone works as a teacher's assistant at a local elementary school and relies on her tight-knit family and community for support.

Social Support and Community Resources:

1. Strong Family Support: Simone's family provides her with a solid network of support. Her mother and sister, who reside nearby, provide assistance with daily responsibilities, emotional support, and childcare. Simone's stress levels are lowered by her family's support, which enables her to concentrate on her health and well-being during her pregnancy.
2. Community-Based Doula Program: A community-based doula program in Simone's neighborhood offers free prenatal, birth, and postpartum support. Simone is paired with a culturally competent doula who provides information, advocacy, and emotional support during her pregnancy and childbirth. Simone's doula offers support services including continuity of care, making sure her voice

is heard at her prenatal and postnatal appointments, and assists her in navigating the healthcare system.

3. Black Maternal Health Coalition: Simone's community has a Black Maternal Health Coalition that works to address the unique challenges that are faced by Black mothers. The coalition seeks to improve maternal health outcomes and promote health equity by planning advocacy campaigns, educational workshops, and support groups on a monthly basis. Through her participation with the coalition, Simone gains a sense of belonging and empowerment by developing connections with other Black mothers who share similar experiences.
4. Faith-Based Support Network: As an active church member, Simone benefits from the support of her faith-based community. The church provides expectant and new mothers with spiritual guidance, prayer support, and practical assistance through its mothers' ministry. This faith-based network helps Simone with maintaining a positive outlook and teaches her effective coping skills to manage the challenges of pregnancy and motherhood.
5. Community Health Center: Simone receives prenatal care at a local community health center that prioritizes culturally competent care for women of color. The health center has a team of diverse healthcare providers who are trained in cultural competency and provide respectful, patient-centered care. The facility provides a wide range of services including mental health assistance, nutrition counseling, and childbirth education classes.

The Outcome

Simone has a healthy pregnancy due to the help of her family, community, and culturally competent maternal medical services. Throughout her prenatal care and childbirth experience, Simone feels as though she has been heard, acknowledged, appreciated, and supported. Simone's access to culturally inclusive resources and strong social support system assists in mitigating the effects of stress and promoting favorable outcomes for maternal health. Simone’s pregnancy goes to full term, she gives birth to a healthy baby, and feels confident in her ability to continue to navigate the challenges of motherhood with the ongoing support of her family and community.

Reflective Overview

Simone's experience demonstrates the crucial role that social support and community resources play in increasing maternal health equity among Black women. Simone benefits from a strong family support system, a community-based doula program, the Black Maternal Health Coalition, a faith-based network, and a culturally competent community health center, all of which contribute to her well-being throughout her pregnancy and into motherhood. These resources assist in countering the effects of systematic racism, discrimination, stress associated with living in an underserved community, and other socioeconomic variables that contribute to maternal health disparities.

ADVOCACY AND POLICY: DRIVING CHANGE FOR BLACK MATERNAL HEALTH

The ongoing discrepancies in maternal health outcomes among Black women in the United States emphasize the critical need for advocacy and legislative actions to address this public health issue. Advocates, researchers, and policymakers play crucial roles in increasing awareness about these disparities. They also work to develop evidence-based solutions and promote systemic change to improve Black maternal health outcomes.

The Black Maternal Health Momnibus Act, which was presented to Congress in 2021 by the Black Maternal Health Caucus, is one of the most progressive maternal health policy efforts in recent years. The Momnibus Act seeks to increase Black women's access to high-quality, culturally competent healthcare by addressing the social determinants of maternal health (Black Maternal Health Caucus, 2021). The act includes provisions to expand Medicaid coverage for postpartum care, invest in community-based organizations, and allocate funds for research to better understand and address maternal health disparities.

The Momnibus Act also focuses on advocacy efforts to expand access to doula care and midwifery services, which have been shown to improve maternal health outcomes and reduce disparities for Black women (Kozhimannil et al., 2013; Suarez, 2020). Reduced rates of preterm birth, cesarean delivery, and postpartum depression have been linked to the ongoing, culturally competent assistance that doulas and midwives provide during pregnancy, childbirth, and the postpartum period. Advocates for doula and midwifery care have called for increased Medicaid reimbursement for doula and midwifery services, and the integration of these providers into standard maternity care models (Kozhimannil et al., 2013).

The Maternal CARE Act, which was introduced in 2019, aims to reduce racial disparities in maternal health outcomes. Through the act, funding is allocated for implicit bias training for healthcare providers, establishing a grant program to support community-based organizations, and improving data collection and research on maternal health disparities (H.R.2902, 2019). Additional policy efforts have focused on undertaking concerns related to paid family leave, affordable housing, and access to nutritious foods, acknowledging the impact of these social and economic factors on maternal health outcomes (Taylor et al., 2022).

Black women's voices have been amplified and legislative change has been sparked by advocacy groups such as the National Birth Equity Collaborative and the Black Mamas Matter Alliance. These organizations conduct community-based research, policy advocacy, and public education initiatives to increase awareness of the maternal health epidemic impacting women of color and support evidence-based solutions. They also provide support and resources for Black women and families, and work to build coalitions across sectors to advance maternal health equity (Black Mamas Matter Alliance, n.d.; National Birth Equity Collaborative, n.d.).

While there have been improvements in recent years, there is a need for continued progress in addressing the persistent disparities in maternal health outcomes for Black women. Ongoing advocacy and policy initiatives must focus on Black women's perspectives and experiences, while also working to eliminate the structural racism and prejudice that contribute to these inequities. Communities can make strides toward maternal health equity for Black women in the United States by implementing community-based solutions, the expansion of access to high-quality culturally competent care, and address the social determinants of health.

Case Study Six: Tanya's Advocacy for Policy Change to Address Black Maternal Health Disparities

Tanya, a 33-year-old African American woman, is a public health researcher and advocate who is dedicated to addressing the maternal health crisis affecting Black women in her community. Motivated by her own experiences and those of her family members, Tanya decides to take action to promote policy changes that can improve maternal health outcomes for Black women. She recognizes that her unique perspective and expertise can contribute to the growing movement to prioritize Black maternal health and promote health equity.

Advocacy and Policy Initiatives

1. The Black Maternal Health Caucus: Tanya has joined the Black Maternal Health Caucus, a congressional group whose goals are to bring attention to the Black maternal health crisis to Congress and advance legislative measures that would enhance maternal health outcomes. Her participation in the caucus contributes to advocating for policy and systemic change to shape laws that attempt to increase access to high-quality, culturally-appropriate care, and address the social determinants of maternal health that impact Black women.
2. Community-Based Participatory Research: Tanya works with a research team to conduct participatory community-based research and collect information on the needs and experiences of Black women in her community. She also collab-

orates with local organizations, healthcare providers, and community members to identify key challenges and potential solutions. Tanya's research efforts and community partnerships help inform policy recommendations and advocacy efforts at the local and state levels.

3. Medicaid Expansion and Reimbursement: Given that many maternal health complications can arise long after delivery, Tanya advocates for the expansion of postpartum Medicaid coverage to last from 60 days to one year. She also aims to secure increased Medicaid reimbursement rates for midwives, doulas, and community health workers, who play a critical role in providing culturally competent care and support to Black women during and after pregnancy.
4. Implicit Bias Training and Workforce Diversity: Tanya collaborates with healthcare facilities and professional groups to provide mandatory implicit bias training for healthcare providers. She emphasizes the significance of identifying and correcting unconscious biases that contributes to racial disparities in maternal healthcare. Additionally, Tanya advocates for programs to increase diversity in the healthcare workforce, specifically in the fields of obstetrics and gynecology.
5. Social Determinants of Health: Acknowledging the multifaceted impact of social and economic factors on maternal health, Tanya works in conjunction with legislators and community organizations to tackle the social determinants of health. She supports policies that promote access to secure and affordable housing, nutritious food options, transportation, and education.

The Outcome

Through Tanya's advocacy efforts and the collective work of the Black maternal health community, important legislative improvements are made. There is additional funding for community-based organizations, research, and healthcare workforce training. Medicaid coverage is expanded to cover postpartum care for one year, and reimbursement rates for midwives and doulas are increased. Healthcare organizations mandate implicit bias training, and efforts to diversify their workforce start to gain momentum. Tanya's efforts can serve as a blueprint for gradual, yet successful advocacy and policy changes related to maternal health outcomes for Black women.

Reflective Overview

Tanya's story demonstrates the power of advocacy and policy change in addressing the maternal health disparities faced by Black women. Tanya assists with advancing Black maternal health and health equity by participating in community-based research, interacting with key stakeholders, and advocating for specific policy initiatives. This case study highlights the importance of addressing the social determinants of maternal health, expanding access to quality and culturally competent pregnancy care, and dismantling systemic racism within the healthcare system at the policy level. While progress continues to be made, ongoing lobbying and legislative efforts are crucial to ensure that Black women receive the support and resources they need to achieve optimal maternal health throughout their prenatal, birth, and postnatal care.

SUMMARY OF INTERVENTIONS AND POLICY RECOMMENDATIONS

Addressing the social determinants of Black maternal health requires a comprehensive, multi-level approach that involves healthcare providers, policymakers, community organizations, and Black women themselves. The interventions and policy ideas outlined below are designed to enhance the health equity and maternal health outcomes specifically for Black women:

1. Expand Access to Quality Healthcare: Ensure that Black women have access to comprehensive, culturally sensitive prenatal and postpartum care by extending insurance coverage, increasing provider diversity, and investing in culturally diverse community health centers. (Howell et al., 2018).
2. Handle Implicit Bias in Healthcare: Create policies and procedures to decrease prejudice in healthcare environments and emphasize implicit bias training for healthcare providers. (Hoffman et al., 2016).
3. Invest in Community-Based Programs: Support and expand community-based programs that provide education, resources, and support for Black mothers including doula services, home visiting programs, and peer support groups (Tandon et al., 2013).
4. Promote Socioeconomic Equity: Implement policies that reduce poverty, increase access to education and job opportunities, and provide support for Black families, such as paid family leave, affordable childcare, and living wage laws (Mehra et al., 2019).
5. Address Environmental Disparities: Collaborate with community organizations and policymakers to improve access to safe and affordable housing, increase the availability of healthy food options in underserved communities, and reduce exposure to environmental toxins (Mendez et al., 2016).
6. Invest in Research and Data Collection: Advocate for research focusing on the social factors influencing Black maternal health and assessing the impact of measures aimed at reducing these inequalities. Enhance data collection and analysis to provide a thorough insight into and track patterns of maternal health results for Black women (Howell et al., 2018).

CONCLUSION

The social determinants of Black maternal health are complex and deeply rooted in the historical legacy of slavery, systemic racism, and ongoing discrimination. Addressing these disparities requires a comprehensive, multi-level approach that recognizes the intersectionality of race, gender, and socioeconomic status in shaping maternal health outcomes. By implementing targeted interventions and policies that address access to quality healthcare, socioeconomic inequities, chronic stress, racism, environmental factors, and social support, the United States can work towards achieving health equity and improving maternal health outcomes for Black women.

Moving forward, it is essential to prioritize Black women's voices and experiences when developing and implementing interventions and policies. Involving Black women as active collaborators in research, program development, and policy creation, can increase the chances that solutions are culturally sensitive and cater to the specific needs and obstacles encountered by tnot his demographic. Furthermore, continued research and data collection are necessary to monitor the progress and evaluate the effectiveness of interventions over time. Ultimately, addressing the social determinants of Black maternal health are both public health and social justice issues. By recognizing and dismantling the systemic barriers that perpetuate health inequities, communities throughout the country can create a more equitable and just society that values the health and well-being of all mothers and their families.

REFERENCES

Bailey, Z. D., Krieger, N., Agénor, M., Graves, J., Linos, N., & Bassett, M. T. (2017). Structural racism and health inequities in the USA: Evidence and interventions. *The Lancet*, *389*(10077), 1453-1463. https://ajph.aphapublications.org/doi/pdf/10.2105/AJPH.2014.302200

Bashir, S. A. (2002). Home is where the harm is: Inadequate housing as a public health crisis. *American Journal of Public Health*, *92*(5), 733–738. DOI: 10.2105/AJPH.92.5.733 PMID: 11988437

Black, A. R., Murry, V. M., Cutrona, C. E., & Chen, Y. (2009). Multiple roles, multiple lives: The protective effects of role responsibilities on the health functioning of African American mothers. *Women & Health*, *49*(2-3), 144–163. DOI: 10.1080/03630240902915051 PMID: 19533507

Black Mamas Matter Alliance. (n.d.). *Our work*. https://blackmamasmatter.org/our-work/

Braveman, P., Heck, K., Egerter, S., Dominguez, T. P., Rinki, C., Marchi, K. S., & Curtis, M. (2017). Worry about racial discrimination: A missing piece of the puzzle of Black-White disparities in preterm birth? *PLoS One*, *12*(10), e0186151. DOI: 10.1371/journal.pone.0186151 PMID: 29020025

Crear-Perry, J., Correa-de-Araujo, R., Lewis Johnson, T., McLemore, M. R., Neilson, E., & Wallace, M. (2021). Social and structural determinants of health inequities in maternal health. *Journal of Women's Health*, *30*(2), 230–235. DOI: 10.1089/jwh.2020.8882 PMID: 33181043

Dunkel Schetter, C., Schafer, P., Lanzi, R. G., Clark-Kauffman, E., Raju, T. N., & Hillemeier, M. M. (2013). Shedding light on the mechanisms underlying health disparities through community participatory methods: The stress pathway. *Perspectives on Psychological Science*, *8*(6), 613–633. DOI: 10.1177/1745691613506016 PMID: 26173227

Gadson, A., Akpovi, E., & Mehta, P. K. (2017). Exploring the social determinants of racial/ethnic disparities in prenatal care utilization and maternal outcome. *Seminars in Perinatology*, *41*(5), 308–317. DOI: 10.1053/j.semperi.2017.04.008 PMID: 28625554

Gavin, N. I., Gaynes, B. N., Lohr, K. N., Meltzer-Brody, S., Gartlehner, G., & Swinson, T. (2005). Perinatal depression: A systematic review of prevalence and incidence. *Obstetrics and Gynecology*, *106*(5), 1071–1083. DOI: 10.1097/01.AOG.0000183597.31630.db PMID: 16260528

Geronimus, A. T., Hicken, M., Keene, D., & Bound, J. (2006). "Weathering" and age patterns of allostatic load scores among blacks and whites in the United States. *American Journal of Public Health, 96*(5), 826–833. DOI: 10.2105/AJPH.2004.060749 PMID: 16380565

Giurgescu, C., Misra, D. P., Sealy-Jefferson, S., Caldwell, C. H., Templin, T. N., Slaughter-Acey, J. C., & Osypuk, T. L. (2015). The impact of neighborhood quality, perceived stress, and social support on depressive symptoms during pregnancy in African American women. *Social Science & Medicine, 130*, 172–180. DOI: 10.1016/j.socscimed.2015.02.006 PMID: 25703670

Hoffman, K. M., Trawalter, S., Axt, J. R., & Oliver, M. N. (2016). Racial bias in pain assessment and treatment recommendations, and false beliefs about biological differences between blacks and whites. *Proceedings of the National Academy of Sciences of the United States of America, 113*(16), 4296–4301. DOI: 10.1073/pnas.1516047113 PMID: 27044069

Howell, E. A. (2018). Reducing disparities in severe maternal morbidity and mortality. *Clinical Obstetrics and Gynecology, 61*(2), 387–399. DOI: 10.1097/GRF.0000000000000349 PMID: 29346121

Howell, E. A., Egorova, N. N., Balbierz, A., Zeitlin, J., & Hebert, P. L. (2018). Site of delivery contribution to black-white severe maternal morbidity disparity. *American Journal of Obstetrics and Gynecology*. Advance online publication. DOI: 10.1016/j.ajog.2016.05.007 PMID: 27179441

H.R.2902 – Maternal CARE Act. 116th Congress (2019-2020) (2019, May 22). https://www.congress.gov/bill/116th-congress/house-bill/2902

Kozhimannil, K. B., Hardeman, R. R., Attanasio, L. B., Blauer-Peterson, C., & O'Brien, M. (2013). Doula care, birth outcomes, and costs among Medicaid beneficiaries. *American Journal of Public Health, 103*(4), e113–e121. DOI: 10.2105/AJPH.2012.301201 PMID: 23409910

Marmot, M., & Allen, J. (2014). Social determinants of health equity. *American Journal of Public Health, 104*(4), 517–519. DOI: 10.2105/AJPH.2014.302200 PMID: 25100411

Mehra, R., Keene, D. E., Kershaw, T. S., Ickovics, J. R., & Warren, J. L. (2019). Racial and ethnic disparities in adverse birth outcomes: Differences by racial residential segregation. *SSM - Population Health, 8*, 1–10. DOI: 10.1016/j.ssmph.2019.100417 PMID: 31193960

Mendez, D. D., Thorpe, R. J., Amutah, N., Davis, E. M., Walker, R. E., Chapple-McGruder, T., & Bodnar, L. (2016). Neighborhood racial composition and poverty in association with pre-pregnancy weight and gestational weight gain. *SSM - Population Health*, *2*, 692–699. Advance online publication. DOI: 10.1016/j.ssmph.2016.09.008 PMID: 29349180

National Birth Equity Collaborative. (n.d.). *National Birth Equity Collaborative (NBEC): General Operating Support.* https://www.commonwealthfund.org/grants/national-birth-equity-collaborative-nbec-general-operating-support

National Partnership for Women and Families. (2023, Nov). *Black women's maternal health: A* multifaceted *approach to addressing persistent and dire health disparities.* https://nationalpartnership.org/report/black-womens-maternal-health/

Nuru-Jeter, A., Dominguez, T. P., Hammond, W. P., Leu, J., Skaff, M., Egerter, S., Jones, C. P., & Braveman, P. (2009). "It's the skin you're in": African American women talk about their experiences of racism. An exploratory study to develop measures of racism for birth outcome studies. *Maternal and Child Health Journal*, *13*(1), 29–39. DOI: 10.1007/s10995-008-0357-x PMID: 18463971

Owens, D. C., & Fett, S. M. (2019). Black maternal and infant health: Historical legacies of slavery. *American Journal of Public Health*, *109*(10), 1342–1345. DOI: 10.2105/AJPH.2019.305243 PMID: 31415204

Petersen, E. E., Davis, N. L., Goodman, D., Cox, S., Syverson, C., Seed, K., Shapiro-Mendoza, S., Callaghan, W. M., & Barfield, W. (2019). Racial/ethnic disparities in pregnancy-related deaths - United States, 2007–2016. *MMWR. Morbidity and Mortality Weekly Report*, *68*(35), 762–765. DOI: 10.15585/mmwr.mm6835a3 PMID: 31487273

Prather, C., Fuller, T. R., Jeffries, W. L.IV, Marshall, K. J., Howell, A. V., Belyue-Umole, A., & King, W. (2018). Racism, African American women, and their sexual and reproductive health: A review of historical and contemporary evidence and implications for health equity. *Health Equity*, *2*(1), 249–259. DOI: 10.1089/heq.2017.0045 PMID: 30283874

Roberts, D. (1997). *Killing the black body: Race, reproduction, and the meaning of liberty*. Doubleday Publishing Group.

Suarez, E. A. (2020). Midwifery and Black maternal health: Claiming our power, resilience, and liberation. *Journal of Midwifery & Women's Health*, *65*(5), 655–657. DOI: 10.1111/jmwh.13164

Tandon, S. D., Cluxton-Keller, F., Colon, L., Vega, P., & Alonso, A. (2013). Improved adequacy of prenatal care and healthcare utilization among low-income Latinas receiving group prenatal care. *Journal of Women's Health, 22*(12), 1056–1061. DOI: 10.1089/jwh.2013.4352 PMID: 24117000

Taylor, J., Novoa, C., Hamm, K., & Phadke, S. (2022, May 5). *Eliminating racial disparities in maternal and infant mortality*. Center for American Progress. https://www.americanprogress.org/article/eliminating-racial-disparities-maternal-infant-mortality/

Walker, R. E., Keane, C. R., & Burke, J. G. (2010). Disparities and access to healthy food in the United States: A review of food deserts literature. *Health & Place, 16*(5), 876–884. DOI: 10.1016/j.healthplace.2010.04.013 PMID: 20462784

Washington, H. A. (2006). *Medical apartheid: The dark history of medical experimentation on black Americans from colonial times to the present*. Doubleday Publishing Group.

Watson, H., Harrop, D., Walton, E., Young, A., & Soltani, H. (2019). A systematic review of ethnic minority women's experiences of perinatal mental health conditions and services in Europe. *PLoS One, 14*(1), 1–19. DOI: 10.1371/journal.pone.0210587 PMID: 30695019

ADDITIONAL READINGS

Hunte, R., Klawetter, S., & Paul, S. (2022). "Black nurses in the home is working": Advocacy, naming, and processing racism to improve black maternal infant health. *Maternal and Child Health Journal, 26*(4), 933–940. DOI: 10.1007/s10995-021-03283-4 PMID: 34817758

Karbeah, J. M., Hardeman, R., Katz, N., Orionzi, D., & Kozhimannil, K. B. (2022). From a place of love: the experiences of birthing in a black-owned culturally-centered community birth center. *Journal of Health Disparities Research and Practice, 15*(2), 47-60. https://www.ncbi.nlm.nih.gov/pmc/articles/PMC10237589/

Kemet, S., Yang, Y., Nseyo, O., Bell, F., Gordon, A., Mays, M., Fowler, M., & Jackson, A. (2022). "When I think of mental healthcare, I think of no care." Mental health services as a vital component of prenatal care for black women. *Maternal and Child Health Journal, 26*(4), 778–787. DOI: 10.1007/s10995-021-03226-z PMID: 34519952

Sperlich, M., & Gabriel, C. (2022). "I got to catch my own baby": A qualitative study of out of hospital birth. *Reproductive Health, 19*(43), 1–13. DOI: 10.1186/s12978-022-01355-4 PMID: 35164785

Trye, A., Campbell Oparaji, D., Roche, N., & Gittens Williams, L. (2022). Addressing racial disparities in maternal health: The case for an equity birth plan. *Journal of Health Disparities Research and Practice, 15*(2). https://digitalscholarship.unlv.edu/jhdrp/vol15/iss2/2/

KEY TERMS AND DEFINITIONS

Antenatal Depression: Antenatal depression, often called prenatal depression, is a type of clinical depression that develops during pregnancy. It is distinguished by persistent feelings of sadness, worry, and hopelessness that can impair a pregnant woman's mental well-being and daily functioning.

Congenital: Congenital refers to any ailment, characteristic, or abnormality that exists from birth. Congenital characteristics can be inherited genetically from parents or arise during pregnancy as a result of environmental factors, maternal health disorders, or fetal development complications. Congenital disorders can range from modest cosmetic issues to serious physical or developmental disabilities.

Doula: A doula is a trained professional who gives ongoing physical, emotional, and informational support to mothers before, during, and after pregnancy, ensuring a healthy and satisfying experience. Doulas are not medical professionals and do not provide medical interventions or clinical services. Instead, they offer a variety of non-medical support services.

Eugenics: Eugenics is a pseudoscience that was founded on the false theory that human characteristics such as morality, intellect, and personality are mostly genetic. The scientific community now fully rejects eugenics as unscientific and a violation of human rights.

Food Desert: A food desert is a geographic area where it is difficult for residents to obtain nutritious and affordable food options, especially fresh fruits and vegetables. Food deserts are typically found in low-income communities and are identified by a lack of full-service grocery stores, farmers' markets, and other providers of healthy food.

Green Space: A green space refers to any area of land that is partially or completely covered with grass, trees, shrubs, or other vegetation. Green spaces include natural and synthetic areas such as parks, public gardens, nature reserves, conservation areas, playgrounds, and walking trails.

Implicit Bias: Implicit bias, also known as unconscious bias, refers to unintentional attitudes, prejudices, or preferences that may influence one's perceptions, choices, and behaviors without the person's conscious knowledge. These biases are shaped by individual experiences, societal standards, and cultural conditioning. Implicit bias is commonly linked to characteristics and qualities such as ethnicity, gender, age, or attractiveness.

Imposter Syndrome: Imposter syndrome is a psychological condition that is characterized by self-doubt regarding one's abilities, talents, or achievements. There is a persistent, internalized fear of being exposed as a fraud or "imposter" despite evidence of one's success and external proof of their competence.

Jim Crow Laws: Jim Crow laws were a collection of state and local statutes that legalized racial segregation and discrimination against African Americans in the southern United States from the late 19th century to the 1960s. Jim Crow Laws consisted of segregation of public facilities such as schools, public transportation, water fountains, and restrooms. Jim Crow Laws also enacted restrictive voting laws, employment discrimination, housing discrimination, and prohibiting interracial marriage.

Midwifery: Midwifery is a healthcare profession that specializes in providing care to women throughout pregnancy, childbirth, and the postpartum period. Midwives are trained to provide a wide variety of services including prenatal care and monitoring, education, counseling, assistance during labor and delivery, family planning, and gynecological care.

Racial Battle Fatigue: Racial battle fatigue is a term that describes the psychological, emotional, and physiological strain that is experienced by people of color due to constant exposure to racism and discrimination. The cumulative effects of navigating and coping with daily instances of racial microaggressions, systemic inequalities, and overt racism are emphasized.

Redlining: Redlining is a discriminatory practice in which financial and other services are denied or restricted in specific geographic areas, often based on the racial or ethnic makeup of those communities.

Socioeconomic Status: Socioeconomic status (SES) assesses an individual's or family's social and economic standing in comparison to others. SES is based on a combination of factors such as income, education, occupation, and wealth. SES is a key determinant of health and well- being that impacts access to resources, opportunities, and support systems.

Chapter 2
Navigating Black Maternal Mental Health and Wellbeing:
Perinatal Anxiety and Depression in Black Mothers

Mercedes Jamecia Moore
https://orcid.org/0009-0002-6230-2680
Capella University, USA

ABSTRACT

The crisis of Black maternal mental health is deeply rooted in the historical context of slavery, characterized by reproductive oppression that exploited Black women for economic gain and perpetuated trauma. Despite the abolition of slavery in 1865, the legacy of injustice manifests in contemporary medical racism, affecting Black women's mental health throughout the perinatal period. Research shows Black mothers experience higher rates of perinatal mood and anxiety disorders, compounded by socioeconomic factors, systemic inequities, and cultural stigma. This article emphasizes the urgent need for culturally competent care and systemic change to address these disparities and enhance birth equity for Black mothers.

ORIGINS OF THE BLACK MATERNAL MENTAL HEALTH CRISIS

The Black maternal mental health crisis today is linked to slavery, where Black women were victims of reproductive oppression. Black women were forced to birth children for the purpose of upholding the institution of slavery (Owens & Fett, 2019). Black mothers assumed the inhumane tasks of increasing the slave population through

DOI: 10.4018/979-8-3693-4272-5.ch002

forced reproduction- rather it be rape or breeding farms, while also carrying out physical labor on the plantation (Borrelli et al, 2023). It is important to highlight that Black women were also forced to be the subjects of medical experiments (O'Brien & Rich, 2022). The exploitation of Black women's bodies had economic advances for slave owners and the field of medicine (Owens, 2017). This was an American system that forced Black women to birth children but disregarded them as mothers, inflicting psychological scars and trauma for generations to come (McCarthy, 2024).

Even though slavery was abolished in 1865, its legacy of reproductive oppression is still embedded in American society, in the form of medical racism. America's history of exploiting Black women's bodies has lasting cultural stigma that influences the ideology of medical professionals who treat Black women today (Brown et al, 2021). The inability to learn from our nation's history of atrocious treatment towards Black women is likely to repeat itself without culturally competent screenings and interventions (Almeida et al, 2021).

Prevalence

Medical literature has been prioritizing its focus on the impact of perinatal mood and anxiety disorders (PMADs) on mothers during and after pregnancy; the perinatal period, defined as the time a woman becomes pregnant up to one year postpartum. Research indicates that about 15% of mothers experience anxiety and mood disorders during the perinatal period. In that 15%, 14% are reported as perinatal depression and 13%-21% are reported as perinatal anxiety (Byrnes,2018). This is a major concern affecting mothers across all racial groups, but Black mothers face adversities and disparities that are unique to only them. In comparison to other racial groups, Black women have higher trauma exposure across their lifespan, meaning that they have experienced at least one trauma event (Markin & Coleman, 2023). Furthermore, trauma exposure rate during the perinatal period is 87% for Black women compared to 29%-74% for other women (Policy Center for Maternal Mental Health, 2023). This makes Black women more vulnerable to perinatal anxiety and depression disorders. Specifically, when compared to White women, Black women are more likely experience PMADs (Floyd James et al, 2023; McCarthy, 2024). 29-44% of Black women report experiencing postpartum depression but are the least likely to receive mental health care (Estriplet et al, 2022; Floyd James et al, 2023).

SOCIAL DETERMINANTS AND SYSTEMIC INEQUITIES

The intersection of race and sex presents Black women with disparities such as gender related violence, racism, and sexism. These unique disparities expose

Black women to negative social determinants of health (SDOH). The conditions in the environment where Black women live, learn, work, worship, and age are their SDOH and plays a significant role in their quality-of-life outcomes (Chinn et al, 2020). SDOH along with systemic inequities can be predictors of PMADs in Black mothers (Hernandez et al, 2022).

Socioeconomic Factors such as *income inequality* and *inequities in access to resources* are areas that add to stress for Black mothers. Due to systemic barriers in employment, Black mothers are more likely face financial hardships and experience poverty. Systemic barriers in employment can also lead to Black mothers being *uninsured, limiting access to healthcare*. According to researchers, Black mothers from low socioeconomic backgrounds experienced the worst healthcare quality. Other areas of concerns associated with socioeconomic factors include *limited access to safe and stable living conditions and proper nutrition.*

Racial and Discrimination Factors can have a negative impact on the maternal mental health of Black mothers in general, but especially when navigating the medical system. According to research, Black mothers' experiences with hospital births included: being yelled at, threatened, and ignored when requesting help. Black women reported a loss of autonomy when navigating the maternity care system. This type of treatment from healthcare providers is linked to *implicit bias* and is a clear indicator for the need of *culturally competent care*. Black woman's' experience of culturally incompetent care by healthcare providers can lead to them feeling unsafe and fearful to advocate for themselves, resulting in negative mental health outcomes.

Birth Complications have been a part of Black women's experiences with childbirth at U.S. hospitals and other childbirth clinics. The medical literature suggests that the *disproportionate impact of the pandemic* on Black communities may have only exacerbated this phenomenon. According to the medical literature, Black women are three to four times more likely to die from childbirth complications than White women. A report from the CDC (2021), revealed the maternal mortality rate for Black women as 69.9 deaths per 100,000 live births in the United States. The racial and discrimination factors listed above have been linked to *culturally incompetent treatment from healthcare providers*, making them contributing factors to this maternal mortality rate. It is also important to note that a CDC report (2022) revealed that Black babies were twice as like to die at birth than White babies. According to the CDC (2022), the infant mortality rate for Black babies was 10.9 per 1,000 live births in the United States. The *socioeconomic factors* listed above- *limited access to healthcare and resources* along with *improper nutrition* have been linked to *poor health outcomes and little to no prenatal care*, making them contributing factors to this infant mortality rate. This can be linked to anticipatory anxiety and medical mistrust.

Cultural Stigma regarding mental health in the Black community can also play a role in Black women not being vocal about their mental health needs. Black women are often described as strong because of their self-sacrificing nature and resilience. The *Strong Black Woman* has its origins in slavery and has been reinforced through decades of film, television, and rap music where Black women have been praised for their suffering and ability to be strong and loyal despite past and current stressors. Researcher indicates that the *Strong Black Woman* syndrome has been linked to poor physical and mental health outcomes.

VOICES AND PERSPECTIVES OF BLACK MOTHERS

Three Black mothers shared their birth experience in U.S. hospitals and medical offices. They were all asked to reflect on their experience navigating pregnancy and birth in the medical setting. It is important to add their lived experiences and center their voices on this topic for the purpose of developing strategies and intervention to improve their birth and parenting experiences.

Tina reported that she remembers her third and final pregnancy the most, not because it was the most recent one, but because it was frustrating and painful. Birth year: 2001, Age today: 51

> *"I did not feel informed as to why I had to have a C-Section. I wanted a vaginal birth because I had already done it twice and it was familiar. I went into labor thinking that I was having a vaginal birth because that's what was discussed. But once the doctor changed his mind about it, it felt forced on me. My questions weren't welcomed at all. I was not able to advocate for myself, and my husband did not know what to do. We both were scared. I still believe I am having complications from that c-section, and this was 23 years ago."*

Brittney reported that as a new wife and mother the entire birthing process was traumatic. Birth year: 2023, Age today: 27

> *"Everything happened so fast. I was home and then I was rushed to the hospital by my husband. I had a midwife, and I was supposed to give birth at home. But my baby was breech and never turned. I felt mishandled by the medical staff. I mean they weren't rude or nice, they were cold. I needed warmth because I was emotional. It was my first pregnancy. I said to myself, I will never do this again. Because of their coldness, I was anxious and even had nightmares about that experience for a while." I wish my doctor was Black and if I have another baby, the doctor will be Black."*

Kyra reported that she really had a hard time navigating the doctor's appointments before and after leading up to delivery more than anything. Birth year: 2022, Age today: 34

"More than once the staff assumed I was unmarried and needed WIC benefits. They would ask for my Medicaid card and just make stereotypical comments when I went to appointments by myself. My husband works a lot so for some appointments I went by myself, and I was always uneasy. I had my son and yes, the birthing experience was traumatic, but I think I was already anxious and nervous. I had a c-section, and it was not a part of the plan. I should have spoken up more, but I didn't feel like I could. When I take my son to the doctor, now they're commenting on his size a lot. It's frustrating."

A PATH TO BIRTH EQUITY

The maternal mortality and morbidity rates for Black women have been on the rise for several decades. Black women from higher socioeconomic status with access to quality insurance and resources have not been exempt from these adverse outcomes. There must be a radical path forward designed specifically with the intention of creating birth equity for Black mothers and families. The birth equity framework can be used to develop strategies and interventions to improve maternal mental health because it focuses on rectifying structural racism and social determinants through system-level change. The actionable strategies and interventions below were developed with the birth equity framework in mind.

1. Implement Mandatory Culturally Competent Training & Testing

Every medical/ mental health provider and staff should be required to take classes that teaches them the history reproductive oppression and medical racism, how to address personal bias and implement culturally competent care and tested for proficiency in these competencies. This should be a prerequisite before licensure is issued and mandatory for renewal of the licensure. Every three months, there should be an accountability clinic where medical staff are provided with facts about the maternal mental health crisis. They should be updated with new cases at these clinics and brought up to speed about the disparities. They should leave the clinic with an accountability task plan of action with how to prevent these crises from happening at their hospitals or medical settings. It's not enough just to give Black mothers Black providers everyone must bear the responsibility of creating pathways to birth equity and anti-racist medical care for Black mothers.

2. Eliminate The Top-Down Approach

The top-down approach is not a reflection of person-centered care. It does not center Black mothers and their families and has a negative impact on their birthing experiences. The top-down approach can continue the cycle of mistrust between Black people and their medical providers and create anticipatory anxiety. Doctors are experts at textbook knowledge and procedures but not at knowing each patient's needs. Implementing shared decision-making with Black mothers and their families empowers them and dismantles the provider-patient power struggles. It promotes trust and safety. This is a sure way to prioritize and meet the needs of Black mothers.

3. Develop Culturally Sensitive Screening Tools

Depression and anxiety look different in Black women in comparison to how it may look in White women. Therefore, universal screening tools such as the PHQ-9 or GAD-7 may not always detect these symptoms in Black women (Perez et al, 2023). How could they? There were developed and tested on mostly White women. The Health Pregnancy Stress Scale (HPSS) was created to assess stress in Black mothers from low socioeconomic backgrounds, excluding other disparities that plague Black mothers (Policy Center for Maternal Mental Health, 2023). There needs to be culturally appropriate screening tools developed to assess for all the challenges Black mothers face. One way to create more validated screening tools is to develop and test them with Black mothers as research participants (Feldman & Pattani, 2019; Herrick & Burkhard, 2024). Working directly with Black mothers will help developers account for the language Black people use to describe symptoms of depression because it does not always reflect the universal language (Nelson et al, 2023).

4. Create A Black Maternal Mental Health First Aid Program

This program should be Black women led and accessible through the hospital and available to family members, friends, doulas, medical staff, and others in the mom's life on how to recognize symptoms of depression, anxiety, suicidal ideation, and other symptoms in mothers. Learning will happen in a group format via discussions and exercises centered on maternal mental health. The outcomes of this program will be as follows: learning to recognize when mom may be experiencing mental health challenges, skills & confidence to initiate vulnerable conversations, steps to take to connect mom with a therapist, and ways to also support yourself. This program would include access to licensed mental health therapists, social workers, and peer support workers to wrap around mom and the entire family as they navigate the perinatal period. Level of care would be decided based on culturally sensitive screenings and determine frequency of therapy sessions. This hospital program should also collaborate with local communities and schools expand its reach.

CASE STUDY

Anita and her husband Mike have two children, a 10-year-old daughter and a 7-year-old son. They recently welcomed a baby girl about 3 months ago. Anita has been home with the baby the entire time, while also working from home as an insurance claim attorney. Mike has noticed that Anita has been having mood swings and stating that she's having headaches daily. Mike feels helpless and doesn't know how to express his concern. Anita yelled at their daughter for going to slow when getting ready for school and that's not like her. She's usually calm and patient with the children. Mike's mom is supposed to be retiring soon and stated that she can help with the baby. Mike and Anita both have concerns about daycare so they agreed that the baby would stay at home with Anita for a while. Mike wants to revisit the daycare option, but the conversation has not gone well when tried to bring it up. He sees her working late and barely getting sleep daily. At a follow-up appointment, Mike noticed that Anita was honest on the depression and anxiety screening but her score still reflected that she was doing well. Mike wanted the doctor to pay attention to his wife when asking the questions, but the entire screening was rushed. It did not feel like a safe space to express concerns because the doctor did not seem interested in there being anything wrong with Anita.

CHAPTER QUESTIONS

1. What does the literature say about reproductive oppression and its ties to today's Black maternal mental health and maternal mortality crisis?
2. How does implicit bias influence a medical provider's ability to care for Black mothers?
3. What are some of the unique disparities that Black women experience?
4. How does these unique disparities impact the mental health of Black mothers?
5. How has your thinking about Black mothers' birthing experiences changed since you began reading this text?
6. Given history between Black women and the medical system, why is it important for medical providers to share decision making with them?
7. Based on what you have read, what would you add as an actionable strategy or intervention to improve Black mothers' birthing experience?

REFERENCES

Alhusen, J. L., Bower, K. M., Epstein, E., & Sharps, P. (2016). Racial Discrimination and Adverse Birth Outcomes: An Integrative review. *Journal of Midwifery & Women's Health*, *61*(6), 707–720. DOI: 10.1111/jmwh.12490 PMID: 27737504

Almeida, J., Belanoff, C., & Erbetta, K. F. (2021). The Time has Come for All States to Measure Racial Discrimination: A Call to Action for the Pregnancy Risk Assessment Monitoring System (PRAMS). *Maternal and Child Health Journal*, *26*(1), 7–11. DOI: 10.1007/s10995-021-03160-0 PMID: 33945082

Borrelli, S., Ramasamy, R., Wong, R., & Spiby, H. (2023). Care and support during maternity for mothers affected by modern slavery: A scoping review. *International Journal of Nursing Studies Advances*, *5*, 100139. DOI: 10.1016/j.ijnsa.2023.100139 PMID: 38746591

Bower, K. M., Geller, R. J., Jeffers, N., McDonald, M., & Alhusen, J. (2023). Experiences of racism and perinatal depression: Findings from the pregnancy risk assessment monitoring system, 2018. *Journal of Advanced Nursing*, *79*(5), 1982–1993. DOI: 10.1111/jan.15519 PMID: 36630188

Brown, H. L., Small, M. J., Clare, C. A., & Hill, W. C. (2021). Black women health inequity: The origin of perinatal health disparity. *Journal of the National Medical Association*, *113*(1), 105–113. DOI: 10.1016/j.jnma.2020.11.008 PMID: 33339616

Byrnes, L. (2018). Perinatal mood and anxiety disorders. *The Journal for Nurse Practitioners*, *14*(7), 507–513. DOI: 10.1016/j.nurpra.2018.03.010

Castelin, S., & White, G. (2022). "I'm a Strong Independent Black Woman": The Strong Black Woman Schema and Mental Health in College-Aged Black Women. *Psychology of Women Quarterly*, *46*(2), 196–208. DOI: 10.1177/03616843211067501

Chinn, J. J., Martin, I. K., & Redmond, N. (2020). Health equity among Black women in the United States. *Journal of Women's Health*, *30*(2), 212–219. DOI: 10.1089/jwh.2020.8868 PMID: 33237831

Dagher, R. K., & Linares, D. E. (2022). A Critical Review on the Complex Interplay between Social Determinants of Health and Maternal and Infant Mortality. *Children (Basel, Switzerland)*, *9*(3), 394. DOI: 10.3390/children9030394 PMID: 35327766

Dalsania, A. K., Fastiggi, M. J., Kahlam, A., Shah, R., Patel, K., Shiau, S., Rokicki, S., & DallaPiazza, M. (2021). The relationship between social determinants of health and racial disparities in COVID-19 mortality. *Journal of Racial and Ethnic Health Disparities*, *9*(1), 288–295. DOI: 10.1007/s40615-020-00952-y PMID: 33403652

Estriplet, T., Morgan, I., Davis, K., Perry, J. C., & Matthews, K. (2022). Black Perinatal Mental Health: Prioritizing maternal mental health to optimize infant health and wellness. *Frontiers in Psychiatry, 13*, 807235. DOI: 10.3389/fpsyt.2022.807235 PMID: 35573337

Etowa, J. B., Beagan, B. L., Eghan, F., & Bernard, W. T. (2017). "You feel you have to be made of steel": The strong Black woman, health, and well-being in Nova Scotia. *Health Care for Women International, 38*(4), 379–393. DOI: 10.1080/07399332.2017.1290099 PMID: 28151098

Feldman, N., & Pattani, A. (2019, Dec 6). *Black Mothers Get Less Treatment For Postpartum Depression Than Other Moms. KFF Health News.* https://kffhealthnews.org/news/black-mothers-get-less-treatment-for-postpartum-depression-than-other-moms/_

Floyd James, K., Smith, B. E., Robinson, M. N., Thomas Tobin, C. S., Bulles, K. F., & Barkin, J. L. (2023). Factors Associated with Postpartum Maternal Functioning in Black Women: A Secondary Analysis. *Journal of Clinical Medicine, 12*(2), 647. DOI: 10.3390/jcm12020647 PMID: 36675575

Hernandez, N. D., Francis, S., Allen, M., Bellamy, E., Sims, O. T., Oh, H., Guillaume, D., Parker, A., & Chandler, R. (2022). Prevalence and predictors of symptoms of perinatal mood and anxiety disorders among a sample of urban black women in the south. *Maternal and Child Health Journal, 26*(4), 770–777. DOI: 10.1007/s10995-022-03425-2 PMID: 35344149

Herrick, C. L., & Burkhard, J. (2024). Black Maternal Mental Health. *Journal of Prenatal & Perinatal Psychology & Health, 38*(1).

Markin, R. D., & Coleman, M. N. (2023). Intersections of gendered racial trauma and childbirth trauma: Clinical interventions for Black women. *Psychotherapy (Chicago, Ill.), 60*(1), 27–38. DOI: 10.1037/pst0000403 PMID: 34843315

Matthews, K., Morgan, I., Davis, K., Estriplet, T., Perez, S., & Crear-Perry, J. A. (2021). Pathways To Equitable And Antiracist Maternal Mental Health Care: Insights From Black Women Stakeholders: Study examines pathways to equitable and antiracist maternal mental health care. *Health Affairs, 40*(10), 1597–1604.

McCarthy, D. (2024). Gendered anti-blackness, maternal health & chattel slavery: OB/Gyn knowledge as a determinant of death of black women. *Social Science & Medicine, 353*, 117038. DOI: 10.1016/j.socscimed.2024.117038 PMID: 38936105

Nelson, T., Ernst, S. C., & Watson-Singleton, N. N. (2023). Perinatal complications, poor hospital treatment, and positive screen for postpartum depressive symptoms among black women. *Journal of Racial and Ethnic Health Disparities*, *10*(3), 1371–1378. DOI: 10.1007/s40615-022-01322-6 PMID: 35513596

O'Brien, E., & Rich, M. (2022). Obstetric violence in historical perspective. *Lancet*, *399*(10342), 2183–2185. DOI: 10.1016/S0140-6736(22)01022-4 PMID: 35691313

Office of Disease Prevention and Health Promotion. (n.d.). Social Determinants of Health—Healthy People 2030 | health.gov. Retrieved November 10, 2023, from https://health.gov/healthypeople/priority-areas/social-determinants-health

Owens, D. C. (2017). *Medical bondage: Race, gender, and the origins of American gynecology*. University of Georgia Press. DOI: 10.2307/j.ctt1pwt69x

Owens, D. C., & Fett, S. M. (2019). Black maternal and infant health: Historical legacies of slavery. *American Journal of Public Health*, *109*(10), 1342–1345. DOI: 10.2105/AJPH.2019.305243 PMID: 31415204

Parker, A. (2021). Reframing the narrative: Black maternal mental health and culturally meaningful support for wellness. *Infant Mental Health Journal*, *42*(4), 502–516. DOI: 10.1002/imhj.21910 PMID: 33470438

Perez, N. B., Melkus, G. D. E., Wright, F., Yu, G., Vorderstrasse, A. A., Sun, Y. V., & Taylor, J. Y. (2023). Latent class analysis of depressive symptom phenotypes among Black/African American mothers. *Nursing Research*, *72*(2), 93–102. DOI: 10.1097/NNR.0000000000000635 PMID: 36729771

Perinatal depression. (n.d.). National Institute of Mental Health (NIMH). https://www.nimh.nih.gov/health/publications/perinatal-depression#:~:text=Perinatal%20depression%20includes%20depression%20that,caring%20for%20themselves%20or%20others

Policy Center for Maternal Mental Health. (2023). Black Maternal Mental Health [Report]. www.policycentermmh.org/black-maternal-mental-health-issue-brief

Tyler, E. T. (2022). Black mothers matter: The social, political and legal determinants of Black maternal health across the lifespan. *Journal of Health Care Law & Policy*, *25*, 49.

Chapter 3
Prevalent Forms of Mental Health Issues and Coping Strategies Amongst Black Women

Najla Abdalla
Northcentral University, USA

ABSTRACT

The chapter summarizes the prevalent types of the mental health issues or problems that are faced by the Black women, particularly during the peripartum and post-partum times of their lives. The coping strategies that are implemented by the Black women to safeguard their mental health are a part of the analysis conducted in the chapter. The overall chapter has provided a clear picture based on the effectiveness of the interventions and the strategies that can be used by healthcare providers for reduction of the issues related to mental health that can be faced by the Black women. The chapter has also provided recommendations for the future changes that can be implemented in the strategies and interventions that can be effective for enhancing the well-being and mental health of the Black women.

INTRODUCTION

New mothers face significant mental-health challenges during peripartum and postpartum periods. Women can face major levels of stress related to the physical and emotional demands related to taking care of their infants which relates to imbalanced negative moods of individuals and parenting outcomes. The following literature review confirms that there is an increase of mental health issues reported by black

DOI: 10.4018/979-8-3693-4272-5.ch003

mothers. Recent studies and articles have shed lights on prevalent forms of mental health challenges and coping strategies. Research has emphasised the unique experiences and coping mechanisms employed by Black women to navigate mental health issues effectively. Understanding these dynamics is crucial for developing targeted interventions and support systems. The study, "A scoping review of the concept of resilience among African American women", it emphasized culturally significant aspects of resilience, such as spirituality, strength, survival, coping strategies, and social support. The results underscore the necessity of defining resilience as a multifaceted concept in upcoming studies involving the African American communities. The study "Black Perinatal Mental Health: Prioritizing Maternal Mental Health to Optimize Infant Health and Wellness" stressed the critical importance of focusing on maternal mental health to enhance infant health and wellness within the Black perinatal population. It underscores the need for targeted support and interventions to address mental health challenges during the perinatal period among Black mothers, ultimately benefiting both maternal and infant well-being. According to the study, "Assessing the impact of telehealth implementation on postpartum outcomes for Black birthing people", it examined the effects of telehealth utilization on postpartum outcomes specifically for Black individuals. The findings shed light on the potential benefits of telehealth in improving postpartum care and outcomes for Black birthing mothers, highlighting the significance of accessible and culturally sensitive healthcare practices in this population. In another study tilted, "Listen to the Whispers before They Become Screams: Addressing Black Maternal Morbidity and Mortality in the United States" delved into the critical issue of Black maternal morbidity and mortality in the U.S. It emphasized the urgent need to address the disparities and challenges faced by Black mothers during pregnancy and childbirth. The findings underlined the importance of early intervention, culturally competent care, and systemic changes to improve outcomes and reduce maternal health inequities within the Black community. By synthesizing insights from these recent studies and, a more nuanced understanding of prevalent mental health issues and coping strategies among Black women can be achieved, paving the way for targeted interventions and support initiatives.

1. Cheryl L. Woods-Giscombe, Karen Patricia Williams, Jamie Conklin, Adam Dodd, Lilian Bravo, Avery M. Anderson, Taleah Frazier, Ganga Bey, Millicent N. Robinson, Barbara J. Warren, Kathy D. Wight, Ashley S. Felix, Cindy M. Anderson, Darryl B. Hood,A scoping review of the concept of resilience among African American women,Archives of Psychiatric Nursing,Volume 46,2023,Pages 107-120,ISSN 0883-9417, https://doi.org/10.1016/j.apnu.2023.04.008. Website:https://www.sciencedirect.com/science/article/pii/S0883941723000456

2. Estriplet T, Morgan I, Davis K, Crear Perry J, Matthews K. Black Perinatal Mental Health: Prioritizing Maternal Mental Health to Optimize Infant Health and Wellness. Front Psychiatry. 2022 Apr 29;13:807235. doi: 10.3389/fpsyt.2022.807235. PMID: 35573337; PMCID: PMC9098970. Website: Black Perinatal Mental Health: Prioritizing Maternal Mental Health to Optimize Infant Health and Wellness - PMC (nih.gov)
3. Kumar NR, Arias MP, Leitner K, Wang E, Clement EG, Hamm RF. Assessing the impact of telehealth implementation on postpartum outcomes for Black birthing people. Am J Obstet Gynecol MFM. 2023 Feb;5(2):100831. doi: 10.1016/j.ajogmf.2022.100831. Epub 2022 Dec 7. PMID: 36496115; PMCID: PMC9726646. Website: Assessing the impact of telehealth implementation on postpartum outcomes for Black birthing people - PMC (nih.gov)
4. Njoku A, Evans M, Nimo-Sefah L, Bailey J. Listen to the Whispers before They Become Screams: Addressing Black Maternal Morbidity and Mortality in the United States. Healthcare (Basel). 2023 Feb 3;11(3):438. doi: 10.3390/healthcare11030438. PMID: 36767014; PMCID: PMC9914526. Website: Listen to the Whispers before They Become Screams: Addressing Black Maternal Morbidity and Mortality in the United States - PMC (nih.gov)

The resilience of new mothers while they face this issue can be enhanced by usage of appropriate coping strategies that are a part of the postpartum period. Coping strategies are highly useful with the stressors and are active in the reduction of stress levels being faced by new mothers. The active strategies of coping are more effective in comparison to the passive strategies based on coping (Dwarakanath et al., 2023). The active strategies based on coping that can be used by the new mothers include reframing, cognitive reappraisal, seeking social support, reframing, and planning for the solutions. Moreover, the passive strategies of coping can include social withdrawal, self-accusation, self-pity, denial, substance use and avoidance. The coping-related strategies that are mainly associated with low levels of perceived stress and resilience can however lead to gaining the negative outcomes related to mental health. Self-care tips can also play an important role in improvement of mental health of the individuals (Dagher, Pérez-Stable & James, 2021).

Tips related to self-care include exercising on a regular basis, eating healthy foods, staying hydrated, prioritizing sleep, practicing the enhancement of gratitude, staying connected with others, and focusing on positive levels of self-esteem. The issues related to poor levels of mental health in women during their pregnancy, and the birth of their children, have increased the health concerns within modern societies. The social aspects related to health have a huge impact on the access that individuals can gain from services based on available healthcare and the overall condition of the economy. The status of black women has been a major reason behind the issues related to poor maternity health which has a major disproportionate impact on these women (Chinn, Martin & Redmond, 2021). This chapter will provide a clear analysis of the effectiveness in different coping strategies and resilience mechanisms that can be implemented by black women dealing with the postpartum issues related to mental health. The challenges related to mental health being faced by black women have been chosen as a part of the analysis in this chapter as it provides detailed information based on the impact of socio-economic status of women's health during pregnancy, as well as after childbirth. The gap related to the development of proper strategies for addressing issues related to mental health of black women during their postpartum period will be addressed effectively in this chapter.

ANALYSIS OF THE PREVALENT MENTAL HEALTH ISSUES AMONG BLACK WOMEN DURING PREGNANCY AND AFTER CHILDBIRTH

Motherhood has proved to be a difficult transition that leads to increased levels of stress in new mothers (Walker and Murry, 2022). However, previous research has been based on the stress levels of new mothers only during the six weeks of the postpartum period. A worsening impact of stress on women during the subsequent few months after childbirth has been a major issue which was not considered effectively as a part of previous research. The maternal stressors have a huge impact on their health, including the aspects of parenting demands, exhaustion, and the changes that have taken place in their bodies. The most widely identified stressors in new mothers are related to overload and lack of proper resources, which have a huge influence on their physical health and mental state. The coping strategies in this case played an important role to ensure that the stressors being faced by the new mothers can be reduced substantially.

The proper management of thoughts and emotions in new mothers is an important strategy that can help in reducing their stress levels. The concerns of working mothers were found to be quite high as the stress levels were also higher in comparison to non-working mothers. The sudden isolation of brought on by motherhood and the loss of their previous lifestyle has caused an increase in stress levels facing new mothers. The coping strategies implemented by women were mainly based on the proactive and reactive approaches. The specific coping strategies that were a part of the postpartum period had a huge influence on the process of maintaining the mental health and stress levels of new mothers. The stressors and coping strategies relating to one another have a huge impact on the postpartum period. The development of scales that are specific to the postpartum period in new mothers has a huge influence on the implementation of coping strategies controlled by them.

The additional demands of motherhood coupled with the already challenging life of adolescence, based on significant levels of physical and emotional transitions, can prove to be quite tough for women (Dwarakanath et al. 2023). Young mothers are faced with higher risks of a negative influence on their mental health as they can face enormous levels of socioeconomic challenges that can include a circumstance of being a single parent with low income. The low-income based Black and the Hispanic women who are a part of the general population are highly likely to suffer due to the issues of postpartum depression. The likeliness of black women initiating postpartum mental healthcare services, and follow-up treatments, is also considered quite low.

The global COVID-19 pandemic led to an increase in the levels of postpartum depression among women as prevalence of the levels were around 34 percent during the pandemic in comparison to 10 percent previously. The risks factors like lower income, along with unemployment and fewer social supports, have a higher negative impact on black women. The increase in the depressive symptoms has been disproportionately high for the pregnant black women as more cases have been reported based on financial strains and concerns related to readily available medical care. The stress levels and issues faced by non-Hispanic women are lower in comparison to the Black and Hispanic women. The increased levels of risk factors, which can predispose the minority mothers, can be highly ineffective for their lives on a long-term basis. Young biracial and black mothers may face higher levels of issues during their postpartum period based on under-reporting of the depressive symptoms during this period and the increased levels of social and structural barriers. The elimination of the barriers related to the external aspects can have a huge impact on the health levels of the individuals. The implementation of coping strategies will be based on the development of appropriate interventions that can help in the maintenance of a healthy pregnancy and in support during the postpartum period.

The economic hardships and psychosocial challenges being faced by the Black and Hispanic women have a huge impact on the postpartum depression levels, which are higher in comparison to other women (Wainaina et al. (2021). These women did not receive effective levels of support from their parents, which proved to be a major reason behind the increased stress and depression they encountered. Forced abortions have also affected the mental status of these new mothers and have led to major issues for them on a long-term basis. The lack of financial support and increased economic hardships had a major negative influence on the mental health of black women. The economic challenges of black women have led to increased postpartum issues of these women. The increased levels of neglect and abandonment, and the stigmatization by the families and friends, proved to be a major issue faced by black women. Backlash from the families and lack of proper care and support have further increased the hardships faced by the black women in Nairobi, Kenya.

Black women have faced the daily challenges of living within the slum environments, resulting in an increased feeling of broken aspirations. Black women also face major levels of social isolation resulting in negative emotions, and increased risks related to postpartum depression. The increased postpartum issues have therefore led the adolescent girls to considering other avenues for releasing their stress levels. The choice of other avenues further led to an increased amount of drugs consumption in these women. Dagher, Pérez-Stable and James (2021) have stated that the mental health-related concerns faced by new mothers in the United States proved to be quite high among the black people in comparison to the white individuals. The increase in depressive symptoms were based on the disparities faced by black women and these outbursts of anger increased after they gave birth. The interventions based on mental health can be based on the development of solutions that can reduce the risks faced by different groups of black women within the United States.

As discussed by Thomas et al. (2021), the people of different color including the black women face disproportionate burden based on the aspects of posttraumatic stress disorder or PTSD and trauma. The pregnant women in this case are facing the most significant levels of stress and risks as the perinatal PTSD can be associated with the child's health and adverse mental health. PTSD is thereby considered to be a disorder that comprises of the discrete symptoms and can influence the health levels of the individuals. The proper adoption of the dimensional understanding based on PTSD can have a positive impact on guiding the selection of proper treatments for black women. Although the trauma and issues faced by pregnant women are quite common for women in the United States, the black women face more significant issues related to the postpartum aspects in comparison to the other women because of the lack of support from the community, unable to request assistance from families. However, some symptoms based on dysphoric arousal were higher among the white women in the United States as compared to black women. Perinatal healthcare is an important factor that can lead to the development of targeted interventions that can be implemented by perinatal women. PTSD is quite common among pregnant women, and this has increased the risks faced by the black women. The PTSD symptoms have a huge influence on the lives of women in the United States and the other countries as well. The severe symptoms related to PTSD have become more evident due to the ethnic and racial differences that exist among women. Chinn, Martin, and Redmond (2021) have stated that, black women within the United States are experiencing substantial levels of improvement in their health in the last few decades. However, the disparities in health care still exist which have been hugely influenced by the economic and social aspects and the conditions faced by black women in different parts of the world. The mortality rates of the black women were quite high in comparison to the other women in the United States. The aspects of ethnicity and race are the major sociocultural constructs that have provided an effective reflection based on the geographic origins, the social histories, and the cultures. The chronic challenges related to discrimination that are experiencesd by-black individuals are important aspects that influenced the mental health of new mothers. Black women faced a major disadvantage based on the implementation of strategies related to perinatal care negatively impacting their health levels.

The mental disorders faced by individuals are not diagnosed properly among the populations within developing countries; this aspect has a disproportionate impact on women (Monaghan et al. 2021). Mental disorders are quite common among new mothers during the postpartum period. The prevalence of these issues has been hugely reported by the women in Ethiopia and were based on proper diagnosis of the postpartum problems. The postpartum disorders related to mental health have thereby influenced the stigmas that are developed against them in the last few decades. The need for the properly supervised and trained staff in the healthcare sector has helped in identifying postpartum in women and referring them to adequate resources. The proper assessment of the stigma related to mental health are important for ensuring that the effective strategies can be implemented for enhancing the health of women during their postpartum period. The presence of the mental illness related to postpartum issues have further increased the prevalence of stigma and have also influenced the maternal health of the individuals. The need for enhancement of the healthcare staff is quite high for ensuring that the postpartum illness of black women can be reduced effectively. Estriplet et al. (2022) have stated that, the mental health in infants is hugely linked to the mental health of new mothers. The birthing persons or mothers face mental health issues during the postpartum period which is an important aspect of the development of a child. The proper identification of economic, social and the cultural disparities faced by black women in their perinatal stages and the experiences of the mothers are important for maintaining their mental health. Proper maintenance of the mental health of infants is also based on the ways by which the health of mothers can be managed.

The disjointed and ineffective systems of healthcare within the developing countries are major factors that have influenced the services being provided to black women. The support that is provided to the black women based on enhanced levels of mental health can be related to the improvement of the healthcare system and the development of infants. The increased structural barriers that are being faced by the black mothers have thereby increased their mental health disorders, issues related to infant health. The black parents can play an important role in supporting the development of infants and the programs related to parent education that can be implemented by the healthcare organizations.

The barriers related to access of mental health care during the pregnancy of black women and the perinatal period have a huge influence on the ethnic minorities of women (Jankovic et al. (2020). The services related to mental health that are provided to the women from ethnic minorities or the Black women can have a positive influence on their future health. The services related to mental healthcare provided to the women belonging to various ethnic groups are quite different from each other. The differences in healthcare services are based on the solutions that can be provided to the Asian, White and the Black African individuals. The community contacts that are attended by black women can thereby have a huge influence on the Black African and the Asian women. Ethnicity of women are thereby considered to be an important aspect that affects the services related to mental health and the solutions that are provided to the women. The access that are provided to different women based on the community mental health-related services is different for the Black women and the women who belong to different minorities. Adeyemo et al. (2020) have stated that PPD or postpartum depression can be considered a major mental health-related disorder that can influence around 10 percent to 15 percent of new mothers in different parts of the world. PPD has a major influence on black mothers, and these can also influence the emotional and cognitive development of children adversely. The socio-demographic factors including age, religion, socio-economic status, unemployment, and education are linked with the issues related to PPD. The factors related to obstetrics, and the infant-related care can lead to the increased issues based on complications in the pregnancy, unhealthy babies, death of infants and the unplanned pregnancies. The high prevalence and increase of PPD among these women have influenced the health levels of women and their overall quality of health as well. Powers et al. (2020) have stated that, the pregnant African American women who are a part of the low-income based urban communities have been influenced by the huge exposure towards trauma and increased risks based on development of the post-trauma related disorders that include the aspects of depression and PTSD or posttraumatic stress disorder.

WAYS USED BY BLACK WOMEN TO COPE WITH THE MENTAL HEALTH ISSUES AND TO PROVIDE RESILIENCE DURING POSTPARTUM PERIOD

Postpartum depression confronted by new mothers has proved to be a major problem related to public health. The attitudes that are depicted by the minority women towards the aspects of postpartum depression and the types of treatment can have a huge influence on the improvement of their health levels. The issues faced by black women due to the increased depression during the postpartum period were. The previous research was related to the extensive analysis of the levels of maternal depression. However, despite the studies, the mental health issues being faced by the women belonging to minorities persist.

Mommy Meltdown was mainly an initiative that was developed for addressing the important aspects of depression within the minority women during their perinatal and the postpartum periods. The issue related to depression faced by the minority women was an important and sensitive aspect that affected the health of minority women. Postpartum depression has been an important issue that is part of the patient populations regardless of race. The white and black women had depicted major levels of comfort based on the increased levels of primary care that are provided to them. However, various research has found that the care provided to black women was not quite adequate as compared to the levels of care that are offered to the white women due to black woman not wanting to leave her neighbourhood for better healthcare. However, currently black women have depicted a receptive nature towards the care that is provided to them based on increased levels of depression. The postpartum depression issues are highly important based on the ways by which the black or African American women are influenced negatively by society. The acceptance of therapy depicted by them is however an important progress that can have a positive influence on their performance levels on a long-term basis. Werchan et al. (2022) stated that, the impact of COVID-19 pandemic was enormous among the perinatal women; this has increased the concerns related to public health. The need for coping strategies has increased considerably due to the pandemic as these strategies can have a positive impact on the mitigation of the issues that are being faced by the infants and women. The women have also reported different behaviours which were related to the reduction of pandemic-based stress and can also have a negative influence on the stress levels. The passive strategies related to coping can be an important aspect that is related to the increase in screen time such as time in front of a computer and intake of comfort foods. The issues related to postpartum stress that are faced by new mothers can increase the importance of coping strategies and the phenotypes, according to Werchan et al. (2022) phenotypes with high levels of passive coping strategies were associated with elevated symptoms of depression, anxiety, and global psychological distress, as well as worsening stress and energy levels, relative to other coping phenotypes. In contrast, phenotypes with high levels of active coping strategies were associated with greater resiliency relative to other phenotypes. The phenotypes based on coping strategies that are implemented by the pregnant women include self-care and social support.

According to Melnyk et al. (2020), the strategies related to prenatal care are quite effective and are used widely within the United States. This helps to improve the health outcomes of women. However, the implementation of prenatal care was not able to significantly reduce the health disparities within minorities. Around two-thirds of the Hispanic and Black women have received the prenatal care during the first trimester of their pregnancy levels. The emotionally distressed experiences that are faced by the black women can lead to the multiple negative outcomes. Around 40 percent to 50 percent of the poor women have depicted various symptoms related to prenatal depression which has a huge influence on the poverty, women who are a part of the minority groups. The Black and Hispanic depressed women have thereby not been able to obtain the proper levels of prenatal care despite the presence of effective strategies regarding this aspect.

Anxiety is a major aspect that has influenced a greater number of women within the general population that have led to inadequate levels of maternal health and the outcomes related to wellbeing of women. The prevalence of the high rates of prenatal anxiety had a negative impact on the increasing anxiety levels of the individuals. The decreased behaviours related to healthy lifestyles of black women are influenced by the aspects of stress, anxiety, and the depressive symptoms. Insan et al. (2022) have stated that, perinatal mental health (PMH) has become a public health-related issues affected pregnant women throughout the world-and has begun crossing the cultural boundaries. However, the presence of PMH conditions can vary in a considerable manner and the disparities can mainly be a part of different societies of the South Asian countries that include Pakistan, India, and Bangladesh. The conditions related to PMH in Global North-West and the different cultural and social norms can be based on the mental and gender health of women. The coping strategies implemented by black women have a huge influence on emphasis that is provided towards the physical symptoms, lack of proper awareness, shame, stigma, and the various other societal aspects. The coping strategies and interventions that can be implemented for reduction of the issues being faced by the black women can thereby be related to a proper understanding that can be gained based on the factors that can increase these issues.

Structural levels of racism can lead to significant levels of inequities that are a part of the maternal and perinatal disorders related to mental health (Matthews et al. (2021). The populations of black mothers and births are mainly burdened by the disjointed levels of systems related to care for the aspects of mental health. The strategies that can be identified and implemented for addressing racism and the inequities within infant and maternal care of mental health are effective for ensuring the issues can be solved on a long-term basis. The prevalence of the experiences related to postpartum depression is quite high in comparison to the other women. The economic and social aspects have thereby increased the issues related to mental health encountered by the black mothers.

Black mothers have also encountered major levels of disparities associated with the lack of appropriate education related to universal mental health. The appropriate practices and strategies that can be implemented for reducing the mental health disorder-linked issues that are being handled by these women can be developed according to the analysis of the problems based on black birthing. The process of reimagining the aspects of maternal mental healthcare-related aspects is important for addressing the crisis of maternal health that is encountered by the black mothers. The value that is provided to the women-led communities can be operative in the development of appropriate strategies that can be effective in development of the proper strategies for reducing the issues of mental health disorders. Floyd James et al. (2024) stated that, the exposure of black women towards stress related to racism that was a part of the postpartum period has proved to be a major indicator of the anxiety disorders and the postpartum mood.

Black women associated with the City of Los Angeles have faced major issues based on increased racism and has had a major negative influence on their postpartum mental health. The society of Los Angeles has depicted huge disparities as black women comprised approximately 9 percent of the overall population and they have faced immense issues based on postpartum mental health levels. The stress based on racism has increased in the daily lives of individuals and has influenced their activities such as shopping or being out in public. The activities related to interpersonal racism are important factors that can affect the perceptions being formed among the individuals related to reduction of the racism issues. Racism-related stress has increased vastly in different countries and has also influenced the development of appropriate coping strategies and mechanisms that can aid in solving the problems of black women during their postpartum period. The symptoms related to PMAD, or perinatal mood and anxiety disorders are related to the increased stressful life-based events, lack of the social support, and the prenatal depression levels. The exposure towards racism-related stress were highest among the black women in comparison to the white women and this exposure has increased the importance of developing strategies or interventions for reducing stress and improving the levels of mental health.

According to Prady et al. (2021), the maternal problems related to mental health during the perinatal period can lead to significant levels of distress and reduced functioning which can have a negative influence on the children as well. The disadvantaged people are mainly facing risks related to increased health inequalities that also include the perinatal aspects of mental health. The implementation of appropriate interventions being developed by the government can thereby be helpful in reducing maternal problems related to mental health. The equity in mental health-related problems can play an important role in ensuring that the appropriate interventions can be effective for the individuals. The hesitancy levels among some of the populations or individuals based on the implementation of solutions that can solve the mental health problems can be more prevalent among black women. The proper identification and effective management of the problems related to perinatal healthcare can also prove to be inequitable for women belonging to the ethnic minorities. Firouzbakht et al. (2022) stated that pregnant women are more vulnerable towards the psychological problems based on adaptive capacities of the coping strategies and the personalities of pregnant women as well.

The increased levels of psychological stress experienced by individuals during their pregnancy can lead to major negative consequences that have a long-term impact on them. The coping efforts can thereby have an impact on the birth outcomes based on reduction of the negative responses related to the cognitive, emotional, physiological, and behavioural aspects. The appropriate responses based on coping can thereby be implemented by the individuals based on their needs which can have a long-term influence on them. The black women or minority women may not be able to use all the different types of coping mechanisms effectively. The seeking of emotional support by individuals can be related to the avoidance strategies that are implemented by the individuals. The pregnant women who have chosen the avoidance of stress levels can readily implement the coping strategies for ensuring that the issues can be resolved effectively.

Anxiety faced by the mothers during their pregnancy can have huge adverse outcomes for the mothers and the infants (Araji et al. (2020). Although many previous studies have mentioned anxiety along with depression, it is a major issue that has influenced the health outcomes of the mothers. The infant outcomes, postpartum maternal outcomes, and the pharmacological treatments have an enormous influence on the focus that is provided towards the high-risk pregnancies. Anxiety can prove to be highly problematic and can impact pregnant patients and their children. The anxiety faced by individuals during pregnancy can thereby lead to a major impact on the women and can provide potential risks for children as well. The improvement of the screening process based on maternal mental health screening and increasing the access towards care can be effective for the mothers to ensure the reduction of depression and anxiety. The proper assessment and diagnosis of anxiety during the post-partum period and pregnancy can be effective for the new mothers to ensure reduction of its impact on their health and the health levels of children as well.

The various avenues of treatment that can be explored by pregnant women can be effective for ensuring that anxiety and stress can be reduced and the negative outcomes on the infants can be stopped as well. Kemet et al. (2022) have stated that black women have been giving birth joyously for centuries, although there is a presence of the disproportionate rates based on the negative perinatal outcomes. The implementation of group-based perinatal care has proved to be quite promising in mitigation of the inequities and the opinions of black women are important for understanding their effectiveness in solving the issues. Black women are provided with federally funded state-wide programs that can be effective in reducing the maternal mental health-related issues. The support that is provided by the group prenatal care is an important tool that can be helpful for black women to reduce the inequities confronting them and can also be effective in reducing the postpartum depression challenging the individuals. The reduction of inequities will also be based on increasing-access of mental healthcare services for black expectant mothers. The prenatal care-related activities are thereby able to provide major benefits to black women for reducing their postpartum depression levels.

WAYS OF ADDRESSING MENTAL HEALTH ISSUES FACED BY BLACK WOMEN DURING POSTPARTUM PERIOD

The postpartum experiences of black women or other women of color have a significant influence on their health and the care that is being provided to the infants as well (Harrell et al. (2022). The reduction of hospital emergencies of black women during their postpartum period can also be possible based on the implementation of postpartum care strategies in the hospitals. The different areas related to appropriate interventions that can be implemented by black women can play an important role in reducing the levels of depression. The aspect of maternal health is highly important for ensuring-the improvement of health in infants, and their future being secured properly as well. The interventions that can be implemented by the healthcare organizations are related to focussing efforts to enhance the continuity of the care and increase-access for black women to receive appropriate healthcare. The proper strengthening of the communication between the providers and patients by the training providers can help in recognition of the unconscious levels of bias. The proper aspect of preparing black women by implementation of the adaptations in teaching materials to an online format and engaging the caregivers of women, throughout pregnancy is an important factor that can improve the levels of social support. Womersley, Ripullone and Hirst (2021) have stated that, healthcare systems have started providing major levels of priority towards the intrapartum and antenatal over the entire postpartum period.

The metabolic diseases and conditions associated with the pregnancy can have a significant impact on the long-term health levels of the individuals. The women belonging to ethnic minority, or the black women categorised in the low socioeconomic groups and-have faced major risks related to the psychiatric and physical complications based on pregnancy in comparison to the white women. The inequalities related to different aspects of coping strategies and interventions were mainly increased due to the lack of accessible education about the risk factors. The proper identification of the approaches that are related to addressing the needs of the black patients is a major responsibility that needs to be fulfilled by the midwives and obstetricians. The improvement of appropriate interventions can be based on the collaboration that is provided by the healthcare professionals from a wide range of specialities. The data collection can be enhanced based on the long-term impact of the psychiatric and metabolic conditions that are related to the postpartum aspects.

The proper optimization of postpartum care has played an important role in highlighting the needs related to management, coordination of care, and the expansion (of what) based on the healthcare-related services after the childbirth (Scott and Davis 2022). The interventions that can be implemented for reducing depression during the postpartum period will be based on implementation of the management, surveillance, and mitigation strategies can prove to be effective for black women. The black woman-person first approach was implemented by the healthcare organizations for ensuring that the strategies can prove to be effective for offering responsive care. The strategies related to democratizing and destigmatizing care has been able to bridge the gaps that can exist between the intent and the levels of impact in the optimization of postpartum care. The proper optimizing of the postpartum care strategies for black women and adolescence can have proper influence on the implementation of appropriate levels of interventions. The levels of equality within postpartum care facing black women are related to the obligatory visits that can be provided to them after giving birth to infants. The safe place that can be provided to the black women and adolescence can have a huge influence on the minority communities based on the reduction of risk factors they might encounter. Alio et al. (2022) stated that the black women have started facing major levels of disparities based on maternal mortality and morbidity as compared to the white women. Different factors can provide major levels of contribution towards the enhancement of disparities that are faced by black women.

The improvement of maternal experiences that can be provided to black women during their postpartum period can play an important role in enhancing the strategies that can be implemented for solving the mental health issues. The communication levels that can be developed between the mother and her provider can have a huge positive impact on the maternal experiences that are offered to black women. The listening sessions that are developed between the mothers and their care providers can thereby play an important role in the development of appropriate interventions and strategies for solving the issues being faced by black women during the postpartum period. The positive experiences that black women can gain during perinatal care can lead to enhancement of the postpartum experiences which can reduce depression and anxiety-related issues. The key aspects that can influence the proper development of strategies for reducing the postpartum issues include communication between mother and provider, social support, systematic factors, and the mental and maternal health.

According to Moore et al. (2021), the issues related to mood or anxiety disorder are common illnesses related to mental health that can occur as a part of perinatal period. The perinatal mental health-related conditions of black women can lead to increased issues being faced by them during the postpartum period. The prevalence of the perinatal conditions related to mental health of black women can be based on the barriers that include bias based on the mental health-based conditions, treatment, and screening the policy-related opportunities that are developed for overcoming the barriers and supporting the reproductive and sexual health can prove to be effective interventions and can help in reducing the depression issues faced by Black women. The coverage can be established based on home visits by the healthcare provider and the programs related to peer support that can be offered to black women. The implementation of effective economic and social policies can be helpful in supporting the families can help in reducing the depression levels of black women. Gonzalez et al. (2021) stated that the aspects of postpartum depression or PPD has been able to influence around 15 percent of new mothers who are a part of the United States. The long-term based adverse influences can be faced by the children and mothers if they are not treated properly. The black women or the women of color have faced the disproportionate and high rates of PPD, and the rates have been around 54 percent.

Latinas have been considered as the groups of individuals who are not always likely to gain support related to their mental health during the postpartum period. The global pandemic has increased the stressful events that are faced by individuals, and these have an increase in levels of depression and anxiety of the Latina and Black women. Latina women hurdled major barriers based on PPD care and the therapy sessions that can be offered to the individuals. The sociocultural barriers being faced by the Latina and Black women are quite based on the interventions that can be implemented for reduction of the depression and anxiety issues.

As argued by Gopalan et al. (2022), the gaps and shortages related to research funding based on the perinatal conditions of mental health have led to the creation of the environment that can be helpful in providing postpartum mental healthcare to the black women. National organizations like the American College of Obstetrics and Gynaecology or ACOG can aim at the development and implementation of appropriate screening strategies for identification of the postpartum and pregnant women who are showing the signs of depression. The issues related to mood disorders can have a negative influence on the families, women, and infants. The primary care physicians or the PCPs and the other providers can play an important role in screening the patients for understanding the issues based on postpartum depression. The implementation of appropriate screening tools can play an important role in understanding the issues related to depression and anxiety during the post-partum period. However, screening can be ineffective alone and can be insufficient for improvement of the clinical outcomes. The implementation of the screening strategies along with the increased awareness based on the perinatal levels of mental health can prove to be highly effective for the strategies being implemented for reducing the issues anxiety and depression. Bains et al. (2023) stated that, the mental illness issues faced by the Black and Asian expectant mothers are higher in comparison to the other women. The researchers have also depicted that the women belonging to the ethnic minorities are less likely to receive the perinatal care from the healthcare professionals. The healthcare professionals who are a part of the journeys of these women have the ability of providing effective perspectives that can be helpful in the development of appropriate strategies that can be implemented for solving the issues related to depression and anxiety that are faced by them. The aspects related to acceptability and accessibility of the mental health services being offered to the Black and Asian women can be related to the ways by which they can address barriers faced by them. The remedies that can be developed and implemented by the healthcare providers for reduction of the inequalities faced by the minority groups.

CONCLUSION AND RECOMMENDATIONS

The issues related to mental health and depression that are burdened by the new mothers can have a huge influence on their overall health aspects and the health of infants as well. The issues faced by black women during their postpartum period are enormous, and these can influence the health of the infants as well. The lack of proper accessibility of the healthcare services for black women and new mothers, belonging to the minority groups, has found to be a major aspect that has further increased the issues facing them. The development of appropriate coping strategies and interventions for reducing the mental health issues of the new mothers or black women can be an important aspect that can affect their development in future. The changes that can thereby be implemented in the strategies will play an important role in ensuring that the future mental health levels can be enhanced properly, and this can also have a positive impact on the infant health. Moreover, the reduction of inequalities within the healthcare services and support that is offered to the pregnant women or new mothers belonging to the minority groups can be effective on a long-term basis for ensuring that their issues can be solved properly.

The recommendations for future improvement of the healthcare support provided to new mothers belonging to the black community are as follows,

- Black women need to be provided with detailed information regarding the importance of the interventions that can be used for reducing the depression and anxiety issues that are faced by them during the postpartum period. The proper provision of information is important for ensuring that the reluctance and hesitant nature of black women can be reduced, and they can access towards the interventions properly.

- Mental health-related support needs to be effectively provided to black women by the healthcare providers who are a major part of their pregnancy journey. The healthcare professionals who are a part of the journeys of Black women have the ability of offering proper insights based on their needs and the appropriate interventions that can be implemented with the aim of reducing their depression and anxiety-related issues.
- Healthcare providers need to play an important role in reduction of the usage of maladaptive coping strategies that are used by black women for reducing the anxiety and depression.
- Culturally Competent Mental Health Services: Encourage the availability of mental health professionals who understand and respect cultural backgrounds and promote training for therapists on racial and cultural issues that may affect treatment.
- Community Support Programs: Develop community-based programs that provide supportive resources for Black mothers, including parenting groups and mental health workshops. Offer peer support systems where mothers can share experiences and coping strategies.
- Advocacy and Policy Change: Support policies aimed at addressing systemic inequalities affecting Black families, including healthcare access and housing. Advocate for mental health awareness campaigns targeting the Black community to reduce stigma.
- Self-Care and Wellness Practices: Encourage the adoption of self-care routines that promote mental health, including mindfulness, exercise, and creative activities and promote the importance of rest and personal time for mothers, emphasizing that self-care is not selfish.
- Education and Resources: Provide education on mental health for mothers, including recognizing the signs of depression and anxiety, and understanding when to seek help. Distribute resources on local mental health services, hotlines, and support networks.
- Inclusive Therapy Options: Promote alternative therapy options that may resonate more with Black mothers, such as art therapy, music therapy, or community healing practices and explore virtual therapy options to increase accessibility, particularly for those in underserved areas.
- Family and Social Support Systems: Encourage strong family ties and connections within communities to provide emotional and practical support and facilitate workshops on building supportive relationships and open communication within families.
- Research and Awareness: Support research focused on the specific mental health needs of Black mothers and the barriers they face. Increase awareness

about the unique challenges of Black motherhood in both healthcare and social settings.

By addressing these challenges and fostering supportive environments, we can help alleviate mental health issues faced by black mothers and promote their overall well-being. Overall, supporting new black mothers is vital not only for their individual health and well-being but also for the broader health of families and communities. It fosters resilience, empowerment, and equality while addressing long-standing disparities that have historically affected black families. By recognizing and addressing the specific needs of black mothers, society can work towards creating an equitable future for all.

REFERENCES

Adeyemo, E. O., Oluwole, E. O., Kanma-Okafor, O. J., Izuka, O. M., & Odeyemi, K. A. (2020). Prevalence and predictors of postpartum depression among postnatal women in Lagos, Nigeria. *African Health Sciences*, *20*(4), 1943–1954. DOI: 10.4314/ahs.v20i4.53 PMID: 34394261

Alio, A. P., Dillion, T., Hartman, S., Johnson, T., Turner, S., Bullock, S., & Dozier, A. (2022). A community collaborative for the exploration of local factors affecting Black mothers' experiences with perinatal care. *Maternal and Child Health Journal*, *26*(4), 751–760. DOI: 10.1007/s10995-022-03422-5 PMID: 35316456

Araji, S., Griffin, A., Dixon, L., Spencer, S. K., Peavie, C., & Wallace, K. (2020). An overview of maternal anxiety during pregnancy and the post-partum period. *Journal of Mental Health & Clinical Psychology*, *4*(4). https://www.mentalhealthjournal.org/articles/an-overview-of-maternal-anxiety-during-pregnancy-and-the-post-partum-period.pdf

Bains, K., Bicknell, S., Jovanović, N., Conneely, M., McCabe, R., Copello, A., Fletcher-Rogers, J., Priebe, S., & Janković, J. (2023). Healthcare professionals' views on the accessibility and acceptability of perinatal mental health services for South Asian and Black women: A qualitative study. *BMC Medicine*, *21*(1), 370. DOI: 10.1186/s12916-023-02978-5 PMID: 37784145

Chinn, J. J., Martin, I. K., & Redmond, N. (2021). Health equity among Black women in the United States. *Journal of Women's Health*, *30*(2), 212–219. DOI: 10.1089/jwh.2020.8868 PMID: 33237831

Dagher, R. K., Pérez-Stable, E. J., & James, R. S. (2021). Socioeconomic and racial/ethnic disparities in postpartum consultation for mental health concerns among US mothers. *Archives of Women's Mental Health*, *24*(5), 781–791. DOI: 10.1007/s00737-021-01132-5 PMID: 33855652

Dwarakanath, M., Hossain, F., Balascio, P., Moore, M. C., Hill, A. V., & De Genna, N. M. (2023). Experiences of postpartum mental health sequelae among black and biracial women during the COVID-19 pandemic. *BMC Pregnancy and Childbirth*, *23*(1), 636. DOI: 10.1186/s12884-023-05929-3 PMID: 37667206

Estriplet, T., Morgan, I., Davis, K., Crear Perry, J., & Matthews, K. (2022). Black perinatal mental health: Prioritizing maternal mental health to optimize infant health and wellness. *Frontiers in Psychiatry*, *13*, 807235. DOI: 10.3389/fpsyt.2022.807235 PMID: 35573337

Firouzbakht, M., Rahmani, N., Sharif Nia, H., & Omidvar, S. (2022). Coping strategies and depression during the COVID-19 pandemic in pregnant women: A cross sectional study. *BMC Psychiatry*, *22*(1), 153. DOI: 10.1186/s12888-022-03792-8 PMID: 35232424

Floyd James, K., Chen, K., Hindra, S. S., Gray, S., Robinson, M. N., Tobin, C. S. T., Choi, K., & Saint Arnault, D. (2024). Racism-related stress and mental health among black women living in Los Angeles County, California: A comparison of postpartum mood and anxiety disorder screening scales. *Archives of Women's Mental Health*, *27*(5), 1–10. DOI: 10.1007/s00737-024-01458-w PMID: 38561564

Gonzalez, C., Ramirez, M., Diaz, A., Duran, M., & Areán, P. (2021). Expanding virtual postpartum mental health care for latina women: A participatory research and policy agenda. *Women's Health Issues*, *31*(2), 96–99. DOI: 10.1016/j.whi.2020.10.005 PMID: 33250342

Gopalan, P., Spada, M. L., Shenai, N., Brockman, I., Keil, M., Livingston, S., Moses-Kolko, E., Nichols, N., O'Toole, K., Quinn, B., & Glance, J. B. (2022). Postpartum depression—Identifying risk and access to intervention. *Current Psychiatry Reports*, *24*(12), 889–896. DOI: 10.1007/s11920-022-01392-7 PMID: 36422834

Harrell, T., Howell, E. A., Balbierz, A., Guel, L., Pena, J., Janevic, T., & Gorbenko, K. (2022). Improving postpartum care: Identifying opportunities to reduce postpartum emergency room visits among publicly-insured women of color. *Maternal and Child Health Journal*, *26*(4), 913–922. DOI: 10.1007/s10995-021-03282-5 PMID: 34982328

House, T. S., Alnajjar, E., Mulekar, M., & Spiryda, L. B. (2020). Mommy meltdown: Understanding racial differences between black and white women in attitudes about postpartum depression and treatment modalities. *Journal of Clinical Gynecology and Obstetrics*, *9*(3), 37–42. DOI: 10.14740/jcgo664 PMID: 33732401

Insan, N., Weke, A., Rankin, J., & Forrest, S. (2022). Perceptions and attitudes around perinatal mental health in Bangladesh, India and Pakistan: A systematic review of qualitative data. *BMC Pregnancy and Childbirth*, *22*(1), 293. DOI: 10.1186/s12884-022-04642-x PMID: 35387619

Jankovic, J., Parsons, J., Jovanović, N., Berrisford, G., Copello, A., Fazil, Q., & Priebe, S. (2020). Differences in access and utilisation of mental health services in the perinatal period for women from ethnic minorities—A population-based study. *BMC Medicine*, *18*(1), 1–12. DOI: 10.1186/s12916-020-01711-w PMID: 32912196

Kemet, S., Yang, Y., Nseyo, O., Bell, F., Gordon, A. Y. A., Mays, M., Fowler, M., & Jackson, A. (2022). "When I think of mental healthcare, I think of no care." Mental Health Services as a Vital Component of Prenatal Care for Black Women. *Maternal and Child Health Journal*, *26*(4), 1–10. DOI: 10.1007/s10995-021-03226-z PMID: 34519952

Kumar, N. R., Arias, M. P., Leitner, K., Wang, E., Clement, E. G., & Hamm, R. F. (2023, Feb). Assessing the impact of telehealth implementation on postpartum outcomes for Black birthing people. *American Journal of Obstetrics & Gynecology MFM*, *5*(2), 100831. DOI: 10.1016/j.ajogmf.2022.100831 PMID: 36496115

Matthews, K., Morgan, I., Davis, K., Estriplet, T., Perez, S., & Crear-Perry, J. A. (2021). Pathways To Equitable And Antiracist Maternal Mental Health Care: Insights From Black Women Stakeholders: Study examines pathways to equitable and antiracist maternal mental health care. *Health Affairs*, *40*(10), 1597–1604. DOI: 10.1377/hlthaff.2021.00808 PMID: 34606342

Melnyk, B. M., Gennaro, S., Szalacha, L. A., Hoying, J., O'Connor, C., Cooper, A., & Gibeau, A. (2020). Randomized controlled trial of the COPE-P intervention to improve mental health, healthy lifestyle behaviors, birth and post-natal outcomes of minority pregnant women: Study protocol with implications. *Contemporary Clinical Trials*, *98*, 106090. DOI: 10.1016/j.cct.2020.106090 PMID: 32745703

Monaghan, S., Akale, M. A., Demeke, B., & Darmstadt, G. L. (2021). Prevalence and stigma of postpartum common mental disorders in the Gurage region of Ethiopia: A mixed-methods observational cohort study. *Frontiers in Psychology*, *12*, 626797. DOI: 10.3389/fpsyg.2021.626797 PMID: 33897534

Moore, J. E., McLemore, M. R., Glenn, N., & Zivin, K. (2021). Policy Opportunities To Improve Prevention, Diagnosis, And Treatment Of Perinatal Mental Health Conditions: Study examines policy opportunities to improve prevention, diagnosis, and treatment of perinatal mental health. *Health Affairs*, *40*(10), 1534–1542. DOI: 10.1377/hlthaff.2021.00779 PMID: 34606359

Njoku, A., Evans, M., Nimo-Sefah, L., & Bailey, J. (2023, Feb 3). Listen to the Whispers before They Become Screams: Addressing Black Maternal Morbidity and Mortality in the United States. *Healthcare (Basel)*, *11*(3), 438. DOI: 10.3390/healthcare11030438 PMID: 36767014

Powers, A., Woods-Jaeger, B., Stevens, J. S., Bradley, B., Patel, M. B., Joyner, A., Smith, A. K., Jamieson, D. J., Kaslow, N., & Michopoulos, V. (2020). Trauma, psychiatric disorders, and treatment history among pregnant African American women. *Psychological Trauma: Theory, Research, Practice, and Policy*, *12*(2), 138–146. DOI: 10.1037/tra0000507 PMID: 31464464

Prady, S. L., Endacott, C., Dickerson, J., Bywater, T. J., & Blower, S. L. (2021). Inequalities in the identification and management of common mental disorders in the perinatal period: An equity focused re-analysis of a systematic review. *PLoS One*, *16*(3), e0248631. DOI: 10.1371/journal.pone.0248631 PMID: 33720994

Scott, K. A., & Davis, D. A. (2022). Destigmatizing and democratizing postpartum care: A "Black woman-person first" approach. *Clinical Obstetrics and Gynecology*, *65*(3), 663–675. DOI: 10.1097/GRF.0000000000000729 PMID: 35723647

Thomas, J. L., Carter, S. E., Schetter, C. D., & Sumner, J. A. (2021). Racial and ethnic disparities in posttraumatic psychopathology among postpartum women. *Journal of Psychiatric Research*, *137*, 36–40. DOI: 10.1016/j.jpsychires.2021.02.030 PMID: 33647727

Wainaina, C. W., Sidze, E. M., Maina, B. W., Badillo-Amberg, I., Anyango, H. O., Kathoka, F., Khasowa, D., & Okoror, C. E. (2021). Psychosocial challenges and individual strategies for coping with mental stress among pregnant and post-partum adolescents in Nairobi informal settlements: A qualitative investigation. *BMC Pregnancy and Childbirth*, *21*(1), 1–11. DOI: 10.1186/s12884-021-04128-2 PMID: 34583684

Walker, L. O., & Murry, N. (2022). Maternal stressors and coping strategies during the extended Postpartum Period: A retrospective analysis with contemporary implications. *Women's Health Reports (New Rochelle, N.Y.)*, *3*(1), 104–114. DOI: 10.1089/whr.2021.0134 PMID: 35136882

Werchan, D. M., Hendrix, C. L., Ablow, J. C., Amstadter, A. B., Austin, A. C., Babineau, V., Anne Bogat, G., Cioffredi, L.-A., Conradt, E., Crowell, S. E., Dumitriu, D., Fifer, W., Firestein, M. R., Gao, W., Gotlib, I. H., Graham, A. M., Gregory, K. D., Gustafsson, H. C., Havens, K. L., & Brito, N. H. (2022). Behavioral coping phenotypes and associated psychosocial outcomes of pregnant and postpartum women during the COVID-19 pandemic. *Scientific Reports*, *12*(1), 1209. DOI: 10.1038/s41598-022-05299-4 PMID: 35075202

Womersley, K., Ripullone, K., & Hirst, J. E. (2021). Tackling inequality in maternal health: Beyond the postpartum. *Future Healthcare Journal*, *8*(1), 31–35. DOI: 10.7861/fhj.2020-0275 PMID: 33791457

Woods-Giscombe, C. L., Williams, K. P., Conklin, J., Dodd, A., Bravo, L., Anderson, A. M., & Hood, D. B. (2023). A scoping review of the concept of resilience among African American women. *Archives of psychiatric nursing*, 46, 107-120. DOI: 10.1016/j.apnu.2023.04.008

Chapter 4
Perinatal Anxiety and Depression in Black Mothers

Mercedes Jamecia Moore
https://orcid.org/0009-0002-6230-2680
Capella University, USA

ABSTRACT

Black women were forced to birth children for the purpose of upholding the institution of slavery. Black mothers assumed the inhumane tasks of increasing the slave population through forced reproduction- rather it be rape or breeding farms, while also carrying out physical labor on the plantation. America's history of exploiting Black women's bodies has lasting cultural stigma that influences the ideology of medical professionals who treat Black women today. Specifically, when compared to White women, Black women are more likely experience PMADs. 40% of Black women reported experiencing postpartum depression, more than double that was reported from the general population. Black women from higher socioeconomic status with access to quality insurance and resources have not been exempt from these adverse outcomes. There must be a radical path forward designed specifically with the intention of creating birth equity for Black mothers and families.

ORIGINS OF THE BLACK MATERNAL MENTAL HEALTH CRISIS

The Black maternal mental health crisis today is linked to slavery, where Black women were victims of reproductive oppression. Black women were forced to birth children for the purpose of upholding the institution of slavery. Black mothers assumed the inhumane tasks of increasing the slave population through forced

DOI: 10.4018/979-8-3693-4272-5.ch004

reproduction- rather it be rape or breeding farms, while also carrying out physical labor on the plantation. It is important to highlight that Black women were also forced to be the subjects of medical experiments. The exploitation of Black women's bodies had economic advances for slave owners and the field of medicine. This was an American system that forced Black women to birth children but disregarded them as mothers, inflicting psychological scars and trauma for generations to come.

Even though slavery was abolished in 1865, its legacy of reproductive oppression is still embedded in American society, in the form of medical racism. America's history of exploiting Black women's bodies has lasting cultural stigma that influences the ideology of medical professionals who treat Black women today. The inability to learn from our nation's history of atrocious treatment towards Black women is likely to repeat itself without culturally competent screenings and interventions (Almeida et al., 2021).

Prevalence

Medical literature has been prioritizing its focus on the impact of perinatal mood and anxiety disorders (PMADs) on mothers during and after pregnancy (the perinatal period, defined as the time a woman becomes pregnant up to one year postpartum). Research indicates that about 15% of mothers experience anxiety and mood disorders during the perinatal period. In that 15%, 14% are reported as perinatal depression and 13%-21% are reported as perinatal anxiety (Byrnes, 2018). This is a major concern affecting mothers across all racial groups, but Black mothers face adversities and disparities that are unique to only them. In comparison to other racial groups, Black women have higher trauma exposure across their lifespan, meaning that they have experienced at least one trauma event. Furthermore, trauma exposure rate during the perinatal period is 87% for Black women compared to 29%-74% for other women (Policy Center for Maternal Mental Health, 2023). This makes Black women more vulnerable to perinatal anxiety and depression disorders. Specifically, when compared to White women, Black women are more likely experience PMADs. 40% of Black women reported experiencing postpartum depression, more than double that was reported from the general population (Estriplet et al., 2022). The intersection of race and sex presents Black women with disparities such as gender related violence, racism, and sexism. These unique disparities expose Black women to negative social determinants of health (SDOH). The conditions in the environment where Black women live, learn, work, worship, and age are their SDOH and plays a significant role in their quality-of-life outcomes (Chinn et al., 2020). SDOH along with systemic inequities can be predictors of PMADs in Black mothers.

Social Determinants and Systemic Inequities

Socioeconomic Factors such as *income inequality* and *inequities in access to resources* are areas that add to stress for Black mothers. Due to systemic barriers in employment, Black mothers are more likely face financial hardships and experience poverty. Systemic barriers in employment can also lead to Black mothers being *uninsured, limiting access to healthcare*. According to researchers, Black mothers from low socioeconomic backgrounds experienced the worst healthcare quality. Other areas of concerns associated with socioeconomic factors include *limited access to safe and stable living conditions and proper nutrition.*

Racial and Discrimination Factors can have a negative impact on the maternal mental health of Black mothers in general, but especially when navigating the medical system. According to research, Black mothers' experiences with hospital births included: being yelled at, threatened, and ignored when requesting help. Black women reported a loss of autonomy when navigating the maternity care system. This type of treatment from healthcare providers is linked to *implicit bias* and is a clear indicator for the need of *culturally competent care.* Black woman's' experience of culturally incompetent care by healthcare providers can lead to them feeling unsafe and fearful to advocate for themselves, resulting in negative mental health outcomes.

Birth Complications have been a part of Black women's experiences with childbirth at U.S. hospitals and other childbirth clinics. The medical literature suggests that the *disproportionate impact of the pandemic* on Black communities may have only exacerbated this phenomenon. According to the medical literature, Black women are three to four times more likely to die from childbirth complications than White women (Policy Center for Maternal Mental Health, 2023). A report revealed the maternal mortality rate for Black women as 69.9 deaths per 100,000 live births in the United States (Hoyert, 2022). The racial and discrimination factors listed above have been linked to *culturally incompetent treatment from healthcare providers*, making them contributing factors to this maternal mortality rate. It is also important to note that a CDC report revealed that Black babies were twice as like to die at birth than White babies. According to the report, the infant mortality rate for Black babies was 10.9 per 1,000 live births in the United States (Hoyert, 2022). The *socioeconomic factors* listed above- *limited access to healthcare and resources* along with *improper nutrition* have been linked to *poor health outcomes and little to no prenatal care*, making them contributing factors to this infant mortality rate. This can be linked to anticipatory anxiety and medical mistrust.

Support Networks are extremely important for Black mothers as they navigate the unique disparities associated with maternal mental health. Given the statistics for Black mothers' maternal mortality rates and Black babies infant mortality rates, anticipatory grief and anxiety can negatively impact Black mothers' and their families' mental health. Black mothers face social isolation when navigating maternal care and because of their experiences with *implicit biased healthcare providers* their mental health needs may go *unnoticed and undiagnosed* during the perinatal period. These experiences can create barriers to Black mothers seeking mental health care, leading to them suffering silence, perpetuating the cycle of the *Strong Black Woman*.

Cultural Stigma regarding mental health in the Black community can also play a role in Black women not being vocal about their mental health needs. Black women are often described as strong because of their self-sacrificing nature and resilience. The *Strong Black Woman* has its origins in slavery and has been reinforced through decades of film, television, and rap music where Black women have been praised for their suffering and ability to be strong and loyal despite past and current stressors. Researcher indicates that the *Strong Black Woman* syndrome has been linked to poor physical and mental health outcomes.

Voices and Perspectives of Black Mothers

Three Black mothers shared their birth experience in U.S. hospitals and medical offices. They were all asked to reflect on their experience navigating pregnancy and birth in the medical setting. It is important to add their lived experiences and center their voices on this topic for the purpose of developing strategies and intervention to improve their birth and parenting experiences.

Mom 1 reported that she remembers her third and final pregnancy the most, not because it was the most recent one, but because it was frustrating and painful. Birth year: 2001, Age today: 51

> *"I did not feel informed as to why I had to have a C-Section. I wanted a vaginal birth because I had already done it twice and it was familiar. I went into labor thinking that I was having a vaginal birth because that's what was discussed. But once the doctor changed his mind about it, it felt forced on me. My questions weren't welcomed at all. I was not able to advocate for myself, and my husband did not know what to do. We both were scared. I still believe I am having complications from that c-section, and this was 23 years ago."*

Mom 2 reported that as a new wife and mother the entire birthing process was traumatic. Birth year: 2023, Age today: 27

> *"Everything happened so fast. I was home and then I was rushed to the hospital by my husband. I had a midwife, and I was supposed to give birth at home. But my baby was breech and never turned. I felt mishandled by the medical staff. I mean they weren't rude or nice, they were cold. I needed warmth because I was emotional. It was my first pregnancy. I said to myself, I will never do this again. Because of their coldness, I was anxious and even had nightmares about that*

experience for a while." I wish my doctor was Black and if I have another baby, the doctor will be Black."

Mom 3 reported that she really had a hard time navigating the doctor's appointments before and after leading up to delivery more than anything. Birth year: 2022, Age today: 34

"More than once the staff assumed I was unmarried and needed WIC benefits. They would ask for my Medicaid card and just make stereotypical comments when I went to appointments by myself. My husband works a lot so for some appointments I went by myself, and I was always uneasy. I had my son and yes, the birthing experience was traumatic, but I think I was already anxious and nervous. I had a c-section, and it was not a part of the plan. I should have spoken up more, but I didn't feel like I could. When I take my son to the doctor, now they're commenting on his size a lot. It's frustrating."

A Path to Birth Equity

The maternal mortality and morbidity rates for Black women have been on the rise for several decades. Black women from higher socioeconomic status with access to quality insurance and resources have not been exempt from these adverse outcomes. There must be a radical path forward designed specifically with the intention of creating birth equity for Black mothers and families. The birth equity framework can be used to develop strategies and interventions to improve maternal mental health because it focuses on rectifying structural racism and social determinants through system-level change. The actionable strategies and interventions below were developed with the birth equity framework in mind.

1. Implement Mandatory Culturally Competent Training & Testing

Every medical/ mental health provider and staff should be required to take classes that teaches them the history reproductive oppression and medical racism, how to address personal bias and implement culturally competent care and tested for proficiency in these competencies. This should be a prerequisite before licensure is issued and mandatory for renewal of the licensure. Every three months, there should be an accountability clinic where medical staff are provided with facts about the maternal mental health crisis. They should be updated with new cases at these clinics and brought up to speed about the disparities. They should leave the clinic with an accountability task plan of action with how to prevent these crises from happening at their hospitals or medical settings. It's not enough just to give Black mothers Black providers everyone must bear the responsibility of creating pathways to birth equity and anti-racist medical care for Black mothers.

2. Eliminate The Top-Down Approach

The top-down approach is not a reflection of person-centered care. It does not center Black mothers and their families and has a negative impact on their birthing experiences. The top-down approach can continue the cycle of mistrust between Black people and their medical providers and create anticipatory anxiety. Doctors are experts at textbook knowledge and procedures but not at knowing each patient's needs. Implementing shared decision-making with Black mothers and their families empowers them and dismantles the provider-patient power struggles. It promotes trust and safety. This is a sure way to prioritize and meet the needs of Black mothers.

3. Develop Culturally Sensitive Screening Tools

Depression and anxiety look different in Black women in comparison to how it may look in White women. Therefore, universal screening tools such as the PHQ-9 or GAD-7 may not always detect these symptoms in Black women. How could they? There were developed and tested on mostly White women (Policy Center for Maternal Mental Health, 2023). There needs to be screening tools developed with the cultural nuances of women of color, specifically Black women in mind. One way to create more validated screening tools is to develop and test them with Black mothers as research participants. Working directly with Black mothers will help developers account for the language Black people use to describe symptoms of depression because it does not always reflect the universal language.

4. Create A Black Maternal Mental Health First Aid Program

This program should be Black women led and accessible through the hospital and available to family members, friends, doulas, medical staff, and others in the mom's life on how to recognize symptoms of depression, anxiety, suicidal ideation, and other symptoms in mothers. Learning will happen in a group format via discussions and exercises centered on maternal mental health. The outcomes of this program will be as follows: learning to recognize when mom may be experiencing mental health challenges, skills & confidence to initiate vulnerable conversations, steps to take to connect mom with a therapist, and ways to also support yourself. This program would include access to licensed mental health therapists, social workers, and peer support workers to wrap around mom and the entire family as they navigate the perinatal period. Level of care would be decided based on culturally sensitive screenings and determine frequency of therapy sessions. This hospital program should also collaborate with local communities and schools expand its reach.

CASE STUDY

Anita and her husband Mike have two children, a 10-year-old daughter and a 7-year-old son. They recently welcomed a baby girl about 3 months ago. Anita has been home with the baby the entire time, while also working from home as an insurance claim attorney. Mike has noticed that Anita has been having mood swings and stating that she's having headaches daily. Mike feels helpless and doesn't know how to express his concern. Anita yelled at their daughter for going to slow when getting ready for school and that's not like her. She's usually calm and patient with the children. Mike's mom is supposed to be retiring soon and stated that she can help with the baby. Mike and Anita both have concerns about daycare so they agreed that the baby would stay at home with Anita for a while. Mike wants to revisit the daycare option, but the conversation has not gone well when tried to bring it up. He sees her working late and barely getting sleep daily. At a follow-up appointment, Mike noticed that Anita was honest on the depression and anxiety screening but her score to reflected that she was doing well. Mike wanted the doctor to pay attention to his wife when asking the questions, but the entire screening was rushed. It did not feel like a safe space to express concerns because the doctor did not seem interested in there being anything wrong with Anita.

CHAPTER QUESTIONS

1. What does the literature say about reproductive oppression and its ties to today's Black maternal mental health and maternal mortality crisis?
2. How does implicit bias influence a medical provider's ability to care for Black mothers?
3. What are some of the unique disparities that Black women experience?
4. How does these unique disparities impact the mental health of Black mothers?
5. How has you thinking about Black mothers' birthing experience changed since reading this text?
6. Given history between Black women and the medical system, why is it important for medical providers to share decision making with them?
7. Based on what you have read, what would you add as an actionable strategy or intervention to improve Black mothers' birthing experience?

REFERENCES

Alhusen, J. L., Bower, K. M., Epstein, E., & Sharps, P. (2016). Racial Discrimination and Adverse Birth Outcomes: An Integrative review. *Journal of Midwifery & Women's Health, 61*(6), 707–720. DOI: 10.1111/jmwh.12490 PMID: 27737504

Almeida, J., Belanoff, C., & Erbetta, K. F. (2021). The Time has Come for All States to Measure Racial Discrimination: A Call to Action for the Pregnancy Risk Assessment Monitoring System (PRAMS). *Maternal and Child Health Journal, 26*(1), 7–11. DOI: 10.1007/s10995-021-03160-0 PMID: 33945082

Castelin, S., & White, G. (2022). "I'm a Strong Independent Black Woman": The Strong Black Woman Schema and Mental Health in College-Aged Black Women. *Psychology of Women Quarterly, 46*(2), 196–208. DOI: 10.1177/03616843211067501

Chinn, J. J., Martin, I. K., & Redmond, N. (2020). Health equity among Black women in the United States. *Journal of Women's Health, 30*(2), 212–219. DOI: 10.1089/jwh.2020.8868 PMID: 33237831

Dalsania, A. K., Fastiggi, M. J., Kahlam, A., Shah, R., Patel, K., Shiau, S., Rokicki, S., & DallaPiazza, M. (2021). The relationship between social determinants of health and racial disparities in COVID-19 mortality. *Journal of Racial and Ethnic Health Disparities, 9*(1), 288–295. DOI: 10.1007/s40615-020-00952-y PMID: 33403652

Estriplet, T., Morgan, I., Davis, K., Perry, J. C., & Matthews, K. (2022). Black Perinatal Mental Health: Prioritizing maternal mental health to optimize infant health and wellness. *Frontiers in Psychiatry, 13*, 807235. DOI: 10.3389/fpsyt.2022.807235 PMID: 35573337

Etowa, J. B., Beagan, B. L., Eghan, F., & Bernard, W. T. (2017). "You feel you have to be made of steel": The strong Black woman, health, and well-being in Nova Scotia. *Health Care for Women International, 38*(4), 379–393. DOI: 10.1080/07399332.2017.1290099 PMID: 28151098

Hoyert, D. L. (2022). *Maternal mortality rates in the United States, 2022*. Centers for Disease Control and Prevention. https://www.cdc.gov/nchs/data/hestat/maternal-mortality/2022/maternal-mortality-rates-2022.htm

Policy Center for Maternal Mental Health. (2023). Black Maternal Mental Health [Report]. www.policycentermmh.org/black-maternal-mental-health-issue-brief

Social Determinants of Health - Healthy People 2030 (n.d.). https://health.gov/healthypeople/priority-areas/social-determinants-health

Chapter 5
You Good, Sis?
Analyzing the Role of Individual and Interpersonal Factors on Mental Health in Former Teenage Mothers of Color

Rahmatu Kassimu
https://orcid.org/0000-0002-4597-076X
Dr. K.'s Health Minute, USA

Elizabeth Wachira
https://orcid.org/0000-0003-4219-7545
East Texas A&M Commerce, USA

ABSTRACT

Teenage pregnancy profoundly impacts the life trajectory of a teenage mother and her child, necessitating public health prioritization. Despite decreasing rates, African American and Latina teens still face significantly higher teenage pregnancy rates compared to their white counterparts. This disparity is alarming due to the intersection of social determinants like race, ethnicity, socioeconomic status, and geographical location with poor mental health outcomes. Women of color who were teenage mothers (WCTM) are particularly burdened, reporting higher depressive symptoms during and after pregnancy than their adult and white counterparts. Rooted in Life Course Theory, this study examined individual and interpersonal factors affecting mental health in WCT Results indicated that factors such as maternal self-efficacy, emotional support, coping strategies, and normative beliefs buffer against anxiety and depression, while high levels of perceived racism and learned helplessness increase these risks. Implications and future research directions are discussed.

DOI: 10.4018/979-8-3693-4272-5.ch005

INTRODUCTION

Teenage pregnancy can profoundly affect the life trajectory of a teenage mother and her child, hence a public health prioritization for research and intervention (Centers for Disease Control and Prevention [CDC], 2021; Winters & Winters, 2012). The teenage birth rate in the United States has steadily declined, although it is still one of the highest in developed nations, from 61.8 to 16.7 births per 1,000 females as of 2019 (CDC, 2021). However, this decline has not been uniform, as specific populations still bear the burden of teenage pregnancy. In 2019, the birth rates for Latina and Black teens were more than twice that of their white counterparts (11.4) at 25.3 and 25.8 per 1,000, respectively.

The impact of teenage pregnancies coupled with these disparities warrants further exploration. Women of color who were teenage mothers [WCTM] bear a significant burden of adolescent pregnancy due to interactions between various social determinants of health, including race, ethnicity, socioeconomic status, geographic location, neighborhood status, and healthcare access (CDC, 2021). For example, geographically, Latina and African American populations tend to be concentrated in states that block access to reproductive health for minors, support abstinence-only sexual health education programs, and have higher poverty rates (Guttmacher Institute, 2017; Wiltz, 2015).

In Texas, the teenage pregnancy rate has also declined, though it lags significantly behind the national average and other states. Texas's teenage pregnancy rate of 23.8 per 1,000 females is ranked ninth in the nation for adolescent births (The Texas Campaign to Prevent Teen Pregnancy, 2021a). One explanation for this disparity is Texas's restrictive laws regarding access to reproductive health for minors, conservative sexual health education, lack of resources, and a burgeoning immigrant population (The National Campaign to Prevent Teen and Unplanned Pregnancy, 2021). Additionally, Texas is ranked number one in the nation for repeat teenage pregnancy. When looking at county data, African Americans and Latina teens had the highest teenage pregnancy rates, up to 133% in some counties, eclipsing the rates of their white counterparts (The Texas Campaign to Prevent Teen Pregnancy, 2021b).

These statistics are particularly alarming because WCTM tend to bear the burden of negative consequences of teenage pregnancy, including poor mental health outcomes. Teenage pregnancy disproportionately affects the mental health status of women of color due to dynamic interactions and intersections between the social determinants of health for adolescent pregnancy and poor mental health status (Schuyler Center for Analysis and Advocacy, 2008). African American and Latina teen mothers are more likely to self-report depressive symptoms during and after their pregnancy than their adult and white counterparts (Barnet et al., 2008; Mollborn & Morningstar, 2009). Furthermore, depression, anxiety, and other mental health conditions have been linked to repeat teenage pregnancy, which can aggravate emotional, economic, and social outcomes, creating additional barriers to effective treatment for mental health issues (Biello et al., 2010; Hodgkinson et al., 2010; Schuyler Center for Analysis and Advocacy, 2008). Prevention methods are crucial because poverty can be both a cause and consequence of teenage pregnancy. Additionally, teenage pregnancy can make it difficult for mothers to achieve their full academic potential and affect their children's academic potential.

LITERATURE REVIEW

Teenage Pregnancy and Mental Health in Women of Color

Individual and interpersonal factors interact in a dynamic and ever-changing relationship, affecting an individual's mental health status. These factors do not occur in silos but work collaboratively in additive and subtractive capacities. Teenage pregnancy interacts with multiple aspects of a woman of color's identity, resulting in profound effects on her mental health status. Due to this, it is imperative to mitigate poor mental health status in WCTM because their adverse mental health can also negatively impact their children (Holland et al., 2011; Teti & Gefland, 1991). Huang et al. (2014) found that after controlling for infant development at baseline, maternal depression at six months was associated with more developmental delays in their children at 18 months. Additionally, the authors found that the Sobel test demonstrated that maternal depression was a significant mediator of the relationship between developmental delays and maternal stress. This research indicates the need for health promotion programs that equip teenage mothers with skills while evaluating factors that mitigate negative mental health status. Several individual and interpersonal factors provide a buffering and mediating effect on negative mental health outcomes in WCTM, as discussed below.

Individual Factors

Maternal Self-Efficacy

Maternal self-efficacy refers to a mother's belief that she can effectively navigate the stressors of motherhood while adequately providing care for her child (Teti & Gefland, 1991). Higher levels of maternal self-efficacy are associated with higher perceived levels of social support, particularly from parents, and lower levels of depression and anxiety (Haslam et al., 2006; Leahy-Warren et al., 2012). In WOC, maternal self-efficacy decreases the frequency of anxiety and depression symptoms and parental distress and increases the mother's overall sense of motherhood (Jackson, 2000; Le & Lambert, 2008). Jackson (2000) found that when Black mothers had higher levels of maternal self-efficacy, there were lower levels of parental stress and child behavior problems. Le and Lambert (2008) found that Latina mothers with higher levels of maternal self-efficacy also had lower levels of maternal depression. Lower levels of maternal self-efficacy have also been linked to other factors that affect maternal depression, such as learned helplessness.

Learned Helplessness

Learned helplessness is a feeling of powerlessness due to repeat failures and traumatic events characterized by feelings of shame and fixed mindsets (Quinless & Nelson, 1988). Differences in attribution style for stressful events between WOC and their white counterparts lead to learned helplessness manifesting differently. However, this factor still contributes to negative mental health outcomes. A high level of learned helplessness has been shown to hinder a woman's ability to constructively cope with trauma and psychological and physical distress constructively, increasing her risk of developing depression and anxiety as well as the severity of these illnesses (Bargai et al., 2007). WOC are also more likely to experience traumatic and violent events such as domestic abuse, which make them more vulnerable to poor mental health, exacerbated by their unwillingness to seek treatment after such events (CDC, 2021; Women of Color Network, 2006). This unwillingness can serve as a coping strategy for WOC, but its effects differ by woman.

Coping Strategies

Coping strategies refer to the specific actions an individual takes to mitigate the effects of stressful life events (Carver, 1997). Coping strategies are individual-specific and are widely varied. They can involve active coping, emotional support, instrumental support, and positive reframing. Coping strategies among women of color are complex and multidimensional. They are more likely to use faith-based coping, counseling, both informal and formal, emotional coping, task-oriented coping, and avoidance, which have been associated with poor mental health outcomes (Gilmore et al., 2013; Moreno & Cardemil, 2013; Ward et al., 2009). Additionally, unhealthy coping styles such as avoidant coping, detachment methods, and outbursts have been associated with severe levels of depression in teenage mothers of color. Panzarine et al. (1995) found that participants coded in their Severe Depression group were more likely to avoid their child when stressed, engage in avoidance coping, have angry outbursts, and have detached coping. These mothers also believed that they had lower levels of emotional support. These perceived lower levels of emotional support are rooted in interpersonal factors.

Interpersonal Factors

Emotional Social Support

Emotional social support refers to support received from outside sources in the forms of sympathy, love, and empathy (Glanz et al., 2008). Adequate emotional social support is associated with lower levels of depression and anxiety among women of color (Norris & Mitchell, 2014; Siegel & Brandon, 2014). Kim et al. (2014) found that mothers who received low levels of social support after the births of their children were five times more likely to develop postpartum depression. Additionally, higher levels of emotional social support are associated with higher maternal self-efficacy and competence levels, decreased depressive symptoms, and an overall sense of well-being among teenage mothers of color (Black et al., 2002; Cox et al., 2008). Cox et al. (2008) found that interactions between maternal self-efficacy and social support provide protective benefits for mental health status in teenage mothers of color. The level of social support received may depend on the normative beliefs of those in the teenager's close social circle.

Normative Beliefs

Normative beliefs refer to how an individual believes their social circle perceives an issue. When an individual feels that they are accepted or rejected in their social circle due to an aspect of their identity, it can significantly affect their mental health. However, these normative beliefs can be complex and specific to communities. Teenage pregnancy is associated with long-held norms and is governed by beliefs about the timing of behavior. Influences on these norms vary by socioeconomic status and community ethnic composition. Childs et al. (2015) found that in African American adolescent girls, normative beliefs about teenage pregnancy manifested negatively, with the girls believing it would bring shame to their families, limit their economic prospects for the future, and tarnish their reputations. Conversely, Latina participants with a high sense of familialism and an intense desire to be a parent positively associated teenage pregnancy with happiness (Rocca et al., 2010). However, other interpersonal factors can affect mental health status in WOC.

Perceived Racism

Perceived racism is an individual's belief they have been mistreated by a person or in a situation due to their race or ethnicity (Dailey, 2008). Perceived discrimination can come in many forms, including being mistreated, being called names, or being denied services due to the color of one's skin (Keith et al., 2010). This can profoundly affect identity development, and prolonged exposure can lead to psychological distress and poor mental health outcomes. Racial discrimination is associated with anxiety, depression, psychological distress, hopelessness, loneliness, negative self-esteem, social and emotional difficulties, and suicide (Neblett et al., 2016; Sellers et al., 2006). For African American youth, discrimination is associated with anxiety, depression, and unhealthy coping strategies (Gaylord-Harden & Cunningham, 2009; Neblett et al., 2016). Additionally, in Latina youth, perceived racism has been associated with poor academic performance, low self-esteem, higher depressive symptoms, and risk-taking behaviors (Rios-Salas & Larson, 2015; Toomey et al., 2013).

Theoretical Foundation

Women of color who were teenage mothers (WCTM) experience dynamic interactions between dimensions of their identity and their status as mothers. Life course theory or life course perspective (LCP) contains constructs that can be utilized to understand the impact of teenage pregnancy in WOC. LCP is a developmental theory with constructs that allow for the longitudinal analysis of how events can affect the trajectory of a person's life (Hutchinson, 2014). Constructs of the theory include cohort, transition, role changes, life events, and trajectory. In the current study, the cohort was defined as African American and Latina women in Texas who gave birth to a child between the ages of 15-19 and did not have a mental health illness diagnosis before their pregnancy. The transition is the change from the role of teenager alone to teenage mother. The life event is the pregnancy during adolescence. The trajectory is the path of the teen's life since they became pregnant.

While several studies have attempted to examine factors that promote positive mental health outcomes in women of color who were teenage mothers, none have taken a multi-level approach (Brown et al., 2012; Hodgkinson et al., 2010; Shanok & Miller, 2007). Such an approach is critical because factors do not occur in silos and often have reciprocal relationships that can be missed if examined singularly. Utilizing a multi-level, inclusive approach guided by the life course perspective, this study attempts to analyze the effects of individual and interpersonal factors on mental health status in women of color who were teenage mothers. The authors hypothesize that the independent variables will be related to one another and, when analyzed together, will create more models that comprehensively predict MHS in WCTM.

METHODOLOGY

Population and Sampling

For this study, the priority population was limited to teenage mothers who were African American or Latina, were from Texas, had given birth to their child between the ages of 15 and 19, and were the primary caregivers for their child. The population was defined this way to reduce inaccurate data that may have resulted from confounders, such as abortion, miscarriage, or death of a child. As a part of screening procedures, participants were asked questions that assessed the limiting factors and asked about mental diagnoses received before pregnancy. If participants did not meet qualifications, they were excluded. Due to the number of variables, a fixed linear regression g*power model for 95% power with a significance level of 0.05 determined that the optimal number of participants would be 98. However, a sample size of 140 was chosen to account for possible missing values and incomplete survey submissions.

This study was conducted with approval from the investigator's Institutional Review Board [IRB]. Participants were provided with digital informed consent documents that detailed the risks of participating in the survey, such as emotional discomfort, fatigue, and loss of confidentiality. Measures were put in place to minimize these risks, such as options for the participant to save their process and return and links to mental health services and providers in their area.

Data Collection Procedures

Participants were recruited through convenience snowball sampling using both online and offline measures. Advertisements were purchased and run on Facebook and Instagram, including a culturally relevant image, the study's purpose, and eligibility criteria. These ads targeted African American and Latina women in Texas who were 20 years of age or older. The advertisement and accompanying image were posted in social media groups and organizations that served the priority population, and participants were offered the option to refer others to the study. While online recruitment was the most accessible form of recruitment, most of the participants were garnered through organizations and referrals. Participants who clicked on the online link were directed to an online questionnaire that first had the informed consent and eligibility questions hosted by the PsychData website.

Instrumentation

To adequately and accurately measure the variables proposed in this study, several scales were adopted and adapted to create a cohesive 75-item scale titled the *WCTM Individual and Interpersonal Factor Scale.* The first four items of the scale are screening questions to determine the participant's eligibility for the study. Table 1 contains a detailed description of each scale, its corresponding numbers in the newly created scale, key information such as adaptations and Cronbach alphas, and corresponding variables. All sub-scales had been previously tested for reliability and validity to measure their specific constructs, but they had not previously been combined as they have in the current study. An overall Cronbach's alpha was not run because the heterogeneous nature of the independent variables would violate the assumptions of the test. However, each sub-scales' Cronbach's alpha is reported in Table 1.

Measures

Pre-Pregnancy Mental Health Status

Pre-Pregnancy Mental Health Status was defined as the mental health status of a participant before they became pregnant as a teenager. The Hospital Anxiety Depression Scale [HADS] was used to determine mental health status prior to pregnancy. This self-assessment tool, developed by Zigmond and Snaith (1983), delineates the difference between depression and General Anxiety Disorder (GAD) (McDowell, 2006). It has also been tested outside of hospital settings and has been found both reliable and valid. The scale contains questions that pertain specifically to depression and GAD. Scores on each scale are summed, and a score of eight or higher on either has been proven to be a valid cutoff for the probability of either condition (McDowell, 2006). When tested in populations outside of a hospital, the scale produced a Cronbach's alpha of .80 and, in the current study, produced a Cronbach's alpha of .82.

Table 1. WCTM Individual and Interpersonal Factor Scale Subscales Details

Variable	Scale Name	Cronbach Alpha	Item Numbers	Changes
Exclusion Criteria	Author Created	NA	1-4	NA
Pre-Pregnancy Anxiety/Depression	Hospital Anxiety and Depression Scale	.82	5-19	NA
Learned Helplessness	Learned Helplessness Scale	.86	19-23	Originally 5 points Likert scale, changed to 4 points.
Coping Strategies	Brief COPE	.87	24-31	Originally Likert switched to True/ False Questions
Normative Beliefs	Author Created	.66	32-36	
Emotional Social Support	Interpersonal Support Evaluation List- Brief	.81	37-40	Originally 5 points Likert scale, changed to 4 points. Verbiage of some of the questions was changed for enhanced comprehension.
Perceived Racism	PEDQ- CV	.90	41-47	Originally 5 points Likert scale, changed to 4 points.
Maternal Self-Efficacy	Maternal Self-Efficacy	.93	48-52	NA
Post-Pregnancy Anxiety/Depression	Hospital Anxiety and Depression Scale	.89	53-66	NA
Demographics	Author Created	.77	67-75	NA

Individual Level Factors

Learned Helplessness

Learned Helplessness was defined as a feeling of powerlessness due to traumatic events or repeated failure. This variable was scored using five items from Quinless and Nelson's (1998) Learned Hopelessness Scale. Items from the scale were measured using a four-point Likert scale and scored accordingly to yield a Learned Hopelessness Scale that was between 4 and 20. Higher scores indicated higher levels of learned hopelessness. These items were found to be highly reliable (5 items; α=.86).

Coping Strategies

Coping Strategies was defined as the actions a person takes to negate or navigate the effects of stressful or traumatic events. These items were scored using eight items from Carver's (1997) COPE Scale-Brief scale. For this study, active coping, instrumental support, emotional support, and positive reframing were used to generate a composite Coping Strategies score. Carver's original scale utilized a Likert scale, but the present study only examined if the intended variable was present or absent. The Likert Scale was paired down from 4 points to a two-point True or False scale. Composite scores could range from 8 to 16. Higher scores indicated high levels of coping strategies. The eight items were found to be highly reliable (8 items; α=.87).

Maternal Self-Efficacy

Maternal Self-Efficacy was defined as a participant's belief that they could successfully complete maternal tasks. This variable was scored using five items from Teti & Gefland's (1991) *Maternal Self-Efficacy Scale*. These items were measured with a four-point Likert Scale to yield a composite Maternal Self-Efficacy score that ranged from 5 to 20. Higher scores indicated higher levels of maternal self-efficacy. Items from this scale were determined to be highly reliable (5 items; α=.93)

Interpersonal Factors

Normative Beliefs

Normative Beliefs were defined in this study as the level of acceptability of teenage pregnancy in the participants' social circle. The items were developed specifically for this study as no suitable scale was available. These items were tested for internal reliability and validity after the pilot administration of the completed scale and yielded a Cronbach's alpha of .66. This indicates a moderate level of internal consistency. These items were measured using a four-point Likert scale to yield a composite score that ranged from 5 to 25. A lower scale indicated that the participant believed that the social acceptability of teenage pregnancy in their social circles was low.

Emotional Social Support

Emotional Social Support was defined as outside support received as expressions of empathy and love (Glanz et al., 2008). This variable was scored using four items from Cohen and Hoberman's (1983) *Interpersonal Support Evaluation List*. While this scale was developed to assess multiple types of emotional support, this study specifically examined appraisal emotional support. These items were highly reliable and assessed using a four-point Likert scale that was scored and coded to yield a composite scale between 4 and 16 (4 items; α=.81).

Perceived Racism

Perceived Racism was defined as an individual's belief that mistreatment in a situation was based on their race (Dailey, 2008). This variable was scored using seven items from Brondolo et al.'s (2005) Perceived Ethnic Discrimination Questionnaire Community Version. The originally scored items used a five-point Likert scale, but the neutral option was removed for this study. These items yielded composite scores between 7 and 35 and were found to be highly reliable (7 items, α=.90).

Mental Health Status

To measure the dependent variable, Mental Health Status, the participants retook the Hospital Anxiety and Depression [HADS] scale to measure their current mental health status. Scale scores for these items were evaluated using criteria set forth by Zigmond and Snaith (1983) for the probability of illness using the presence of symptoms. These items were the same as those utilized at the beginning of the scale to determine Pre-Pregnancy Mental Health Status, but the Cronbach alpha of these items was higher (.82 versus .89). This increase is likely due to recall bias in the pre-pregnancy version of the questions compared with present state.

Current SES

Current SES was defined as a covariate in this study and was determined through a combination of descriptive variables, including education level, household income level for the past 12 months before taxes, and governmental aid received. The questions about the types of governmental aid received were summed up and reverse-scored before being combined with the education and household income questions to generate a current SES score. These scores ranged from 3 to 18 and yielded a Cronbach's alpha of .77.

Treatment of Data

Before data analysis was conducted using the Statistical Package for the Social Sciences [IBM SPSS], data was cleaned to remove invalid data and duplicates, and a plan was made to assess incomplete data. Responses that did not meet inclusion/

exclusion criteria but did not begin the survey or meet criteria and did not finish more than 65% of the survey were removed.

Creation of Variables Prior to Data Analysis

The independent variables were scored, summed, and reverse-scored to generate six variables: Learned Helplessness, Maternal Self-Efficacy, Coping Strategies, Perceived Racism, Emotional Support, and Normative Beliefs. The pre-pregnancy version of the HADS questions was used to create a Pre-Pregnancy Anxiety score and a Pre-Pregnancy Depression score. Mental Health Status was calculated and coded in three different ways. Sum scores on the current iteration of the HADS generated Post-Pregnancy Anxiety and Post-Pregnancy Depression scores. These sum scores were then converted into dichotomous Low/High Possibility of Anxiety or Depression variables using the literature-supported cutoffs for each scale. Finally, the Pre and Post-Anxiety and Depression scores were subtracted to create Change in Anxiety and Change in Depression variables.

Demographics

Frequency testing was conducted to determine the demographic composition of the sample. Demographic variables were also tested for differences in Mental Health Status. Additionally, ANOVAs with Tukey posthoc tests were run to determine statistical differences between the six independent variables.

Research Question and Hypotheses Testing

Pearson's correlation, paired T-test, and regression models were used to evaluate this study's research questions and hypotheses. Pearson's correlation was run to determine if there were any significant relationships between the independent variables and Changes in Depression and Changes in Anxiety scores. A paired T-test was run to determine if there was a statistically significant difference in the means of the Pre-and Post-Pregnancy Anxiety and Depression scores. Multiple regression models were run to determine if the sum-scored independent variables predicted the dependent variable and whether Current SES would change that relationship.

For testing the independent variable against the continuous version of the dependent variable, a linear regression was run with just the variables first, then run again, plus the covariate of Current SES using pairwise deletion to handle missing data. Next, a bivariate logistic regression was run using the dichotomous categorical version of the dependent variable, first with the I.V.s alone and then with the covariate added. This generated four different models (two for linear regression and two for bivariate logistic regression), which were run against the Post-Pregnancy Anxiety scores and Post-Pregnancy Depression scores separately. The linear regression Model 1 (M1) predicted the continuous form of Mental Health Status from the I.V.s. In contrast, Model 2 (M2) predicted a continuous form of Mental Health Status from the I.V.s while controlling for Current SES. These models were then repeated for the bivariate logistic regression analysis, with Model 3 (M3) predicting the dichotomous form of Mental Health Status from the I.V.s alone and Model 4 (M4), which attempted to predict the dichotomous form of Mental Health Status from the IVS while controlling for Current SES. Finally, M1 and M2 were also run to determine if the I.V.s could predict Change in Depression scores and Change in Anxiety scores.

RESULTS

During the six-month span of the study, 297 responses were collected; however, after data was cleaned for invalid responses, 147 valid responses remained. Of the 147 responses, some lacked information for specific demographic categories, a breakdown of which is provided in Table 2. The majority of participants in the study were between the ages of 20 to 29 (72.7%), African American (49.7%), educated at a level of "Some college, no degree," or lower (79%), with a total household income in the last 12 months before taxes as $75,000 or lower (91.3%). Most of the participants gave birth to their first child at 18 (22.4%), and most had one or two children (63.2%). The mean for Current SES was 8.96, with a standard deviation of 3.07, indicating that participants had a low to middle-level current SES.

Table 2. Frequencies and Percentages for Categorical Demographic Variables

Variable	Frequency	Percent	Cumulative Percent
Age (in years)			
20 to 24	48	32.7	34.5
25 to 29	53	36.1	72.7
30 to 34	15	10.2	83.5
35 to 39	10	6.8	90.6
40 to 44	9	6.1	97.1
45 and older	4	2.7	100.0
Total	139	94.6	

continued on following page

Table 2. Continued

Variable	Frequency	Percent	Cumulative Percent
Race/Ethnicity			
African American	73	49.7	52.5
Hispanic	64	43.5	98.6
Other	2	1.4	100.0
Highest Level of Education Achieved			
Some high school, no diploma	16	10.9	11.6
High school diploma or equivalent	44	29.9	43.5
Some college, no degree	49	33.3	79.0
Bachelors Degree	19	12.9	92.8
Graduate Degree	8	5.4	98.6
Professional Degree	2	1.4	100.0
Total	138	93.9	
Total Household Income Level Before Taxes over the Last 12 Months			
Less than $25,000	49	33.3	35.5
$25,000 to $34,999	40	27.2	64.5
$35,000 to $49,999	19	12.9	78.3
$50,000 to $74,999	18	12.2	91.3
$75,000 to $99,999	9	6.1	97.8
$100,000 to $149,999	2	1.4	99.3
$150,000 or more	1	.7	100.0
Total	138	93.9	
Age at Birth of First Child (in years)			
			(continued)
15	16	10.9	11.7
16	30	20.4	33.6
17	29	19.7	54.7
18	33	22.4	78.8
19	29	19.7	100.0

continued on following page

Table 2. Continued

Variable	Frequency	Percent	Cumulative Percent
Total	137	93.2	
Number of Total Children			
1	42	28.6	30.9
2	44	29.9	63.2
3	29	19.7	84.6
4	15	10.2	95.6
5	5	3.4	99.3
Over 5	1	.7	100.0
Total	136	92.5	
Mental Health Illness Diagnosis			
Yes	7	4.8	5.0
No	123	83.7	93.5
If Yes, Please specify	9	6.1	100.0
Total	139	94.6	
Anxiety Status Post Pregnancy			
Low possibility of Anxiety	45	30.6	36.0
High possibility of Anxiety	80	54.4	100.0
Total	125	85.0	
Depression Status Post Pregnancy			
Low possibility of depression	63	42.9	50.0
High possibility of depression	63	42.9	100.0
Total	126	85.8	

Note. Frequencies that do not equal N=147 or percentages that do not = 100 indicate missing data

Based on how respondents answered the post-pregnancy mental health status questions, 64% of the participants scored as having a High Possibility of Anxiety, and 50% scored as having a High Possibility of Depression. However, only 5% of the participants reported having a mental health diagnosis. A Cross Tabulation revealed that 41% (n=48) of participants with complete data had comorbidities and belonged to both the High Possibility of Anxiety and High Possibility of Depression groups.

Paired sample t-test results showed that participants displayed a significant increase in their Depression scores following their teenage pregnancies from 3.86 ± 3.429 to 6.97 ± 4.950, an increase of 3.114 ± 4.791. Similarly, the participants displayed a significant increase in their Anxiety scores post-pregnancy from 5.41 ± 4.007 to 8.91 ± 4.720, an increase of 3.492 ± 4.915. Additionally, Mann-Whitney U Tests mainly found no significant relationships between the dichotomous form of the Mental Health Status variable and the demographic variables. However, these tests indicated that the Age of Birth of First Child was significantly higher in participants who scored in the Low Possibility of Depression group than those in the Higher Possibility of Depression group ($U = 1471.0, p = .021$). Furthermore, the Number of Total Children was also statistically lower in the Low Possibility of Depression group, indicating that the older a participant was when she gave birth and the lower number of children she had, increased her odds of scoring in the Low Possibility of Depression group.

Pearson correlation results showed significant positive and negative relationships between the six independent variables, as reported in Table 3. Most relationships were weak to moderate, but the only variables that did not indicate any level of relationship were between Normative Beliefs and Learned Helplessness ($r = -.154, p = .072$).

Table 3. Pearson's Product Moment Correlations among Independent Variables

	Learned Helplessness	**Coping Strategies**	**Normative Beliefs**	**Emotional Support**	**Perceived Racism**
Coping Strategies	**-.265****				
Normative Beliefs	-0.154	.399**			
Emotional Support	-.326**	.453**	.319**		
Perceived Racism	.244**	-.225**	-.365**	-.369**	
Maternal Self-Efficacy	-.447**	.422**	.474**	.475**	-.475**

** Correlation is significant at the 0.01 level (2-tailed).

When the means of the independent variables were compared with the dichotomous versions of the Mental Health Status for Anxiety, the Post Pregnancy Anxiety High/Low (PPAS) variable means significantly differed for all independent variables except for Coping Strategies ($F(1,119) = 2.796, p = .097$) and Normative Beliefs ($F(1,120) = 1.291, p = .258$). The High Possibility of Anxiety group had significantly higher means for Perceived Racism ($F(1,117) = 9.636, p = .002$) and Learned Helplessness ($F(1,119) = 5.905, p = .017$), indicating that participants with higher scores for these variables were more likely to be placed in the

High Possibility of Anxiety Post-Pregnancy Group. Additionally, participants in the High Possibly of Anxiety Group had significantly lower means for Emotional Support ($F(1,121) = 8.969$, $p = .003$) and Maternal Self-Efficacy ($F(1,121) = 13.550, p = < .001$), indicating that participants who scored lower on these variables had higher chances of being placed into High Possibility of Anxiety group.

When the same test was run to determine differences in Post Pregnancy Depression High/Low (PPDS) membership, differences were found for all six variables. The Low Possibility of Depression group had significantly higher means for Emotional Support ($F(1,123) = 12.19, p = < .001$), Maternal Self-Efficacy ($F(1,122) = 17.66, p = < .001$), Coping Strategies ($F(1,120) = 17.66, p = < .001$), and Normative Beliefs ($F(1,120) = 14.79, p = < .001$), indicating that these variables served as buffers decreasing that participants' odds of being placed in the High Possibility of Depression group. Similarly, these participants also had significantly lower means for Perceived Racism ($F(1,118) = 15.83, p = < .001$) and Learned Helplessness ($F(1,120) = 10.58, p = < .001$), indicating that lower scale scores for these variables also buffered against a participants' likelihood of being placed in the High Possibility of Depression Group.

Research Question and Hypotheses Testing

Model 1

To test the research question and hypotheses, four different models were run against the Post-Pregnancy Anxiety Scores and Post-Pregnancy Depression Scores in their continuous and dichotomous forms, the completed results of which are reported in Tables 4 and 5. When M1 was run to predict Post-Pregnancy Anxiety Scores using the independent variables, a significant regression equation was determined ($F(6,117) = 7.309, p = < .001$), with an Adjusted R^2 of .235. Perceived Racism ($p = < .001$), Maternal Self-Efficacy ($p = .011$), and Normative Beliefs ($p = .031$) proved to be significant to the overall model. High scores for Normative Beliefs and Perceived Racism increased PPAS, but high Maternal Self-Efficacy scores decreased PPAS.

When M1 was run to predict the Post-Pregnancy Depression Scores (PPDS) using the independent variables, a significant regression equation was found ($F(6,122) = 23.500, p = < .001$), with an Adjusted R^2 of .513. Perceived Racism ($p = .001$) and Maternal Self-Efficacy ($p = < .001$) proved to be statistically significant to the overall model, indicating that higher Maternal Self-Efficacy Scores reduced PPDS, but PPDS increased with higher Perceived Racism scores.

Model 2

Model 2 (M2), also a linear regression model, predicted the continuous form of the Mental Health Status from the I.V.s while controlling for Current SES and found a significant regression equation of ($F(7,116) = 6.212, p = < .001$), with an Adjusted R^2 of .229. Upon controlling for Current SES, Normative Beliefs ($p = .036$), Maternal Self-Efficacy ($p = .014$), and Perceived Racism ($p = .003$) proved statistically significant to the overall model. After controlling for Current SES, PPAS decreased as Maternal Self-Efficacy scores increased and Normative Beliefs and Perceived Racism scores decreased.

When M2 was run to predict PPDS from the independent variables while controlling for Current SES, a significant regression equation was found ($F(7,121) = 20.964, p = < .001$), with an Adjusted R^2 of .522. After controlling for Current SES, higher Perceived Racism ($p = < .001$) scores resulted in higher PPDS, while higher Maternal Self-Efficacy ($p = < .001$) scores resulted in lower PPDS scores.

Model 3

These models were then repeated for the bivariate logistic regression analysis with Model 3 (M3) predicting the group membership in the High and Low groups for the Possibility of Anxiety and Depression from the I.V.s alone. The model indicated that the interpersonal level independent variables distinguished between those in the Low Possibility of Anxiety and High Possibility of Anxiety groups ($X2 = 14.446$, $p = .025$ with $df = 6$). A Nagelkerke's R^2 of 0.171 indicated a weak relationship between independent variable predictors and the anxiety groups. The overall success of the model was 61.5% (23.7% for Low Possibility and 81.7% for High Possibility). None of the independent variables were significant to the overall model.

M3 indicated that the interpersonal level independent variables distinguished between a Low Possibility of Depression and a High Possibility of Depression group membership ($X2 = 56.981, p = < 0.001$ with $df = 6$). A moderate relationship was indicated between the predictors and the Depression groups with a Nagelkerke's R^2 of 0.539. The overall success of the model was moderate to high at 81.8% (78.9% for High Possibility and 84.9% for Low Possibility). Maternal Self-Efficacy was the only variable found to be a significant predictor of the overall model ($p = < .001$). An Exp(B) of Maternal Self-Efficacy of 0.673 indicated that for every increase in Maternal Self-Efficacy, the overall depression score decreased, increasing the odds a participant would be categorized as Low Possibility of Depression.

Model 4

Model 4 (M4) attempted to predict the dichotomous form of the Mental Health Status variable from the I.V.s while controlling for Current SES. The model indicated that the individual-level factors significantly distinguished between the Low and High Possibility of Anxiety Groups ($X2 = 15.566, p = < .001$ with $df = 7$). A weak relationship was indicated between the predictor variables and the anxiety groups with a Nagelkerke's R^2 of 0.186. The overall model had a success percentage of 66.4% (82.6% for High Possibility and 36.8% for Low Possibility). None of the independent variables significantly contributed to the overall model after controlling for Current SES.

M4 indicated that the individual-level independent variables were statistically significant in distinguishing group membership between those with a Low Possibility of Depression and those with a High Possibility of Depression ($X2 = 55.331, p = < .001$ with $df = 7$). A moderate relationship was indicated between the predictor variables and the Depression groups with a Nagelkerke's R^2 of 0.535. The overall model had a success percentage of 80.6% (78.6% for High Possibility and 82.7% for Low Possibility). After controlling for Current SES, Maternal Self-Efficacy remained a significant predictor of the overall model; however, no other predictor was significant. The Exp(B) of Maternal Self-Efficacy of 0.682 indicated that for every increase in Maternal Self-Efficacy, the overall depression score decreased, thus increasing the odds a participant would be categorized as Low Possibility of Depression.

Table 4. Predicting Anxiety and Change in Anxiety with Individual Factors, Interpersonal Factors, and Socioeconomic Status

	M1: W/O Control PPAS	M2: W/ Control PPAS	M3: Dichotomous W/O Control OR PPAS	M4: Dichotomous W/ Control OR PPAS	M1: W/O Control Change in Anxiety	M2: W/ Control Change in Anxiety
Learned Helplessness	0.073	0.074	1.028	1.003	-0.214	-0.239
Coping Strategies	-0.198	-0.197	1.012	0.989	-0.005	-0.21
Maternal Self-Efficacy	-0.323*	-0.323*	0.889	0.916	-0.348*	-0.324*
Normative Beliefs	.236*	0.236*	1.098	1.066	-0.002	-0.021
Emotional Support	-0.093	-0.093	0.915	0.904	0.008	0.003
Perceived Racism	0.160**	0.160**	1.055	1.051	0.115	0.117*

continued on following page

Table 4. Continued

	M1: W/O Control PPAS	M2: W/ Control PPAS	M3: Dichotomous W/O Control OR PPAS	M4: Dichotomous W/ Control OR PPAS	M1: W/O Control Change in Anxiety	M2: W/ Control Change in Anxiety
Socioeconomic Status		.004		0.908		-0.101
Constant	10.764	10.711	0.601	2.343	9.175	10.536
Range of N	124-142	124-142	109	107	122-144	122-144
Adjusted R2	0.273	0.273			0.104	0.099
Pseudo R2			0.171	0.186		

*p < .05 **p < .01

Model 1 and Change Scores

Finally, M1 and M2 were also run to determine if the independent variables could predict Change in Depression scores and Change in Anxiety scores, the results of which are also reported in Tables 4 and 5. M1 found a significant regression equation ($F(6,115) = 3.332, p = .005$), with an Adjusted R^2 of .104. Maternal Self-Efficacy (p=.015) proved to be statistically significant to the overall model, indicating that there was a smaller change from pre- to post-pregnancy anxiety scores the higher a participant's Maternal Self-Efficacy Score was.

M1 found a significant regression when predicting Change in Depression scores from the independent variables ($F(6,118) = 4.914, p = < .001$), with an Adjusted R^2 of .159. Higher Perceived Racism scores predicted a larger Change in Depression scores, while higher Maternal Self-Efficacy scores predicted a smaller Change in Depression scores

Model 2 and Change Scores

M2 was proven statistically significant in predicting the Change in Anxiety from independent variables when controlling for Current SES ($F(7,114) = 2.900, p = .008$). After controlling for Current SES, Perceived Racism (p=.049) and Maternal Self-Efficacy (p=.028) proved to be statistically significant to the overall model. Higher Perceived Racism scores resulted in larger changes in pre- to post-pregnancy anxiety scores, while higher Maternal Self-Efficacy scores resulted in smaller changes.

M2 was proven statistically significant in predicting the Change in Depression from independent variables when controlling for Current SES ($F(7,117) = 4.457, p = < .001$), with an Adjusted R^2 of .163. Only Perceived Racism was determined to be significant to the overall model after controlling for Current SES, indicating that a higher Perceived Racism (p=.013) score resulted in a larger change between pre- and post-pregnancy Depression scores.

Table 5. Predicting Depression and Change in Depression with Individual Factors, Interpersonal Factors, and Socioeconomic Status

	M1: W/O Control PPDS	M2: W/ Control PPDS	M3: Dichotomous W/O Control OR PPDS	M4: Dichotomous W/ Control OR PPDS	M1: W/O Control Change in Depression	M2: W/ Control Change in Depression
Learned Helplessness	0.061	0.014	1.071	1.042	-0.153	-0.199
Coping Strategies	-0.203	-0.233	0.815	0.806	-0.162	-0.191
Maternal Self-Efficacy	-0.544**	-0.501**	0.673**	0.682**	-0.273*	-0.231
Normative Beliefs	.047	0.011	1.00	0.992	-0.073	-0.108
Emotional Support	-0.094	-0.104	1.044	1.061	-0.010	-0.019
Perceived Racism	0.139*	0.142**	1.059	1.061	0.135*	0.138*
Socioeconomic Status		-0.189		0.926		-0.183
Constant	15.400	17.942	6.896	8.018	10.011	12.468
Range of N	129-144	129-144	110	108	125-144	125-144
Adjusted R2	0.536	0.548			0.159	0.163
Pseudo R2			0.539	0.535		

*p < .01 ***p* <. 001

DISCUSSION AND IMPLICATIONS

The data analysis in this study revealed several significant relationships that provided insight into individual and interpersonal factors that affect mental health status in women of color who were teenage mothers (WCTM). Regression models found that the independent variables predicted mental health status in WCTM with statistical significance for Post-Pregnancy Anxiety Scores, Post-Pregnancy Depression Scores, Low/High Anxiety group membership, Low/High Depression group membership, Change in Anxiety Score, and Change in Depression Score. Statistical analysis indicated that all the independent variables were correlated with each other with relationships ranging from weak to moderate strengths indicating that the assumption that these variables interact and affect each other and do not occur in silos was correct. For example, this finding was supported by literature that indicates that Coping Strategies, Maternal Self-Efficacy, and Emotional Support buffer against feelings of helplessness (Bargai et al., 2007; Cohen & McKay, 1984). A participant was statistically more likely to be placed in the High Possibility of Anxiety group if their Learned Helplessness and Perceived Racism scores were high but their Maternal Self-Efficacy, Emotional Support, and Coping Strategies scores were low. However, participants were statistically more likely to be placed in the Low Possibility of Depression group if their Learned Helplessness and Perceived Racism scores were low, while their Normative Beliefs, Emotional Support, Maternal Self-Efficacy, and Coping Strategies scores were high. This result substantiated previous results that indicated higher levels of helplessness are associated with higher levels of racism (Vines et al., 2006). Additionally, these variables affected the participants' changes in mental health status scores. A participant's difference between Pre-and Post-Pregnancy Depression Scores was smaller with higher Normative Beliefs, Coping Strategies, and Maternal Self-Efficacy scores but higher with higher Perceived Racism scores. Similarly, the difference in a participant's Pre-and Post-Pregnancy Anxiety Score was smaller with higher Normative Beliefs and Maternal Self-Efficacy scores but larger with higher Perceived Racism scores.

Further statistical testing revealed that PPAS increased with higher Normative Beliefs and Perceived Racism scores but decreased with higher Maternal Self-Efficacy scores, indicating that Maternal Self-Efficacy acted as a buffer for PPAS, but Normative Beliefs and Perceived Racism exacerbated PPAS. These relations remained even after controlling for Current SES. PPDS increased with higher Perceived Racism scores but decreased with higher Maternal Self-Efficacy scores, and these relationships remained after controlling for Current SES. Furthermore, Current SES proved to be a complex factor. In WCTM, low SES can be a potential predictor of teen pregnancy, heighten the risks associated with teenage pregnancy, and be an outcome of teenage pregnancy (Biello et al., 2010; Hodgkinson et al., 2010; Kearney & Levine, 2012; Schuyler Center of Analysis and Advocacy, 2008).

Implications

It is estimated that 21% of U.S. adults (18.4% Latino and 17.3% African American) experience some form of mental illness, with 5.6% experiencing severe mental illness (NAMI, 2021). The findings of this study are mostly consistent with the current literature that examines factors that promote and exacerbate mental health status in WCTM. These findings are important considering that 42.9% of the sample reported scores that placed them in the High Possibility of Depression group, and 54% reported scores that placed them in the High Possibility of Anxiety group. These percentages are higher than the national prevalence for both depression (6.7%) and anxiety (18.1%), indicating a serious issue for WCTM (Anxiety and Depression Association of America, 2022; Kessler et al., 2005). Additionally, for those with complete data to compare, 41% of the sample had comorbidity for anxiety and depression, scoring in the High Possibility groups for both Anxiety and Depression.

The risk of developing a mental illness increases exponentially when a child enters adolescence. Approximately 50% of chronic mental illnesses begin by age 14, and 75% will begin before the individual turns 24 (Corcoran, 2016; NAMI, 2021). This risk is exacerbated for WCTM because many of the social determinants of health for teenage pregnancy intersect, making it difficult to determine the direction of causality (Hodkinson et al., 2014). It is difficult to determine if an individual's pregnancy is a result of these determinants, which then increase the teenager's risk for poor mental health outcomes, or if poor mental health outcomes proceeded the pregnancy and were made worse by the pregnancy. However, in the current study, participants experienced marked increases in their mean Anxiety and Depression scores from Pre-Pregnancy to Post-Pregnancy. There may be unqueried factors that affected this increase, as well, but research supports the assertion that this increase is the result of psychological stress that accompanies the life role change from adolescent to mother and caregiver as stated by the constructs of LCP (Hodgkinson et al., 2014; Mollborn & Morningstar, 2009).

Premises of the Life Course Theory were supported in this study as the participants experienced changes in roles, responsibilities, and trajectory as a result of the event: their pregnancy. The poorer mental health outcomes can result from reconciliation stress, which occurs when the teenager attempts to reconcile the duties of their new role as a mother with their duties as a teenager. Participants who were older at the time of birth of their first child were statistically more likely to have a low possibility of depression. The event of childbirth at a younger age disrupts the natural aging process and causes transitions and role changes that the teenager may not be mentally equipped to handle (Mirowsky & Ross, 2002; Mollborn & Morningstar, 2009).

Future Directions and Practice Applications

These results indicate the need for multi-level and multi-faceted health promotion programs that target teenagers before they become pregnant and provide continued, long-term support after giving birth. This study focused on Texas, which is ranked 9th in the nation for teenage pregnancy, but there are several states ranked higher or lower where their residents of color experience similar social determinants of health, making them more likely to experience a teenage pregnancy and poor mental health outcomes. These states will likely also need health education programs that deter teenage pregnancy and promote positive mental health outcomes. Therefore, research to evaluate individual and interpersonal factors in WCTM in other states in the United States is needed, as geographical location can shape health outcomes (Guttmacher Institute, 2017; Wiltz, 2015). This study found that maternal self-efficacy was determined to be the most significant predictor and buffer against poor mental health outcomes in WCTM. Therefore, studies should be conducted to determine what factors promote the development and sustainability of maternal self-efficacy in WCTM. Lastly, future studies should be conducted to really parse out the barriers to seeking mental health treatment in WCTM. These studies could determine specificities that can be addressed with tailored health promotion programs. These recommendations will be further expanded upon below.

Multi-Level Health Promotion Programs

Developing comprehensive health promotion programs is essential to addressing the unique challenges faced by teenage mothers of color. These programs should encompass a range of services from pre-pregnancy education to long-term post-pregnancy support. For example, integrating comprehensive sexual education into school curricula can inform young women about contraception and the risks of teenage pregnancy, which can empower them to make informed decisions about their reproductive health. Additionally, post-pregnancy support groups can provide ongoing mental health resources and parenting education, creating a supportive community for young mothers. Culturally tailored programs, which respect and incorporate the cultural norms of African American and Latina communities, can improve the relevance and effectiveness of these initiatives. For example, a health promotion program in Texas could include culturally specific parenting workshops that address the unique social and familial expectations of these communities. Policymakers should advocate for comprehensive sexual education and secure funding to sustain these maternal health programs, ensuring they are accessible to all who need them.

Improving Maternal Self-Efficacy

Increasing maternal self-efficacy among former teenage mothers can significantly improve both mental health and parenting outcomes. One effective approach is to establish mentorship programs that pair young mothers with experienced mentors who can offer guidance, support, and encouragement. For example, a mentorship program might connect teenage mothers with older women who have successfully navigated similar challenges, providing a model of resilience and effective parenting. Skills training workshops can further bolster self-efficacy by teaching practical parenting techniques, stress management, and self-care strategies. In addition, creating peer support networks where mothers can share experiences and solutions in a non-judgmental environment can reinforce their confidence and sense of community. Policymakers should support community-based initiatives by providing grants and resources for these programs and advocate for the integration of maternal self-efficacy training in public health and welfare programs. Such measures would help to institutionalize support for young mothers, making it a standard part of maternal health services.

Addressing Perceived Racism and Discrimination

Mitigating the negative impacts of perceived racism on mental health is essential for supporting teenage mothers of color. This can be achieved by implementing anti-discrimination training for healthcare providers, educators, and community leaders to help them understand the effects of racism and how to provide inclusive support. For example, healthcare institutions could offer regular workshops on cultural competence and implicit bias, helping staff to recognize and counteract discriminatory behaviors. Creating safe spaces, such as community centers or support groups, where young mothers can access resources without fear of discrimination or judgment is another effective strategy. Additionally, launching advocacy and awareness campaigns that highlight the impact of racism on mental health can foster a broader understanding and drive societal change. Policymakers should advocate for stronger anti-discrimination laws and ensure that resources and support services are equitably distributed, prioritizing communities with high rates of teenage pregnancy and systemic disadvantages. These actions can help create a more inclusive and supportive environment for young mothers of color.

Promoting Positive Coping Strategies

Encouraging healthy coping strategies is necessary for helping teenage mothers of color manage the stresses associated with pregnancy and motherhood. Providing mental health workshops that teach techniques like mindfulness, problem-solving, and emotional regulation can equip young mothers with the tools they need to handle stress effectively. For example, community centers could offer weekly sessions on mindfulness practices or resilience training tailored to the needs of young mothers. Increasing access to counseling services, especially for those who are culturally competent and understand the unique challenges faced by these mothers, is also vital. Collaborating with faith-based organizations to offer support services that align with the spiritual and cultural values of the community can further reinforce these coping strategies. Policymakers should increase funding for mental health services that focus on coping skills and integrate these practices into school and community programs. These efforts can build resilience among young mothers, helping them to navigate the challenges of motherhood more effectively.

Improving Emotional and Social Support

Strengthening emotional and social support systems can reduce the risk of depression and anxiety among teenage mothers of color. Developing family engagement programs that foster a supportive home environment is a key strategy. For example, workshops that teach family members how to support young mothers can help create a more understanding and nurturing home life. Community partnerships that provide a network of support, including access to childcare, housing, and educational opportunities, can also significantly benefit young mothers. Establishing resource centers that offer comprehensive services, from mental health care to educational resources, can provide a one-stop shop for support, making it easier for mothers to access the help they need. Policymakers should advocate for the expansion of these social support programs and ensure that they are well-funded and accessible to all young mothers, particularly in underserved communities. These measures can help to create a more supportive and resource-rich environment for teenage mothers and their families.

Research and Evaluation

Continuous evaluation and improvement of programs and policies based on emerging research and community needs are essential for effectively supporting teenage mothers of color. Conducting regular research to assess the effectiveness of existing programs can help identify areas for improvement. For example, community organizations could collaborate with local universities to conduct longitudinal studies on the outcomes of support programs for young mothers. Collecting and analyzing feedback from participants ensures that programs are meeting their needs and making a positive impact. Using this data to make informed adjustments can keep programs relevant and effective. Policymakers should advocate for increased funding for research on the mental health and well-being of teenage mothers of color and promote evidence-based policy-making. Grounding policies in rigorous research and best practices allows stakeholders to better support young mothers and improve their mental health outcomes.

LIMITATIONS

This study had several limitations. The data was gathered through a self-administered online survey, which may have resulted in prevarication and recall bias. For some of the participants, years had passed since they had given birth, so their mental health status prior to the birth of their child may have been difficult to recall accurately. Additionally, as mental health status is stigmatized in both the African American and Latino communities, participants may not have answered truthfully for fear of judgment. Furthermore, as this sample was gathered through snowball sampling, it may not be generalizable to other populations of WCTM.

REFERENCES

Bargai, N., Ben-Shakhar, G., & Shalev, A. Y. (2007). Posttraumatic stress disorder and depression in battered women: The mediating role of learned helplessness. *Journal of Family Violence*, *22*(5), 267–275. DOI: 10.1007/s10896-007-9078-y

Barnet, B., Liu, J., & DeVoe, M. (2008). Double jeopardy: Depressive symptoms and rapid subsequent pregnancy in adolescent mothers. *Archives of Pediatrics & Adolescent Medicine*, *162*(3), 246–252. DOI: 10.1001/archpediatrics.2007.60 PMID: 18316662

Biello, K. B., Sipsma, H. L., & Kershaw, T. (2010). Effect of teenage parenthood on mental health trajectories: Does sex matter? *American Journal of Epidemiology*, *172*(3), 279–287. DOI: 10.1093/aje/kwq128 PMID: 20576756

Black, M. M., Papas, M. A., Hussey, J. M., Dubowitz, H., Kotch, J. B., & Starr, R. H. (2002). Behavior problems among preschool children born to adolescent mothers: Effects of maternal depression and perceptions of partner relationships. *Journal of Clinical Child and Adolescent Psychology*, *31*(1), 16–26. DOI: 10.1207/S15374424JCCP3101_04 PMID: 11845646

Brondolo, E., Kelly, K. P., Coakley, V., Gordon, T., Thompson, S., Levy, E., Cassells, A., Tobin, J. N., Sweeney, M., & Contrada, R. J. (2005). The perceived ethnic discrimination questionnaire: Development and preliminary validation of a community version 1. *Journal of Applied Social Psychology*, *35*(2), 335–365. DOI: 10.1111/j.1559-1816.2005.tb02124.x

Brown, J. D., Harris, S. K., Woods, E. R., Buman, M. P., & Cox, J. E. (2012). Longitudinal study of depressive symptoms and social support in adolescent mothers. *Maternal and Child Health Journal*, *16*(4), 894–901. DOI: 10.1007/s10995-011-0814-9 PMID: 21556696

Carver, C. S. (1997). You want to measure coping but your protocol is too long: Consider the brief COPE. *International Journal of Behavioral Medicine*, *4*(1), 92–100. DOI: 10.1207/s15327558ijbm0401_6 PMID: 16250744

Centers for Disease Control and Prevention. (2021). *About teen pregnancy.* Reproductive Health: Teen Pregnancy. https://www.cdc.gov/vitalsigns/teenpregnancy/index.html

Childs, G. D., Knight, C., & White, R. (2015). Never-pregnant African American adolescent girls' perceptions of adolescent pregnancy. *Journal of Pediatric Nursing*, *30*(2), 310–320. DOI: 10.1016/j.pedn.2014.08.012 PMID: 25236337

Cohen, S., & Hoberman, H. M. (1983). Positive events and social supports as buffers of life change stress. *Journal of Applied Social Psychology*, *13*(2), 99–125. DOI: 10.1111/j.1559-1816.1983.tb02325.x

Cohen, S., & McKay, G. (1984). Social support, stress and the buffering hypothesis: A theoretical analysis. In Baum, A., Taylor, S. E., & Singer, J. E. (Eds.), Vol. 4, pp. 253–267). Handbook of Psychology and Health. Erlbaum., DOI: 10.4324/9781003044307

Cox, J. E., Buman, M., Valenzuela, J., Joseph, N. P., Mitchell, A., & Woods, E. R. (2008). Depression, parenting attributes, and social support among adolescent mothers attending a teen tot program. *Journal of Pediatric and Adolescent Gynecology*, *21*(5), 275–281. DOI: 10.1016/j.jpag.2008.02.002 PMID: 18794023

Dailey, D. (2008). Conceptualizing perceived racism and its effect on the health of African- Americans: Implications for practice and research. *Journal of National Black Nurses' Association. Journal of National Black Nurses' Association*, *19*, 73–80. DOI: 10.1177/1054773808314636 PMID: 18807782

Gaylord-Harden, N. K., & Cunningham, J. A. (2009). The impact of racial discrimination and coping strategies on internalizing symptoms in African American youth. *Journal of Youth and Adolescence*, *38*(4), 532–543. DOI: 10.1007/s10964-008-9377-5 PMID: 19636726

Gilmore, A. D., Osho, G. S., & Heads, A. B. (2013). Stress, anxiety, depression and psychological responses among African Americans: Empirical investigation and coping strategies. *American Journal of Health Sciences*, *4*(3), 121–130. DOI: 10.19030/ajhs.v4i3.8008

Glanz, K., Rimer, B. K., & Viswanath, K. (2008). *Health behavior and health education: Theory, research, and practice* (4th ed.). Jossey-Bass.

Guttmacher Institute. (2017). *Sex and HIV education.* State Laws and Policies. https://www.guttmacher.org/state-policy/explore/sex-and-hiv-education

Haslam, D. M., Pakenham, K. I., & Smith, A. (2006). Social support and postpartum depressive symptomatology: The mediating role of maternal self-efficacy. *Infant Mental Health Journal*, *27*(3), 276–291. DOI: 10.1002/imhj.20092 PMID: 28640472

Hodgkinson, S., Beers, L., Southammakosane, C., & Lewin, A. (2014). Addressing the mental health needs of pregnant and parenting adolescents. *Pediatrics*, *133*(1), 114–122. DOI: 10.1542/peds.2013-0927 PMID: 24298010

Hodgkinson, S. C., Colantuoni, E., Roberts, D., Berg-Cross, L., & Belcher, H. M. (2010). Depressive symptoms and birth outcomes among pregnant teenagers. *Journal of Pediatric and Adolescent Gynecology*, *23*(1), 16–22. DOI: 10.1016/j.jpag.2009.04.006 PMID: 19679498

Holland, M. L., Yoo, B. K., Kitzman, H., Chaudron, L., Szilagyi, P. G., & Temkin-Greener, H. (2011). Self-efficacy as a mediator between maternal depression and child hospitalizations in low-income urban families. *Maternal and Child Health Journal*, *15*(7), 1011–1019. DOI: 10.1007/s10995-010-0662-z PMID: 20706866

Huang, C. Y., Costeines, J., Kaufman, J. S., & Ayala, C. (2014). Parenting stress, social support, and depression for ethnic minority adolescent mothers: Impact on child development. *Journal of Child and Family Studies*, *23*(2), 255–262. DOI: 10.1007/s10826-013-9807-1 PMID: 24653641

Hutchison, E. D. (2014). *Dimensions of human behavior: Person and environment* (5th ed.). SAGE Publications.

Jackson, A. P. (2000). Maternal self-efficacy and children's influence on stress and parenting among single black mothers in poverty. *Journal of Family Issues*, *21*(1), 3–16. DOI: 10.1177/019251300021001001

Kearney, M. S., & Levine, P. B. (2012). Why is the teen birth rate in the United States so high and why does it matter? *The Journal of Economic Perspectives*, *26*(2), 141–166. DOI: 10.1257/jep.26.2.141 PMID: 22792555

Keith, V. M., Lincoln, K. D., Taylor, R. J., & Jackson, J. S. (2010). Discriminatory experiences and depressive symptoms among African American women: Do skin tone and mastery matter? *Sex Roles*, *62*(1-2), 48–59. DOI: 10.1007/s11199-009-9706-5 PMID: 21151821

Kessler, R. C., Chiu, W. T., Demler, O., & Walters, E. E. (2005). Prevalence, severity, and comorbidity of 12-month DSM-IV disorders in the National Comorbidity Survey Replication. *Archives of General Psychiatry*, *62*(6), 617–627. DOI: 10.1001/archpsyc.62.6.617 PMID: 15939839

Kim, T. H., Connolly, J. A., & Tamim, H. (2014). The effect of social support around pregnancy on postpartum depression among Canadian teen mothers and adult mothers in the maternity experiences survey. *BMC Pregnancy and Childbirth*, *14*(1), 162. DOI: 10.1186/1471-2393-14-162 PMID: 24884410

Le, H. N., & Lambert, S. F. (2008). Culture, context, and maternal self-efficacy in Latina mothers. *Applied Developmental Science*, *12*(4), 198–201. DOI: 10.1080/10888690802388136

Leahy-Warren, P., McCarthy, G., & Corcoran, P. (2012). First-time mothers: Social support, maternal parental self-efficacy and postnatal depression. *Journal of Clinical Nursing, 21*(3-4), 388–397. DOI: 10.1111/j.1365-2702.2011.03701.x PMID: 21435059

McDowell, I. (2006). *Measuring health: A guide to rating scales and questionnaires* (3rd ed.). Oxford University Press. DOI: 10.1093/acprof:oso/9780195165678.001.0001

Mirowsky, J., & Ross, C. E. (2002). Depression, parenthood, and age at first birth. *Social Science & Medicine, 54*(8), 1281–1298. DOI: 10.1016/S0277-9536(01)00096-X PMID: 11989963

Mollborn, S., & Morningstar, E. (2009). Investigating the relationship between teenage childbearing and psychological distress using longitudinal evidence. *Journal of Health and Social Behavior, 50*(3), 310–326. DOI: 10.1177/002214650905000305 PMID: 19711808

Moreno, O., & Cardemil, E. (2013). Religiosity and mental health services: An exploratory study of help seeking among Latinos. *Journal of Latina/o Psychology, 1*(1), 53–67. DOI: 10.1037/a0031376

National Alliance on Mental Illness. (2022). *Mental health by the numbers.* About Mental Health. https://www.nami.org/mhstats

Neblett, E. W.Jr, Bernard, D. L., & Banks, K. H. (2016). The moderating roles of gender and socioeconomic status in the association between racial discrimination and psychological adjustment. *Cognitive and Behavioral Practice, 23*(3), 385–397. DOI: 10.1016/j.cbpra.2016.05.002

Norris, C. M., & Mitchell, F. D. (2014). Exploring the stress-support-distress process among Black women. *Journal of Black Studies, 45*(1), 3–18. DOI: 10.1177/0021934713517898

Panzarine, S., Slater, E., & Sharps, P. (1995). Coping, social support, and depressive symptoms in adolescent mothers. *The Journal of Adolescent Health, 17*(2), 113–119. DOI: 10.1016/1054-139X(95)00064-Y PMID: 7495822

Quinless, F. W., & Nelson, M. A. M. (1988). Development of a measure of learned helplessness. *Nursing Research, 37*(1), 11–15. DOI: 10.1097/00006199-198801000-00003 PMID: 3340571

Reeves, W. C., Pratt, L. A., Thompson, W., Ahluwalia, I. B., Dhingra, S. S., McKnight-Eily, L. R., ... & Safran, M. A. (2011). Mental illness surveillance among adults in the United States. DOI: 10.15585/mmwr.su6003a1

Ríos-Salas, V., & Larson, A. (2015). Perceived discrimination, socioeconomic status, and mental health among Latino adolescents in US immigrant families. *Children and Youth Services Review, 56*, 116–125. DOI: 10.1016/j.childyouth.2015.07.011

Rocca, C. H., Doherty, I., Padian, N. S., Hubbard, A. E., & Minnis, A. M. (2010). Pregnancy intentions and teenage pregnancy among Latinas: A mediation analysis. *Perspectives on Sexual and Reproductive Health, 42*(3), 186–196. DOI: 10.1363/4218610 PMID: 20887287

Schuyler Center for Analysis and Advocacy. (2008). *Teenage births: Outcomes for young parents and their children.* http://www.scaany.org/documents/teen_pregnancy_dec08.pdf

Sellers, R. M., Copeland-Linder, N., Martin, P. P., & Lewis, R. H. (2006). Racial identity matters: The relationship between racial discrimination and psychological functioning in African American adolescents. *Journal of Research on Adolescence, 16*(2), 187–216. DOI: 10.1111/j.1532-7795.2006.00128.x

Shanok, A. F., & Miller, L. (2007). Stepping up to motherhood among inner-city teens. *Psychology of Women Quarterly, 31*(3), 252–261. DOI: 10.1111/j.1471-6402.2007.00368.x

Siegel, R. S., & Brandon, A. R. (2014). Adolescents, pregnancy, and mental health. *Journal of Pediatric and Adolescent Gynecology, 27*(3), 138–150. DOI: 10.1016/j.jpag.2013.09.008 PMID: 24559618

Teti, D. M., & Gelfand, D. M. (1991). Behavioral competence among mothers of infants in the first year: The mediational role of maternal self-efficacy. *Child Development, 62*(5), 918–929. DOI: 10.2307/1131143 PMID: 1756667

The National Campaign to Prevent Teen and Unplanned Pregnancy. (2021). *Texas data.* Power to Decide. https://thenationalcampaign.org/data/state/texas

The Texas Campaign to Prevent Teen Pregnancy. (2021a). *Teen birth in Texas.* https://txcampaign.org/research-data/teen-birth-in-texas/

The Texas Campaign to Prevent Teen Pregnancy. (2021b). *Disparities.* https://txcampaign.org/research-data/disparities/

Toomey, R. B., Umaña-Taylor, A. J., Updegraff, K. A., & Jahromi, L. B. (2013). Ethnic identity development and ethnic discrimination: Examining longitudinal associations with adjustment for Mexican-origin adolescent mothers. *Journal of Adolescence, 36*(5), 825–833. DOI: 10.1016/j.adolescence.2013.06.004 PMID: 24011098

Vines, A. I., Baird, D. D., McNeilly, M., Hertz-Picciotto, I., Light, K. C., & Stevens, J. (2006). Social correlates of the chronic stress of perceived racism among Black women. *Ethnicity & Disease*, *16*, 101. DOI: 10.1016/j.eatdis.2006.01.009 PMID: 16599356

Ward, E. C., Clark, L. O., & Heidrich, S. (2009). African American women's beliefs, coping behaviors, and barriers to seeking mental health services. *Qualitative Health Research*, *19*(11), 1589–1601. DOI: 10.1177/1049732309350686 PMID: 19843967

Wiltz, T. (2015, Mar 3). *Racial, ethnic disparities persist in teen pregnancy rates.* The PEW Charitable Trusts. https://www.pewtrusts.org/en/research-and-analysis/blogs/stateline/2015/3/03/racial-and-ethnic-disparities-persist-in-teen-pregnancy-rates

Winters, L. I., & Winters, P. C. (2012). Black teenage pregnancy. *A Dynamic. SAGE Open*, *2*(1), 2158244012436563. Advance online publication. DOI: 10.1177/2158244012436563

Women of Color Network. (2006). *Domestic violence.* Women of Color Network Facts and Stats Collection: Communities of Color. https://www.doj.state.or.us/wp-content/uploads/2017/08/women_of_color_network_facts_domestic_violence_2006.pdf

Zigmond, A. S., & Snaith, R. P. (1983). The hospital anxiety and depression scale. *Acta Psychiatrica Scandinavica*, *67*(6), 361–370. DOI: 10.1111/j.1600-0447.1983.tb09716.x PMID: 6880820

Chapter 6
The Maternal Mental Health of Black Women Working

Jennifer J. Edwards
Renewell Foundation, USA

ABSTRACT

Black women working suffer disproportionate maternal mental health challenges compared to other working women. It is important to have this very valuable conversation about mental health for working Black women who are pregnant, and who are thinking about becoming pregnant. Maternal mental health and coping are directly influenced by social support, partner support, and the environment that she is in. Considering maternal mental health among workplace recruitment tools is a beneficial approach to elevate the experience of women, Black women, and mothers in the workplace. Innovative workplaces who value DEIB can design intentional programming in support of the maternal mental health of Black women, including crafting supportive benefits packages. Assessing and addressing the forces that fight against Black women working is essential to support mental health and maternal mental health. There is no sustainable professional success without stable maternal mental health.

INTRODUCTION

Black women working suffer disproportionate maternal mental health challenges compared to other working women. It is important to have this very valuable

DOI: 10.4018/979-8-3693-4272-5.ch006

conversation about mental health for working Black women who are pregnant, and who are thinking about becoming pregnant.

Research suggests that Black, Hispanic, and Asian women are more likely to experience depressive symptoms than White women. For example, according to Howell et al. (2005), African-American women have an adjusted odds ratio of 2.16 for reporting postpartum depressive (PPD) symptoms, compared to white women – two times more likely. Furthermore, from 2010 to 2021, the rate of PPD increased by 60% among Whites, 110% among Hispanics, 140% among Blacks, and 280% among Asian/Pacific Islanders (Getahun et al., 2023). Approximately 15% of women diagnosed with postpartum depression receive treatment. While undertreatment of postpartum depression is prevalent in the general population, Black women are even less likely to initiate treatment for postpartum depression (Policy Center for Maternal Mental Health, 2023).

Workplaces have an opportunity to consider how maternal mental health can be included as part of their benefit offerings for staff. Maternal health in this discussion encompasses the health of mothers with perinatal lived experiences. This discussion centers women, and while non-male gender identities are present in modern families, they may not be represented fully in the available data for this discussion. We are specifically uplifting Black women working, not to the detriment of others who work and are parents.

When a Black woman's environment is not supportive of her health needs, it becomes more difficult for her to make the appropriate health decisions she may need to make. She may delay or feel apprehensive about getting screened for things like depression, anxiety, or other mental health challenges for example. Then as a result, the woman suffers in silence. As the woman continues to suffer in silence for months and sometimes years at a time this suffering can then be exacerbated by what should be a joyful time of pregnancy. Her preexisting, untreated clinical conditions can potentially get worse.

CULTURAL CONTEXT

References to Black women includes women who are African American, African Caribbean, and Afro Latino ethnicities in the United States. Black is a racial identifier that encompasses many ethnic identifiers and Black women are not a monolith. Social values consist of the attitudes that persons of a culture hold toward moral and personal issues as learned through socialization, including health and disease; and social customs represent social values in the form of cultural actions, rituals, and communication rules (Chen, 1989). We can acknowledge in this safe literary space that we have knowledge, attitudes, and beliefs of our respective cultures that may differ, yet that we can honor what is special about each other. Our priorities relating to business, personal performance, and personal life may not be the same.

The subjective norms pertaining to women in in Black cultures have the potential to affect maternal mental health attitudes and workplace performance, communications, and coping based on the level of empowerment the women may feel (Jones, 2011). This discussion is evidence-based and also largely from the perspective of an African-American woman, mother, and researcher. There are considerations, opportunities, insights, and innovation that can pivot the maternal mental health experience for all Black women working.

We must be careful not to *anthropomorphize* clinical conditions by referencing things like "Black cancer" or "Black mental health" – cancer and mental health should not be racialized and are not people. The medical sociology of those experiences, however, is indeed intricate and impacted by race-related experiences. Adding a racial identifier to the disease or to the illness implies that the condition cannot be separated from the woman or healed. Maternal mental health is guided by genetics. It is guided by environment. It is guided by personal attitudes and beliefs as well. We cannot consider maternal mental health for Black women working without understanding the history and medical sociology behind the mental health journey In the Black community, mental health is still very much a stigmatized topic that has undercurrents of blame and shame. Black women deserve appropriate levels of wraparound support so they can restore, health, and thrive in the workplace, community, and families.

The United States is among the worst countries to live in as a pregnant working mother. The United States has the worst paid maternity leave allowance among all Organization for Economic Co-operation and Development (OECD) measured countries, at zero months of paid maternity leave. On average across the 38 OECD countries, paid maternity leave lasts for 18.5 weeks, but it can range from 43 weeks in Greece to none in the United States, although some states within the U.S. do offer paid maternity leave (OECD, 2024). These findings do not reflect paternity leave, adoption, or other related policies. Paternity and partner birth leave timeframes tend to be significantly shorter.

THE HIGH IMPACT BLACK WOMAN WORKING

Women lead approximately half of households as the primary income earner, with Black women most often leading married households in comparison to other racial groups (Goodman et al., 2021). As modern families evolve and consist of more working women, Black women in the workplace come highly credentialed and highly experienced. Mental health becomes an utmost concern for the high impact Black woman working. Challenges relating to mental health are compounded by family and caregiving responsibilities. Black women notoriously face microaggressions in the workplace, where some not all of us may acknowledge that there is racism in the workplace. Experiences of support by allies are also present and real many times. Based on our multinational Black cultures and our histories, we may have differing definitions of racism. A woman may say she has to explain herself more, persuade people more often, and justify her presence and ideas more. However, she may not define that as racism, sexism, or ageism. Others would affirm that race-based biases that require a Black woman to prove herself more than anyone else is absolutely racism in the workplace.

Pervasive microaggressions and racism over time can lead to mental health conditions, including anxiety and depression and hopelessness. When that is added to being a mother or becoming a mother, maternal mental health can suffer. Systemic racism is a root cause of health inequities and worse health outcomes (CDC, 2024). It is essential that workplaces take responsibility for an aspect of these unspoken and very damaging dynamics. Some workplaces have gone so far as to state they are anti-racist workplaces. Other workplaces have robust diversity, equity, inclusion, and belonging (DEIB) initiatives. Others have eliminated these programs entirely. Workplaces must recognize that they are active contributors and change agents that can support the mental health of Black women working.

The pregnancy journey can be challenging, particularly as women are getting pregnant at older ages, introducing more risk for complications at an advanced maternal age (Cleveland Clinic 2024). There are philosophical debates around whether or not a woman should work while pregnant, or if she should work while being a mom, and what roles the mother's partner should have in the journey. What is clear, what is known, and what is proven is that burnout is real. And if a woman is burned out, she cannot be of service to herself, her family or her workplace.

Maternal mental health and coping are directly influenced by social support, partner support, and the environment that she is in. Work-life integration may be more attainable for some than others, and burnout is more likely for some than others. This underscores why establishing boundaries, building a village or support in our age of long-distance extended families, and having personal awareness of capacity remains imperative.

Workplace Politics and Pressures

Organizational support for Black women working in the U.S. and all mothers must happen now through policies and executive leadership champions. According to the Society for Human Resource Management (2022), "The message that taking parental leave is important must come from the top and be reinforced throughout the organization." Organizational culture and climate directly influence the maternal mental health experience of Black women working. How supportive is the workplace of pregnant mothers, expecting families, and parents?

Social forces actively create and shape patterns of disease, and these forces connect social interactions and human activities to health outcomes, including those relating to maternal mental health (Link et al., 2008; Libby, Fallon, and Jarris, 2008). Social systems – like organizational politics in the workplace – influence the health status of persons through constructs of power and marginalization, thereby creating health inequities and disparities. For example, that race-based microaggressions in the workplace can iteratively – repeatedly and relentlessly - affect mental health of those who experience them in the absence of effective coping tools, mindfulness, boundaries, and human resources support. Social systems are represented in the societal hierarchies and institutions of a culture, such as the healthcare system (Chen, 1989).

Untreated workplace-related anxiety in a woman is absolutely compounded once a woman is pregnant. Pregnancy is a time of joy and also stress for many; and unchecked mental health conditions can make the journey traumatizing at the most and difficult. It is valuable for workplaces to consider the perinatal season as a special season of support for Black women. During the perinatal journey, there are physical symptoms and experiences that affect the Black woman working. Working mommy brain is a very real phenomenon, common though not a clinical diagnosis (Baylor, Scott, & White, 2023). If a woman returns to work too quickly, she may still be experiencing this postpartum brain fog while also trying to be productive in the workplace. In general, fatigue is also very important to be aware of. Flexibility in workplace schedules can support reducing fatigue that parents in the postpartum period might be experiencing. Black women working mothers need rest and restoration too.

It should be noted that a woman's experience as a salaried employee could be very different from an hourly employee's experience. As an hourly employee, workplace benefits will differ, access to parental leave, and health benefits will differ, where some part-time employees may not have access to these benefits at all.

SUPERVISORY SUPPORT

Anecdotally, nuanced dynamics can emerge when a woman may or may not report to a supervisor who has children. Supervisors who have children, particularly in a similar age group, may more understanding than supervisors who do not have children in similar age groups. If a supervisor has children who might be older, there is a tendency to have forgotten what the haste and hustle and bustle of the younger years with children might have been like. There may be a disconnect and lack of understanding and lack of flexibility concerning workload and workplace accommodations. This can be further compounded in the presence of race-based practices that result in lack of understanding or accommodation of requests for the Black woman working, akin to the trend that biases can perpetuate negative treatment of minorities pain complaints (Association of American Medical Colleges, 2020), for example.

It is, however, an excellent pairing when a supervisor is empathetic or in a similar stage of life with children of a similar age as there can be a higher level of spoken and unspoken understanding. These factors are largely uncontrollable in the hiring and employment experience, however, the nuanced dynamics do make a difference relating to organizational climate, resulting pressures, or flexibility. These elements directly link to maternal mental health and work-life balance and integration. Work-life integration represents an acknowledgement that rarely are all things balanced equally at the same time. However, there are various aspects of life that come together that are integrated beautifully into a picture of work, life, community, family, and self for the Black woman working.

SHANICE'S CASE STUDY: PERSONAL ADVOCACY FOR THE BLACK WOMAN WORKING

It is essential for a Black woman working to be her own personal advocate in the workplace. For this case study, we will consider a married Black woman who is pregnant with her first child. The woman's name is Shanice (pseudonym), and Shanice is not aware of workplace practices relating to pregnant and expecting mothers and parents. Shanice works at a large state university and Shanice had a supervisor who is not a mother. Shanice did have a flexible work schedule, however, there was a lack of clarity offered within the departmental level around what her benefits are relating to pregnancy and the perinatal period. During that time, her supervisor, the department chair, did not offer any resources.

Lack of Awareness

The lack of resources provided to Shanice did not seem to be intentional or malicious. However, in reflecting on the experience, Shanice was still left with no proactive information from her employer about pregnancy and perinatal benefits and leave expectations. At her employer, there is an unspoken culture of taking limited time off during the semester at her university. Shanice was feeling the pressures, particularly in this workplace and in an academic environment. Further, she put an extensive amount of pressure on herself because of her own attitudes toward work and performance that had already affected her mental health.

Shanice may have had Family and Medical Leave Act (FMLA) paperwork that was filed in her workplace, however, additional leave was not part of discussions with the employer's human resources office. This may have been due to lack of awareness on Shanice's part in terms of knowing what to even ask about these benefits. As a somewhat early careerist, she was proceeding with the inaccurate perception that her workplace was providing all the information she needed to know.

Case Question

1. What are three questions that Shanice could have asked her supervisor to empower herself and be her personal advocate during her pregnancy and postpartum experience?

The Need for Boundaries for Maternal Mental Health

There was an unfortunate gap in resources, education, and awareness in Shanice's particular case. Colleagues did step in to teach the last couple of weeks of Shanice's class for that semester. She, however, was in the hospital still checking the online learning management system because an automated exam was being delivered the same day that she gave birth. Whether due to unspoken pressures for success in an academic environment or her own pressures for being present for her students, Shanice worked on the day she gave birth.

Benefits Offered

While Shanice was able to take six weeks off through FMLA, no proactive discussion from her employer occurred to inform her she could leverage short-term disability after any paid leave or other time off had been exhausted. Shanice was not aware of her full slate of options as a Black woman working.

Case Questions

1. What are five questions that Shanice could have asked human resources to empower herself and be her personal advocate during her pregnancy and postpartum experience?
2. What resources can Shanice seek the next time she's having a child?

WORKPLACE CAPACITY SUPPORTING BLACK WOMEN WORKING

Considering maternal mental health among workplace recruitment tools is a beneficial approach to elevate the experience of women, Black women, and mothers in the workplace. Innovative workplaces who value DEIB can design intentional programming in support of the maternal mental health of Black women, including crafting supportive benefits packages. Information around leave practices, emotional and peer support will take the maternal mental health of Black women working a long way. We have to know and be confident that being a mother at work is not going to penalize us from opportunities, from being promoted, from advancing, or from getting raises. Legal or not, career barriers can be present that exacerbate stress and long-term mental health if unaddressed.

Sample impactful workplace practices identified by Business and Professional Women Foundation (2008) are as follows: future leave self-funded sabbatical for personal purposes, women's forum and process to transition women who have been out of the workforce due to maternity, paid time off bank up to 80 hours, and flexible work schedules.

Designing equitable career pathways is also important for workplaces to support maternal mental health. Workplaces must actively engage in stay surveys to understand the current climate of their staff. Stay surveys offer an opportunity to explore organizational culture, organizational climate, daily practices, and behaviors of staff members among each other (Trailhead Institute, 2023). These stay surveys can be leveraged to explore maternal mental workplace needs and opportunities for staff.

Additionally, ensuring equitable career pathways provides an opportunity to acknowledge the unique circumstances of Black women working. Organizations can develop and design programs relating to leadership competencies and managing stress for Black women, and create a chance to propel Black women forward as thought leaders, where the core of advancement and promotion in the workplace is stable mental health. Assessing and addressing the forces that fight against Black women working is essential to support mental health and maternal mental health. A Black woman is a leader, a staff person, a contributor, a mother, all at the same time. Understanding why she stays – or leaves – a workplace is imperative.

Workplace allies for mothers and families are essential to support maternal mental health and create an organizational culture of empowered mothers and parents. Fathers and non-parents alike can support redistribution of labor and advocate for maternal mental health benefits. Johnson, Worrell, and Chandler (2005) assessed psychological health and empowerment in women specifically pertaining to individual attitudes and behaviors. The researchers stated that empowered women successfully access resources to achieve change. The researchers examined empowerment as a woman's ability to access skills and resources to cope with current and future stress and trauma.

Supporting the mental health journey of Black women working is essential, from acknowledging the emotional toll that pregnancy, and in-vitro fertilization (IVF) treatments, to adoption. Workplaces can consider resources like employee assistance programs (EAPs) that can specifically reinforce maternal mental health. They can highlight that EAPs to support staff on anxiety and depression, postpartum anxiety, postpartum depression, and in extreme cases, post partum psychosis. Workplaces can offer a base of health education information to support employees understanding the value of the EAP sessions and to begin examining their own personal experiences, signs and symptoms to determine whether or not starting with a EAP is a good choice for them. EAPs allow for clients to engage in a series of counseling and therapy sessions with costs initially covered by the employer. The number of sessions is also often limited. However, the EAP offers a pathway to sustained therapeutic care because a relationship with the counselor is built through the initial series of sessions that can be access on a paid basis long-term.

Notably, workplaces can increase capacity by inviting maternal mental health community health workers to offer educational training and resources for staff. The Renewell Foundation is a nonprofit that has curated a free certificate program representing the intersection of maternal health, mental health, and community health work. Maternal mental health solutions do not have to be offered internally, extending capacity through community health workers, trainers, and consultants during designated times of year can be instrumental in improve the maternal mental health climate in the workplace.

Lastly, workplaces can also offer employee resource groups (ERGs) in support of maternal mental health experiences. ERGs are groups of individuals with shared common identities and experiences who get together on a routine basis to talk about their challenges, their successes, opportunities to work together, opportunities to improve the workplace, and to have an impact based on the collective identity that they share together. A workplace ERG that centers motherhood, maternal mental health, or focuses on Black women are all peer support options that can help empower and equip Black women working. ERG origins are in equity-related initiatives, and participating mothers gain increased confidence, resilience, and resolve to press forward in life and work.

CONCLUSION

Challenges in one area of life can affect other areas of life. Mental health as a mother intricately relates to mental health as an employee. For example, global economic pressures absolutely impact grocery expenses and influence a possible overarching level of stress that also affect work.

When toxic and unsupportive workplaces are compounded with the disparities and inequities that Black women and Black mothers experience, worse maternal health and general health outcomes are the result. We must get to the root of why the United States is behind in maternal policies. Political advocates have increased awareness around and developed foundational mechanisms for Congress to support essential topics in maternal health through research and policy.

Workplace policies and practices can absolutely support maternal mental health while remaining comprehensive in addressing core health benefits. Whether a parent has a newborn or has a teen, the experiences of Black women working are disproportionately affected by an organizational culture that might be deficient in valuing diversity, equity, inclusion, and belonging. There is no sustainable professional success without stable maternal mental health. Developing employer benefits and experiences of a workplace is beneficial for supporting the maternal mental health of Black women working.

REFERENCES

Baylor, Scott, & White Health. (2023). *Is mom brain real? Understanding and coping with postpartum brain fog*. https://www.bswhealth.com/blog/is-mom-brain-real

Business and Professional Women Foundation. (2008). *Successful workplaces digest*. https://bpwfoundation.org/wp-content/uploads/2015/02/BPW_Foundation_Successful_Workplaces_Digest.pdf

Centers for Disease Control and Prevention. (2024). *Impact of racism on our nation's health*. https://www.cdc.gov/minority-health/racism-health/index-1.html

Chen, G. M. (1989). Relationships of the dimensions of intercultural communication competence. *Communication Quarterly*, *37*(2), 118–133. DOI: 10.1080/01463378909385533

Cleveland Clinic. (2024). *Advanced maternal age*. https://my.clevelandclinic.org/health/diseases/22438-advanced-maternal-age

Goodman, L., Choi, J. H., & Zhu, J. (2021). *More women have become homeowners and heads of households. Could the pandemic undo that progress?* Urban Institute. https://www.urban.org/urban-wire/more-women-have-become-homeowners-and-heads-household-could-pandemic-undo-progress

Johnson, D. M., Worrell, J., & Chandler, R. K. (2005). Assessing psychological health and empowerment in women: The personal progress scale revised. *Women & Health*, *5*(1), 109–129. DOI: 10.1300/J013v41n01_07 PMID: 16048871

Jones, J. (2010). *Suffering in silence? Intrapersonal communication regarding female empowerment and healthcare access for breast cancer screening in Cape Town*. Publication No.

Libby, P. M., Fallon, M. M., & Jarris, P. E. (2008). Public health practice and health equity: Challenges and opportunities. *Journal of Public Health Management and Practice, 14*(S), S53–S55.

Link, B. G., Northridge, M. E., Phelan, J. C., & Ganz, M. L. (2008). Social epidemiology and the fundamental cause concept: On the structuring of effective cancer screens by socioeconomic status. *The Milbank Quarterly*, *76*(3), 375–402. DOI: 10.1111/1468-0009.00096 PMID: 9738168

Sabin, J. (2020). *How we fail Black patients in pain*. Association of American Medical Colleges. https://www.aamc.org/news/how-we-fail-black-patients-pain

Society for Human Resource Management. (2022). *Leveling the parental-leave playing field.* https://www.shrm.org/topics-tools/news/benefits-compensation/leveling-parental-leave-playing-field

Trailhead Institute. (2023). *Restore: The Colorado blueprint for innovative public health workforce development.* https://trailhead.institute/wp-content/uploads/2023/05/Trailhead-CO-Blueprint-Report-Final-Web.pdf

Organization for Economic Co-operation and Development. (2024). *Paid parental leave: Big differences for mothers and fathers.* https://oecdstatistics.blog/2023/01/12/paid-parental-leave-big-differences-for-mothers-and-fathers/

Chapter 7
Addressing Maternal Mental Health Trauma in Black and Brown Communities: A Culturally Competent and Bioethical Approach

Lena Sharara
Maternal Outcomes for Translational Health Equity Research Lab, Tufts University School of Medicine, USA

Tyra Gravesande
Maternal Outcomes for Translational Health Equity Research Lab, Tufts University School of Medicine, USA

Vickie Dugat
https://orcid.org/0000-0002-7343-8957
Center for Black Maternal Health and Reproductive Justice, Tufts University School of Medicine, USA

Farida Yada
Maternal Outcomes for Translational Health Equity Research Lab, Tufts University School of Medicine, USA

Ndidiamaka Amutah-Onukagha
Department of Public Health and Community Medicine, Tufts University School of Medicine, USA

DOI: 10.4018/979-8-3693-4272-5.ch007

ABSTRACT

Black maternal health disparities remain a critical public health issue, with Black birthing people facing significantly higher rates of maternal mortality and morbidity than their white counterparts. This chapter explores the intersection of bioethics and Black maternal mental health, highlighting ethical considerations in healthcare practices, decisions, and policy. The research delves into systemic factors such as structural racism and discrimination that contribute to these disparities, emphasizing their ethical implications. Key areas of focus include perinatal depression and anxiety, postpartum maternal mental health, and the Edinburgh Postnatal Depression Scale. Additionally, the impact of COVID-19 on mental health and key principles of bioethics – such as autonomy, nonmaleficence, beneficence, and justice – are emphasized. Aimed at healthcare practitioners, policymakers, and researchers, this chapter aims to deepen understanding of ethical dimensions in Black maternal mental health, fostering interventions and policies that promote equitable care and address disparities.

INTRODUCTION

Among Black mothers and birthing people, we see vast disparities that continuously highlight systemic factors such as socioeconomic inequalities, racism, and a lack of social support that exacerbate the risk of these conditions, making it imperative to foster awareness and create inclusive mental health support systems. Perinatal depression and anxiety represent significant health concerns that particularly affect Black mothers and birthing individuals, underscoring the importance of addressing these issues within this demographic. Research has consistently shown that the intersection of maternal mental health and race can lead to mental health disparities, with Black birthing people experiencing higher rates of perinatal mood and anxiety disorders (PMADs) and less access to culturally competent care. Rates of PMADs among Black birthing people continue to increase with rates changing from 9.2% to 22% between 2010 and 2021–a 140% increase (Getahun et al., 2023). This trend underscores the urgent need for early intervention and tailored treatment approaches that consider the unique experiences and stressors faced by black mothers.

Structural racism describes how historical residential segregation and policies affect the distribution of resources and power (*Structural Racism and Discrimination*, n.d.). This uneven distribution influences the risks of pregnancy-related complications and amplifies psychosocial stressors among Black birthing people and their families. It also affects the distribution of health-promoting material goods and resources and socioeconomic opportunities, including access to quality and timely healthcare, health literacy, disposable income, and social capital.

Within this chapter, we will address how maternal mental health encompasses the psychological and emotional well-being of women before, during, and after pregnancy. It is a crucial factor that affects not only the mothers themselves but also the developmental outcomes of their children. We will examine the prevalence of perinatal depression and anxiety disorders among Black birthing individuals, discuss potential systemic failures contributing to these high rates, and explore interventions designed to reduce this prevalence. Additionally, we will discuss the multifaceted issues surrounding maternal mental health, and how these may be compounded by factors such as the COVID-19 pandemic. Finally, this chapter will address questions that align with the theoretical framework of a Black bioethicist from a bioethics perspective. These questions are crucial for gaining an understanding and questioning the narrative surrounding the achievement of fairness for Black birthing people, which is essential for their future progress.

The primary focus of this chapter is to emphasize the importance of incorporating bioethical principles while considering the distinct experiences and needs of Black birthing people. This integration is crucial for attaining health equity and justice in the context of Black maternal mental health. We aim to discuss the need for establishments to secure equitable settings for academics of color, whose specialized knowledge, when combined with that of specialists in other domains, should be given utmost importance by the bioethics community. The cultivation of sustained change necessitates a crucial disposition to engage in proactive measures, particularly in situations where the path ahead remains ambiguous. This implies that to effectively promote anti-racism and reproductive and mental health justice, the field must actively and consistently strive to broaden its goals, approaches, theories, and methodologies.

From a bioethical perspective, healthcare practitioners must strike a balance between upholding autonomy and promoting beneficence. These concepts are explored in greater detail in the Bioethics section of this chapter. This entails responsibly navigating the mother's informed consent process while making important health decisions and actively ensuring the protection of her mental well-being. To cultivate an environment that upholds dignity and facilitates healing during this vulnerable phase, it is crucial to ensure equitable access to mental health resources, implement culturally sensitive care practices, and safeguard patient confidentiality. To promote maternal mental health outcomes, and foster the fundamental connection between mother and child during the early stages of life, it is imperative to give precedence to these ethical considerations.

We hope this chapter provides a comprehensive understanding of the intersections between Black maternal mental health, systemic racism, and bioethics, highlighting the urgent need for equitable and culturally competent care. Through this discussion, we aim to contribute to the ongoing efforts to achieve justice and improved health outcomes for Black mothers and birthing people, ultimately fostering a more inclusive and equitable healthcare system.

* Language Note: Throughout this chapter, the terms "birthing people," "mother," "birthing individuals", and "woman" are used interchangeably to acknowledge the diverse range of individuals who may give birth, recognizing that the experience of childbirth is not limited to those who identify as women.

THE RETROSPECTIVE OF ENSLAVEMENT, MATERNAL HEALTH AND TRAUMA

During the time period of the transatlantic slave trade and within the landscapes of the Antebellum south, the experience of maternity was nothing short of a spine-chilling, daunting experience. According to Marie Jenkins Schwartz, slave owners valued the life of the mother far more than the life of the infant that the enslaved woman carried. In fact, Dr. Joseph P. Logan affirmed the medical principle that the life of the mother was far more important than the continuation of the pregnancy. Although this may sound kindred, slaveowners took pride in ensuring that black enslaved women could have healthy pregnancies and bear children, exercising a slaveowner's power over their slaves (Schwartz 108). Following the transatlantic slave trade, slaveowners became more reliant on black enslaved women's fertility, as they relied on physicians in the antebellum south to tend to enslaved women at birth. Moreover, slaveowners tend to buy as many young, black enslaved women as they can in order to bear children, thus being deemed valuable. Among all of this, slaveowners sought assistance from white physicians for difficult births, infertility, and infant mortality. However, infant mortality in plantation settings remained high, with 50% of enslaved infants stillborn or dying within the first year of life in the South (Owens and Fett 2019). Slaveowners acted quickly if a black, enslaved woman's reproductive health encountered complications, as their future earnings solely depended on whether an enslaved woman could carry to full term and bear children (Schwartz 68). Enslaved women were often subjected to forced pregnancies to increase the slave population, a practice that stripped them of autonomy over their bodies. The pressure to reproduce under strenuous conditions created an environment where maternal health was severely compromised. High fertility rates were demanded, yet the availability of medical care for pregnant enslaved women was abysmally low. Malnutrition, excessive labor, and a lack of prenatal care often led to high incidences of miscarriage, stillbirth, and maternal mortality. Physicians, however, took a liking to tending to enslave women's fertility issues, and continued to experiment on their bodies in order to pinpoint the cause of infertility. Nevertheless, Black enslaved women's bodies were continuously commodified and used as experiments, testing sites, and teaching tools among physicians and white medical schools. In 18th- and 19th-century slave societies, white physicians established their reputations by "medicalizing blackness." (Owens and Fett, 2019).

The trauma associated with these experiences was not merely physical but deeply psychological, leaving lasting scars. Enslaved women faced the constant threat of having their children sold, tearing the very fabric of their family structure. This separation inflicted severe emotional and psychological trauma, affecting not only the mother but also the broader community. The trauma experienced by enslaved mothers extended beyond their loss, embedding itself into the collective memory and cultural psyche of their descendants.

The forced subjugation of enslaved women's reproductive capacities also had long-term consequences for their fertility. The relentless cycle of pregnancy and childbirth, interspersed with physical abuse and inadequate medical support, led to numerous reproductive health issues. Conditions like pelvic inflammatory disease, infections from poor birthing practices, and chronic gynecological problems were rampant. These health issues often persisted into freedom, impacting the fertility and maternal health of subsequent generations. n present times, understanding the historical context of slavery and its impact on maternal health allows for a more comprehensive approach to addressing persistent racial disparities in maternal health outcomes. Studies show that African American women today are more likely to experience complications during pregnancy and childbirth and have higher rates of infant and maternal mortality compared to their white counterparts (Centers for Disease Control and Prevention [CDC], 2020). The intergenerational trauma resulting from slavery's reproductive exploitation continues to echo, manifesting in health disparities influenced by socio-economic determinants, systemic racism, and mistrust in the medical system.

Efforts to improve maternal health outcomes for African American women must therefore acknowledge the historical trauma of slavery. Health interventions should incorporate culturally sensitive care and trauma-informed practices. Addressing systemic inequities in healthcare access, providing comprehensive reproductive health education, and fostering community-based support systems can mitigate some of these adverse outcomes. The legacy of slavery impacts maternal health, fertility, and trauma in profound ways. By acknowledging and addressing these historical and cultural influences, there is potential to improve health outcomes and foster a more equitable healthcare system. Understanding this intricate relationship underscores the importance of a holistic and historically informed approach to maternal health care, aiming to heal past wounds and build a healthier future for all.

A BRIEF ANTHOLOGY OF THE BLACK WOMAN AND BIRTHING PERSON'S EXPERIENCE

Ericka Hart: A Journey through Motherhood as a Black, Queer Parent

Ericka Hart, a sex educator, always dreamed of being pregnant and becoming a parent. But, after being diagnosed with breast cancer in 2014, along with the roadblocks that both queer and trans people face to get pregnant, they did not think that it was possible.

Hart's partner, Ebony, is trans. When they both found out that Hart was pregnant, they were overfilled with joy and emotion. Both Ericka and Ebony went through intrauterine insemination (IUI) approximately three times. But the fourth time was an absolute miracle—almost as if they just created a child out of thin air.

"I'm a sex educator, so I'm constantly inundated with a lot of information about birth. I'm well aware of the rates of maternal mortality for Black people who are pregnant. So I knew that since I live in New York City, which has some of the highest rates in the country, I was absolutely having a home birth," Hart says.

Hart recommended that future Black, Queer or trans parents equip themselves with a lot more resources.

"The process of finding and securing a Black midwife was severely difficult, especially trying to find a Black, queer midwife," Hart says. In New York, the state possesses some of the most racist laws against midwives. There is a plethora of white midwives in the State of New York, but not enough Black, queer, trans or trans-affirming birth workers.

Fortunately, both Hart and Ebony were able to secure a black midwife through another birth worker by the name of Racha Tahani Lawler Queen, CPM, LM.

"I thought, Well, that's a strong recommendation. She was based in Los Angeles at the time, and I live in Brooklyn. I didn't know how it was going to work. But I ended up having a work trip in L.A. so we were able to meet up with Racha and we just hit it off," Hard tells.

Black women in the United States experience unacceptably poor maternal health outcomes, including higher rates of death related to pregnancy or childbirth. At 33 weeks of pregnancy, Hart traveled to upstate New York to visit some friends. However, they began to experience symptoms of nausea and feelings of discomfort. One day, their entire face was swollen, along with their feet and hands. Hart immediately made plans to travel back to the city with their partner in order to take a visit to see their general practitioner. Hart's blood pressure was 150 over 100. The next day, their pressure was 165 over 110.

During an urgent visit to the oncologist, the physician said, "You're pregnant, and your blood pressure is not good. I want you to go to the ER today. You need to call your midwife and get confirmation from her. but I'm just telling you, I really think you need to go to the ER." Ericka consoles their midwife, Racha, as they both coast through this developing yet fearful journey all together. Ericka's partner, Ebony, prepared a hospital bag, which completely concerns Ericka and makes them question what's truly going on in their body.

At the ER, Hart discovers that they developed preeclampsia, a serious pregnancy impediment—which is a red flag that the pregnancy can be fatal for both the baby and the person carrying the child. At the time, Hart's blood pressure had already risen to 175 over 110, even higher than the night prior.

The doctors in the ER explained to both Hart and Eboni that the birth of their child could occur at any time. Their child, East Alice Coltrane Turiyasangitananda, was transverse while lying across Ericka's stomach, a dangerous position for the baby; thus, a cesarean section was required.

"At that moment, I realized the birth plan I had envisioned was not going to happen. I felt like I wasn't even in the room. I know that my body was there, but my mind was somewhere else. My mom is deceased and I was communicating directly with her. As I was talking to my mom, I said, 'I don't know what's going on, but this is not the plan, and I'm going to need your grandchild to get through this." Hart prays to her mother in heaven. By the time Hart arrived at the hospital, it was 3:00 p.m., and at 7:11 p.m., Hart and Ebony had their child.

Ericka says, "From not being able to hold your kid after they're born, to being pregnant one day to not being pregnant the next, these are traumatic events. My trauma was not taken into consideration at all.".

Four days after East's birth, Hart was let go. They had to take blood pressure and pain medicine, and they had to keep monitoring their blood pressure. Hart felt better after awhile, and their blood pressure has returned to normal. The root cause of preeclampsia is unknown. Ericka says, "We can claim that it is typical for Black women to give birth since pregnancy is already stressful on the body and because systems of oppression impose so much stress on all of us, but we actually don't know.".

East's return was also strange. Hart always imagined that becoming a parent would be something they invented on their own, independent of what their own family did. They desired to change a lot of the parenting they received, but I also wanted to keep parts of it.

"Whether it's blackness, gender identity, or sexuality, I want my child to know that none of these things are a barrier," Ericka says.

Hart educates and implores others about the importance of becoming equipped with more than enough resources if you identify as a Black, queer and/or trans parent. There should be a lot more materials that describe what it means to become a parent, including the legal implications of it, for Black queer people who desire to do so.

"How do you legally defend yourself when you have children, especially in a nation that is homophobic? How do you ensure the safety of both you and your child?" Hart asks. The use of affirming pronouns, making no assumptions about people's relationships, and asking questions are also important considerations for medical workers. Don't forget it once they identify that person as their spouse in response to your question, "Who is this person to you?" Remember, a person is their partner and treat them as such the next time you enter the room.

Birth attendants must also be knowledgeable about working with queer and trans people. People with queer and trans identities should not have to educate the midwives themselves on how to perform an IUI, where to receive the supplies or the instruments needed for sperm. It is not just queer trans people who receive IUIs. Birth workers must become familiar with the alternatives to conceiving a child.

PERINATAL DEPRESSION AND ANXIETY

Perinatal depression and anxiety refer to a spectrum of mood disorders that can impact a birthing person anytime from conception through the first year postpartum (Ni et al., 2005). Within the United States, statistics reveal that perinatal mood and anxiety disorders (PMADs) affect approximately 11-21% of women (Byrnes, 2019), with Black mothers and birthing individuals experiencing these conditions at disproportionately higher rates compared to their white counterparts (Yehudah & Tadros, 2022). Analyzing data from a comprehensive study involving ten thousand pregnant individuals, the Edinburgh Postnatal Depression Scale identified a greater likelihood of screen-positive results among single, young, and less-educated Black birthing individuals enrolled in public health insurance programs (Wisner et al., 2013). In another study examining a group of Black birthing individuals, the prevalence of symptoms of PMAD was found to be 56% (Hernandez et al., 2022). Additionally, when postpartum Black women report mental health concerns, they are less likely to receive follow-up care than their white counterparts. A lack of follow-up care can result in long-term negative health consequences for the birthing person and their family (Hernandez et al., 2022). These alarming disparities can be attributed to various intersecting stressors, including socioeconomic inequalities, systemic racism, and a lack of culturally competent care (Watson & Hunter, 2015). The compounding effects of these stressors exacerbate feelings of isolation and amplify the risks of perinatal mood disorders among Black birthing individuals. Additionally, environmental challenges, ranging from elevated crime rates to exposure to environmental toxins, coupled with limited access to essential resources such as nutritious food and stable housing, further intensify the burdens faced by Black mothers. These challenges are notably accentuated due to the historical occurrences of residential redlining and segregation, which have perpetuated systemic disparities in housing, education, and healthcare access (Mendez et al., 2013).

Difficulties with perinatal mood and anxiety disorders (PMADs) during pregnancy can often be predicted by instances of adverse childhood experiences (ACEs), such as physical, emotional, and sexual abuse. These traumatic experiences in childhood can have profound and lasting effects on mental health, specifically increasing the likelihood of developing PTSD and depression during pregnancy (Atzl et al., 2019). The impact of ACEs on maternal mental health is particularly significant considering that studies show these experiences are more prevalent among low-income Black women (Mersky et al., 2021).

The cumulative impact of these stressors escalates the levels of chronic stress experienced by Black birthing individuals, consequently heightening their susceptibility to adverse pregnancy outcomes, including birthing trauma, preeclampsia, and preterm birth (Traylor et al., 2020). Additionally, evidence shows that stress experienced by the mother during pregnancy can lead to an excess amount of corticotropin-releasing hormone (CRH) and cortisol reaching the fetal brain, which could alter the developing personality of the child and predispose them to conditions such as ADHD and depression (Weinstock, 2005). These physiological changes can have long-term implications on the mental and physical health of the child, further perpetuating cycles of disadvantage and health disparities. The compounded effects of these stressors necessitate a multifaceted approach to addressing maternal and fetal health. This includes not only immediate medical interventions but also long-term strategies aimed at dismantling the systematic barriers that contribute to chronic stress. Addressing these disparities necessitates the implementation of structural support systems tailored to meet the unique needs of Black mothers and birthing individuals. Such support systems could involve increased access to prenatal and postnatal care, mental health services, and community support programs. Additionally, there is a critical need for healthcare providers to receive training in cultural competence to ensure they can adequately support and advocate for Black birthing individuals. Policies and initiatives that aim to reduce socioeconomic disparities, combat systemic racism, and promote health equity are essential in crafting a more just and supportive environment for Black mothers and their children.

An intervention with demonstrated efficacy is the integration of doulas, or birthing companions, into birth teams. By offering social and emotional support before, during, and after labor, doulas play an indispensable role in mitigating the isolation and anxiety often experienced by Black birthing individuals. Furthermore, doulas serve as advocates, navigating instances of implicit bias within healthcare settings and facilitating clear communication between clinicians and patients, thereby, promoting shared decision-making and informed consent (Carvalho et al., 2022). Through a series of in-depth interviews, researchers Arteaga et al. (2023) found that Black birthing people felt that a doula's contribution to their birthing experience goes beyond the realm of clinical care. Participants in the study recognized that doulas provided a unique level of emotional support, comfort, and a sense of community that they did not experience with medical professionals. Many participants compared their relationship with their doula to that of a family member, emphasizing the bond and level of trust that was established (Arteaga et al., 2023). This level of familiarity and trust is particularly important in the context of childbirth, where Black birthing people feel vulnerable and need comprehensive support. The participants expressed that having a doula allowed them to openly share their fears, concerns, and thoughts without hesitations, something they felt was often lacking in interactions with medical staff. This open communication is vital for ensuring that the birthing persons' needs and preferences are fully understood and respected, leading to a safer and more positive experience.

In addition to doula care, the establishment of support groups in the form of sister circles provides another avenue for Black birthing individuals to foster community and cultivate essential coping strategies (Somerville et al., 2023). Sister circles, rooted in cultural traditions and kinship networks, offer a culturally competent approach to connection and support, addressing the unique social and emotional needs of Black mothers (Neal-Barnett et al., 2011). Sister circles have been established in educational and professional spaces, providing Black women and girls an opportunity to gather and provide support for each other in environments that may otherwise feel unwelcoming (Neal-Barnett et al., 2011). In a healthcare setting, sister circles referred to as *Prime Time Sister Circles* (PTSC) were implemented (Gaston et al., 2007). Researchers used these circles to examine their efficacy in reducing risk factors such as poor nutrition, stress, and low activity levels. Over 12 months, researchers tracked these risk factors and observed an increase in yearly mammograms, blood pressure checks, utilization of stress management strategies, and consumption of nutritious foods (Gaston et al., 2007).

Expanding upon these community-based initiatives holds promise for enhancing maternal well-being and resilience among Black birthing individuals, ultimately fostering healthier outcomes for both mothers and their newborns. Finally, the utilization of music therapy has been investigated as a means to reduce stress and anxiety in pregnant individuals, yielding results that demonstrate a decrease in stress and anxiety levels, as measured by the Edinburgh Postnatal Depression Scale (Chang et al., 2008). A study conducted in China examined the effects of music therapy on pregnant women on bed rest due to having high-risk pregnancies. In this randomized study, participants in the intervention group were placed in a room where they listened to various classical music pieces as well as Chinese folk music (Yang et al., 2009). The findings revealed that these music listening sessions significantly reduced anxiety among high-risk pregnant individuals, suggesting that music has a soothing and anxiety-relieving influence (Yang et al., 2009). Moreover, the incorporation of both classical and Chinese folk music reflects a culturally sensitive approach to therapy, recognizing the importance of cultural familiarity and personal preference in the effectiveness of such interventions. Furthermore, it is essential for researchers to also focus on conducting studies within Black communities, utilizing culturally competent music that is tailored to resonate with the cultural backgrounds and experiences of Black birthing individuals. Embracing this culturally tailored approach holds significant promise as a method for addressing chronic stress within this demographic, improving maternal mental health and overall well-being.

EDINBURGH POSTNATAL DEPRESSION SCALE (EPDS)

When assessing the effectiveness of interventions aimed at enhancing Black maternal mental health, researchers often turn to established measurement tools such as the Edinburgh Postnatal Depression Scale (EPDS), a widely recognized screening instrument for postpartum depression (Cox et al., 1987). While the EPDS serves as a valuable resource in identifying maternal mental health concerns, it is important to critically evaluate its suitability in capturing the nuanced experiences of Black mothers. Over time, researchers have questioned the cultural validity of such measuring, designing projects to examine whether they adequately encompass the diverse range of symptoms and expressions of distress prevalent among Black populations (Oliver-Williams and Viruell-Fuentes, 2021). To gain a deeper understanding of the mental health challenges faced by Black mothers, there's a pressing need to broaden our assessment methods. This entails not only acknowledging the limitations of existing tools but also, embracing innovative approaches that better align with the experiences of Black birthing individuals. Specifically, recent investigations focusing on low-income Black birthing individuals have shed light on the limitations of using screening scales such as the EPDS within this demographic. While these tools continue to be valuable for identifying cases of perinatal depression and anxiety, their efficacy is only improved when adjustments are made to the scale cutoffs, particularly within marginalized communities (Chaudron et al., 2010). The EPDS consists of 10 statements that ask patients to reflect on whether they have experienced specific symptoms of PMADs over the past seven days (Shrestha et al., 2016). If patients score above a certain threshold, they are recommended for follow-up. While there is no universally recognized cutoff score, the most commonly used thresholds are greater than 10 and greater than 13 (Levis et al., 2020). By lowering the cutoff point for intervention, the EPDS becomes more sensitive to the unique challenges faced by Black birthing people and encourages early and more rapid intervention. However, the challenge lies in determining the appropriate threshold for identifying PMADs among Black birthing individuals.

In a recent study investigating the sensitivity of the EPDS to the unique needs of this population, it was found that even scores as low as 10 may overlook factors such as discrimination stress, systematic racism stress, and partner abuse stress (Sroka et al., 2023). This study emphasizes the need to adopt more comprehensive assessment methods, which can be accomplished by either integrating a behavioral health model or using federally funded programs to ensure a more accurate detection of perinatal mental health concerns (Sroka et al., 2023). This underscores the importance of tailoring screening protocols to address the unique needs and experiences of Black mothers. By doing so, we can enhance the accuracy of mental health assessments and ensure equitable access to appropriate care and support.

Additionally, a study by Lee King (2012) suggests that the statements in the EPDS may not resonate with low-income, non-Hispanic Black birthing people in the same way they do with other groups. The study's findings indicate that these individuals are more likely to experience anhedonia, or an inability to feel pleasure, rather than postpartum depression (Lee King, 2012). This highlights the necessity of developing culturally sensitive screening tools that can accurately capture the mental health experiences of diverse populations. The recognition that different populations may exhibit distinct symptoms and experiences of mental health conditions calls for a more inclusive approach to both research and clinical practice. Moreover, this approach can help bridge the gap in mental health outcomes and contribute to a more equitable healthcare system that recognizes and responds to the diverse experiences of all birthing people.

In addition to traditional screening methods, researchers have developed an innovative tool called *Listening to Women and Pregnant and Postpartum People (LTWP),* representing a forward-looking alternative to in-person assessments (Witcraft et al., 2024). This technology, delivered via phone/text software, offers a discreet and accessible platform for individuals to express their mental health concerns. By providing this avenue, LTWP is able to mitigate the potential for judgment and stigma that some patients may experience when confronted with questions about their mental well-being. This has the potential to enhance the convenience of screening and create a safe environment for individuals seeking assistance with their mental health during the perinatal period (Witcraft et al., 2024). This advancement is particularly significant for Black communities, where although mental health stigma is on the decline (Nelson et al., 2022), Black women still lack adequate mental health research and support (Carrington, 2006).

By incorporating perspectives from diverse cultural backgrounds and considering the unique sociocultural factors influencing maternal mental health, researchers can develop more nuanced and culturally sensitive measures. Moreover, advancing our understanding of maternal mental health outcomes among Black mothers requires a commitment to longitudinal research. This is particularly important for the long-term health and well-being of Black individuals because by tracking individuals over extended periods, researchers can uncover the long-term impacts of perinatal depression and anxiety on both maternal and child health outcomes. Through comprehensive longitudinal studies, we can determine the complex interplay between maternal mental health, child development, and long-term health trajectories, providing valuable insights into the multifaceted nature of perinatal mental health concerns (Woods-Giscombé et al., 2015).

COVID-19

The repercussions of the COVID-19 pandemic have profoundly exacerbated the various challenges confronting Black mothers and birthing individuals. With a disproportionately higher concentration of people of color living in densely populated and historically segregated urban centers, the impact of the pandemic has been disproportionately severe within Black communities. Studies have indicated that COVID-19 has led to elevated rates of diagnosis, more severe illness presentations, and a mortality rate among Black individuals that is 3.4 times higher than that of their white counterparts (Carvalho et al., 2022). Financially, Black women were disproportionately affected by the pandemic, experiencing a significant impact on their employment status. This demographic faced higher rates of job loss and reduced working hours compared to other groups, exacerbating existing economic disparities (Gur et al., 2020). Many Black women also faced significant challenges in securing affordable housing, dealing with the stress of potential eviction due to housing instability and landlord harassment (Versey & Russell, 2023). Along with this, studies conducted worldwide have reported that the circumstances surrounding COVID-19 have led to a gradual increase in symptoms of depression and anxiety among pregnant individuals (López-Morales et al., 2021). The unprecedented stressors brought about by the pandemic, such as social isolation, financial instability, and heightened health concerns, have compounded the emotional and psychological burdens faced by expectant mothers.

Beyond its direct health effects, the global pandemic has exposed the systemic shortcomings in healthcare systems' responsiveness to maternal mental health needs, particularly within Black communities (Paremoer et al., 2021). Studies indicate that during the pandemic, Black and brown birthing individuals were less likely to schedule postpartum care than their white counterparts (Mi et al., 2022). In addition, hospital policies during the pandemic often restricted companions from being present with pregnant women to limit COVID-19 transmission. Although these measures were essential for controlling the spread of the virus, this could have long-term mental health consequences for Black birthing women who were unable to have a companion or doula by their side (Gausman & Langer, 2020). The absence of supportive figures during labor and delivery can intensify feelings of isolation and stress, potentially impacting both immediate and long-term mental health outcomes for these women (Çankaya & Can, 2021).

The lack of access to adequate postpartum care further exacerbates the risk of untreated PMADs, contributing to long-term health consequences for both the birthing individuals and their children. The disruption of maternal care services, coupled with heightened anxiety surrounding finances and health risks, has further compounded the vulnerabilities faced by Black individuals during the perinatal period. The resultant state of heightened isolation and uncertainty has significantly exacerbated the prevalence of perinatal depression and anxiety among Black mothers and birthing individuals.

In response to these pressing challenges, initiatives such as Maternal Trauma Responsiveness among Black and Brown Birthing People have emerged as crucial avenues for addressing the unique needs of marginalized communities (Price et al., 2017). Trauma-informed care encourages healthcare providers to be mindful of trauma symptoms and to create environments that minimize the risk of triggering patients during their care. This includes implementing practices that prioritize giving birthing people as much autonomy and choice as possible in their care experiences (Choi et al., 2020). These initiatives are founded on the recognition of the complex trauma histories and stressors disproportionately experienced by individuals of color. By integrating this understanding into healthcare practices, these initiatives aim to cultivate a more informed and sensitive approach to care delivery, with the overarching objective of mitigating the factors contributing to perinatal depression and anxiety within Black communities. Through targeted interventions and systemic reforms, these initiatives strive to dismantle the structural barriers impeding access to equitable maternal mental health care for Black mothers and birthing individuals. By fostering a healthcare environment that is attuned to the diverse needs and experiences of marginalized communities, these efforts represent critical steps toward achieving health equity and justice within the realm of perinatal mental health.

One particular instance of trauma-informed care aimed at improving maternal mental health and birthing outcomes is the B'More Fit for Healthy Babies intervention in Baltimore City (Tuck et al., 2017). This initiative recognized that elevated levels of obesity during pregnancy, which disproportionately affect Black birthing individuals and contribute to heightened mortality rates, are often caused by factors such as chronic stress (Proper et al., 2013), and environmental challenges such as neighborhood safety concerns (Gómez et al., 2004). To combat these issues, the intervention began with an analysis involving focus groups to identify issues hindering Black birthing people from accessing nutritious food and engaging in physical activity. Subsequently, researchers developed a tailored program equipped with more applicable weight loss strategies, while also advocating for policy changes within Baltimore's health departments to enhance city services (Tuck et al., 2017). By integrating these approaches, the B'More Fit for Healthy Babies intervention exemplifies a holistic strategy that not only helps lower health risks but also addresses underlying social determinants of health, which are further defined in the *Bioethics* section of this chapter.

BIOETHICS

Bioethics serves as a compass for guiding fair and respectful treatment within the realm of healthcare, illuminating the ethical concerns surrounding postpartum maternal mental health. In this context, various ethical dimensions come to the forefront, particularly the assessment and management of perinatal mental health disorders. Bioethics, as a field, prioritizes the understanding and advocacy of ethical issues in the realms of medicine, life sciences, and associated technologies. Ethical principles are crucial for specific approaches to strategic thinking and ethical decision-making in the fields of medicine and life sciences. The analysis of policies that necessitate intentional and morally upright thinking are centered around the bioethical principles of nonmaleficence, beneficence, principles of justice, and respect for autonomy. Every day in the field of bioethics, healthcare professionals, scientists, researchers and philosophers encounter challenging decisions that are influenced by both moral and biological factors. Among its central principles are respect for autonomy, nonmaleficence, beneficence, and justice (Beauchamp and Childress, 2001). These principles have direct applications to postpartum maternal mental health.

Autonomy

Respecting autonomy involves honoring a new mother's decisions about her treatment options during the perinatal period, even when they diverge from medical or familial expectations. This principle is especially crucial for Black birthing individuals, who often face systemic biases and pressures that can undermine their autonomy. When Black birthing individuals are put in positions that compromise their autonomy and decisions are made without their consultation, they are at a significantly higher risk of experiencing birth-related posttraumatic stress disorder (PTSD) symptoms (Lathan et al., 2023). The perinatal period is a particularly vulnerable time for birthing people, and the ability to make informed and autonomous decisions about their care is fundamental to their psychological and emotional well-being. Black birthing individuals frequently encounter situations where their preferences are overlooked or dismissed by healthcare providers, leading to feelings of powerlessness and mistrust (Altman et al., 2020). This lack of respect for their autonomy can exacerbate the trauma associated with childbirth, contributing to long-term mental health issues. To mitigate these risks, healthcare professionals need to actively engage Black birthing individuals in discussions about their care. This involves providing information about healthcare options, acknowledging cultural and personal concerns, and supporting their decisions.

Nonmaleficence

Nonmaleficence requires healthcare professionals to work to minimize harm to patients actively. This involves the direct prevention of physical harm and the avoidance of psychological and emotional damage. One key aspect of nonmaleficence is the avoidance of stigmatization, which can have profound negative effects on patients' mental and emotional well-being. Stigmatization in healthcare settings can lead to a range of detrimental outcomes, including decreased patient trust in medical professionals, reduced willingness to seek care and the exacerbation of existing conditions due to neglect or inadequate treatment. Research on Black birthing people has shown that racialized pregnancy stigma contributes to poorer maternal and infant health outcomes. This stigma leads to a reduction in the quality of healthcare received, diminished social support, and adverse psychological health, all of which negatively impact both mothers and their babies (Mehra et al., 2020).

In addition to avoiding stigmatization, nonmaleficence requires the provision of appropriate, evidence-based care. This means that healthcare providers must remain informed about the latest medical research and clinical guidelines to ensure that their practices are grounded in the best available evidence. Providing evidence-based care involves making well-informed decisions about treatment options, considering the potential risks and benefits, and avoiding interventions that are unlikely to benefit the patient or could cause unnecessary harm. Nonmaleficence extends to the systemic level, requiring that healthcare institutions implement policies and practices that minimize harm across the patient population. This includes creating safe and supportive environments, ensuring equitable access to care, and addressing social determinants of health that may contribute to harm. The phrase "social determinants of health" refers to a set of conditions identified by the World Health Organization as influential in creating health inequalities. These conditions encompass where people are born, grow, live, work, and age. Examples include financial stability, employment status, educational opportunities, food and housing security, early childhood development, and access to quality healthcare (*Social Determinants of Health*, n.d.). These factors influence the distribution of resources and power, thereby impacting the health of Black birthing people.

Beneficence

Beneficence compels the healthcare community to actively enhance the well-being of postpartum women by providing comprehensive support and early intervention when necessary. For Black birthing individuals, this principle underscores the importance of implementing tailored, culturally competent care strategies that address the unique challenges they face. Healthcare providers must actively work to create an environment where these individuals feel supported and understood, offering resources that range from early access to mental health services to support networks.

To ensure that Black birthing individuals receive comprehensive and culturally competent care, several key interventions are recommended. First, regular and mandatory cultural competency training for healthcare providers is important. This training should focus on understanding and addressing the unique needs and challenges faced by a Black birthing individual. It should cover implicit bias, historical context, and effective communication strategies to ensure that providers can offer empathetic and informed care. Second, it is crucial to prioritize the recruitment and retention of a diverse healthcare workforce that reflects the communities they serve. Employing Black healthcare professionals and support staff can significantly enhance trust and improve patient-provider relationships, making Black birthing individuals feel more understood and supported. Finally, developing individualized care plans tailored to the cultural, social, and personal preferences of each individual is critical. This approach involves actively incorporating the patient's input and respecting their autonomy in all decision-making processes, ensuring that their unique needs and preferences are honored. By implementing these interventions, healthcare providers can create a more inclusive and supportive environment that promotes the well-being of Black birthing individuals.

Justice

Lastly, justice demands that all mothers, regardless of their socioeconomic status or racial and ethnic background, have equitable access to mental health resources. This principle insists on the removal of barriers that disproportionately affect disadvantaged and marginalized communities, ensuring that quality care is not a privilege but a fundamental right. For Black birthing individuals, who often face systemic racism and discrimination within the healthcare system, justice requires targeted interventions to address these disparities. This includes increasing the availability of culturally competent mental health professionals, expanding community-based support programs, and implementing policies that promote health equity.

Respectful Maternity Care

The implementation of these bioethics principles has led to the creation of guidelines by the World Health Organization, known as "respectful maternity care" (Bohren et al., 2020). These guidelines were developed in accordance with human rights-based approaches and were heavily influenced by the women's rights movement. The WHO recommends that these guidelines be applied to all birthing individuals. The aim is to ensure that maternity care is provided in a manner that upholds key ethical and human rights principles. This includes maintaining the autonomy of birthing individuals, and ensuring they have the freedom to make informed choices about their care without coercion. It also involves safeguarding them from harm and mistreatment, ensuring that they are treated with dignity and respect throughout the childbirth process. Finally, the guidelines stress the importance of privacy and confidentiality, recognizing that birthing individuals have the right to a private and secure environment where their personal and medical information is protected (Bohren et al., 2020).

One significant concern regarding respectful maternity care is that its implementation varies depending on the interpretation and cultural context of each health facility. To address this variability, Shakibazadeh et al., (2018) conducted a synthesis and qualitative analysis of 67 studies in 32 countries. Their research produced a list of twelve domains that characterize an evidence-based approach for implementing the WHO guidelines. These twelve domains are as follows: 1) Being free from harm and mistreatment, 2) Maintaining privacy and confidentiality, 3) Preserving women's dignity, 4) Prospective provision of information and seeking informed consent, 5) Ensuring continuous access to family and community support, 6) Enhancing quality of physical environment and resources, 7) Providing equitable maternity care, 8) Engaging with effective communication, 9) Respecting women's choices that strengthen their capabilities to give birth, 10) Availability of competent and motivated human resources, 11) provision of efficient and effective care, 12) Continuity of care (Shakibazadeh et al., 2018). These domains serve as a comprehensive framework to guide healthcare providers in delivering respectful and effective maternity care, aligning with the WHO's vision for universal and equitable treatment of all birthing individuals.

MOTHERS AT CROSSROADS: BIOETHICAL CHALLENGES IN CULTURALLY DIVERSE SETTINGS

When it comes to maternal health and the problems of cultural competency that follow, it is imperative to challenge these narratives, however, through an ethical lens that further enunciates why maternal health is considered a public health crisis and needs undivided and devoted attention. The conflict between biomedical ethics and traditional cultural practices frequently leads to conflicting perspectives on childbirth procedures, prenatal care, and postpartum practices. This is a fundamental issue. For example, in certain cultures, the presence of traditional birth attendants or specific rituals during childbirth may be prioritized over medically recommended interventions, such as using anesthesia or performing cesarean sections. This cultural preference can result in ethical dilemmas for healthcare providers, who must balance the necessity of ensuring the safety and well-being of both mother and child with respect for cultural traditions. Furthermore, language barriers further complicate informed consent processes, making it difficult to guarantee that patients comprehend the medical advice or procedures that are presented to them.

The Case of Angela Carder: Maternal Fetal Issues and Principles of Informed Consent

This case involves Angela Carder, a pregnant woman with terminal cancer, who was faced with the decision of whether to undergo treatment to prolong her life or prioritize her own comfort. Angela's husband, mother, and physicians agreed that her comfort should be the primary concern, but legal counsel and a judge became involved to determine the best interests of the fetus. Despite Angela's clear indication that she did not want a cesarean section, the judge ruled in favor of the procedure to give the fetus a chance at life. The fetus did not survive, and Angela passed away two days later. This situation raises ethical questions regarding the rights and autonomy of the pregnant woman, the best interests of the fetus, and the role of legal intervention in medical decisions (Practical Bioethics 2021). During the hearing, legal counsel was also appointed to represent Mrs. C, and her fetus, and the judge invited the District of Columbia Corporation Counsel to participate. The lawyer for the hospital opened the proceeding, stating that the patient and her family wanted no intervention if the patient died. The hospital sought declaratory relief from the court to direct the hospital on what to do with the fetus, whether to intervene and save its life (Practical Bioethics 2021). The lawyer for the fetus expressed the view that the fetus was probably viable at twenty-six weeks, and the court's task was to balance the interests of the fetus with whatever life is left for the mother. Ms. C's lawyer argued that she opposed surgical intervention to remove the fetus. Her attending physician testified that Ms. C had agreed to have the child at twenty-eight weeks but did not want the fetus delivered earlier due to the higher odds of a major handicap at twenty-six weeks gestation. A neonatologist testified hypothetically, having no direct involvement with the mother or the family, and strongly supported intervention on the basis that survival and morbidity are "very difficult to predict." The patient's mother testified that the previous day, after her daughter was informed that her condition was terminal, she only wanted to die, just to get her out of this pain. The lawyers' arguments focused on the best interests of the fetus and Ms. C's terminal condition. The lawyer for the fetus argued that the state's obligation to rescue a potential life from a dying mother was the decisive consideration. The judge issued his opinion orally, finding that the fetus had a 50 to 60 percent chance to survive and a less than 20 percent chance for serious handicap. He concluded that it was not an easy decision to make, but given the choices, the court is of the view that the fetus should be given an opportunity to live. After the hearing, Dr. Hamner informed Ms. C of the decision to perform a cesarean section without her consent. Ms. C was on a ventilator but could mouth agreement. The court reconvened upon learning that Ms. C was awake and communicating. The chief of obstetrics, Alan Weingold, reported a recent discussion with the patient in which she "clearly communicated" and understood who Dr. Hamner was. Counsel for the District of Columbia suggested that her current refusal did not change anything because the entire proceeding had been premised on the belief that she was refusing to consent. The cesarean section was performed, and the nonviable fetus died approximately two hours later. Ms. C, now confronted with both recovery from major surgery and the knowledge of her child's death, died approximately two days later.

The issue regarding the case of Angela Carder was the fact that her right to informed consent was violated, as well as her right to bodily autonomy. Informed consent is an important component of the maternal health paradigm due to the many health complications that are at stake, which could affect the mother or birthing person and the child. Additionally, informed consent must play a role in physician-patient relationships, as this relationship will be critical when making decisions for their care without feeling pressured or making inadequate decisions. Additionally, the autonomy of a mother and her ability to provide truly informed consent can be significantly influenced by the varying cultural and societal norms surrounding childbirth. Specifically, certain communities may place a higher value on medical authority or hold specific beliefs about maternal responsibilities that influence decision-making processes. Advancements in prenatal technology, such as genetic testing and imaging techniques, have exacerbated ethical dilemmas by presenting parents with complex choices regarding potential interventions, without ensuring absolute outcomes. To effectively address these challenges, healthcare providers must adopt a patient-centered approach that prioritizes transparent communication and respects individual values, while also ensuring that all pertinent information is conveyed comprehensively and empathetically. Ultimately, the resolution of these bioethical challenges necessitates systemic initiatives that promote the empowerment of women through education and advocacy, while also cultivating an environment that facilitates shared decision-making between clinicians and expectant mothers.

ADVOCACY FOR BIRTH JUSTICE: BIOETHICS AND POLICY CHANGE FOR CULTURALLY COMPETENT MATERNAL HEALTHCARE

Thinking about the crisis of maternal health among Black women and birthing people within the United States will always remain a scary thought. In historical times, it was deemed within white medical schools that between black women and white women, black women do not experience pain; thus, they do not require as much care or attention as white women do. Consequentially, black women are more likely to report mistreatment and misdiagnoses by their provider, losing their autonomy through it all. Many are more likely to experience coercion and policing of their bodies throughout the entirety of their birthing process. The United States ranks as the worst in maternal care, having the highest rates of maternal mortality compared to other nations (Melillo 2020). To make matters worse, 50 percent of pregnancy-related deaths in the United States occur postpartum. According to the Commonwealth Fund, the United States, along with Canada, have the lowest supply of OBGYNs and midwives, with 12 to 15 providers per 1,000 births. Without a team of maternal health providers such as midwives and OBGYNs, maternal health is in grave danger of experiencing an even greater number of complications and abnormalities.

There was a time when vaginal birth after a cesarean section was a common practice. Between 1980 and 1996, the number of VBACs grew exponentially, practically to 30 percent. However, Black women in the United States are least likely to birth their first child vaginally compared to their white and Latinx counterparts (Oparah and Bonaparte, 158). Over time, hospitals have placed VBAC bans to prevent pregnant people from attempting vaginal births after a cesarean delivery. In July 2014, a Florida woman by the name of Jennifer Goodall had three previous cesarean sections and became pregnant with a fourth child. She sought to have her fourth child by vaginal birth; however, she received a letter from her prenatal care providers stating that they would obtain a court order to perform the procedure with or without her consent. Afterwards, they will report her to the authorities for allegedly endangering her child. Goodall eventually filed a lawsuit by NAPW, gave labor at home and gave her consent to a cesarean at a different hospital (Oparah and Bonaparte 160). Goodall's case eventually became the start of a birth justice revolution, with women and birthing people having full control over their birthing experience and process. VBAC activism and stories such as Goodall's sparked a movement within birth justice, educating pregnant women and pregnant people to make decisions that will support their care in the most adequate way possible while being equipped with tools and resources to support their decisions. In regards to policy changes that are centered on maternal health and caring for the lives of the underrepresented, currently within the United States, US Representatives such as Congresswomen Lauren Underwood (IL-14) and Alma Adams (NC-12) recently celebrated the passing of the 'Black Maternal Health Momnibus' Act in May of 2021. The purpose of this bill is to tackle the issues of maternal mortality among black mothers, as well as eliminate mortality, morbidity, and health disparities among the vulnerable groups who identify as black mothers. In February 2021, according to the US House of Representatives, the Black Maternal Health Momnibus Act was comprised of nine individual bills sponsored by the Black Maternal Health Caucus. The legislation will make efforts in the following areas: Making investments in social determinants of health that contribute towards nutrition, housing and transportation, studying the maternal health risk factors among vulnerable groups such as women veterans, funding community organizations that focus on improving black maternal health outcomes, growing and diversifying the perinatal workforce, improving data collection and qualitative measures to better understand the causes of maternal health crises, investing in maternal care, investing in digital health tools to incentivize high-quality maternity care and innovative payment models of continuity health insurance coverage. Similarly, the Social Determinants for Moms Act is directed towards the federal departments to address the social determinants of maternal health, such as the impact of maternal health outcomes, clinical and nonclinical factors, and economic and social factors. Because of this, the US Department . of Health and Human Services must work and develop a task force in order to tackle the federal efforts on social determinants of maternal health, efforts to support access to free child care during both prenatal and postpartum appointments, addressing social determinants of health and working to eliminate racial and ethnic disparities in maternal health.

Our black and brown women need healthcare professionals who know and/or are willing to take time to learn and understand the black female body. Millions of black women have died. in the hands of those who are supposed to serve, protect and care for us; in actuality, they are the predators of our lives. As open season continues to take out black women, there are a multitude of ways in which society can work towards protecting and keeping our black women safe. As more individuals who don't identify as marginalized individuals become more aware and outraged by racism as a global pandemic, many have taken immediate action to fight the racial implications that black women face on a daily basis. Social media presence with the foundation of digital education, thousands of in-person rallies and peaceful protests, donating millions of dollars to the lost loved ones's families and becoming more vocal towards elected officials. To further alleviate the racial implications of medical treatment and healthcare among black women, one can take the following steps in order to work toward closing the discriminatory gap in healthcare and treatment(s): Recognizing intersectional oppression, demanding reproductive justice and maternal health rights, fighting racial injustice and demanding accountability towards healthcare professionals, the government and elected officials. For further action, more black women and future mothers are encouraged to have doulas and midwives coach them throughout their pregnancies and during childbirth to prevent the medical negligence that hospitals and major clinics create for black women. Lastly, to prevent prevalent health diseases such as cardiovascular diseases, maternal mortality and any other prevalent health disease among black women, it is imperative that, as a society, we work towards mentoring and coaching young black individuals early so that they will have the opportunity to serve within the healthcare field and care for black bodies—bodies that they can understand, feel and attest to personally.

POSTPARTUM MATERNAL MENTAL HEALTH

Postpartum maternal mental health affects not only the immediate well-being of mothers but also the long-term health of their children, demonstrating a critical need for embedding bioethical considerations in maternal health services. A bioethical framework is imperative for aligning the screening protocols and treatment modalities for postpartum maternal mental health with the principles of autonomy, justice, beneficence, and non-maleficence. There is an ethical obligation to consider a mother's autonomy in decisions regarding her mental health care while ensuring that newborns and infants thrive in safe, nurturing environments. The responsibility to diagnose and treat maternal health conditions must be balanced with respect for a mother's right to participate in her own healthcare decisions. To foster an ethical approach to postpartum maternal mental health, ongoing research and policy reformulation are required. The intersection of policy changes and postpartum maternal mental health is an area of critical importance that impacts numerous new mothers annually. Postpartum maternal mental health incorporates various psychological conditions that can emerge during the first year after childbirth, including postpartum depression, anxiety, and psychosis. These conditions may have significant repercussions not just for the mother but for the child as well, including impairing the ability to form a secure mother-infant bond, which is crucial for the child's development.

Despite the known impacts of postpartum mental health disorders, maternal health policies have historically been inadequate in addressing the mental health needs of new mothers. Traditional healthcare policies often prioritize physical recovery from childbirth without integrating mental health considerations transparently and consequently. However, recognition of the importance of mental health has brought about critical shifts in this trend. Policy changes aiming to improve postpartum maternal mental health have manifested in various forms, such as extending healthcare coverage for postpartum care, mandating screening for mental health conditions, improving access to mental health services, and providing education on postpartum conditions for healthcare professionals and patients. For instance, under the Affordable Care Act (ACA) in the United States, policy changes have expanded coverage for mental health and substance use disorder services, including increased access to postpartum care (Schuster et al., 2022). This is crucial because financial burden and a lack of insurance coverage can otherwise be barriers to seeking mental health care. In certain geographies, there is a movement towards legislation that would require maternal mental health screening. For example, New Jersey has led the way with a law requiring healthcare providers to screen new mothers for postpartum depression (Rhodes & Segre, 2013). The impacts of these policy changes can be profound.

By implementing comprehensive mental health evaluations during the postpartum period, healthcare providers can identify and provide timely interventions to mothers experiencing mental health difficulties, thus reducing long-term negative outcomes for both mother and child. Moreover, policy-driven efforts to educate can demystify and destigmatize mental health conditions, thereby encouraging more women to seek help without fear of judgment or repercussions. Ethical challenges evolve with emerging evidence and societal changes, necessitating a flexible yet principled approach to bioethics in maternal health. As the medical community gains a deeper understanding of perinatal mental health, bioethical considerations must also adapt to ensure that the care provided to mothers remains both scientifically sound and ethically justifiable.

CONCLUSION

Improving Black maternal mental health demands a holistic, culturally attuned, and compassionate approach that recognizes and addresses the unique hurdles encountered by Black mothers and birthing individuals. Urgent action is needed to narrow health disparities, encourage trauma-informed care, and establish mechanisms for monitoring advancements in maternal mental health. It is only through sustained, collaborative endeavors that we can truly fortify the mental well-being of Black mothers, nurturing stronger, more resilient families and communities. Despite the persistent challenges of the 21st century, it remains important to press forward in the fight for equity in Black maternal health and to rectify the glaring lack of diversity, equity, and inclusion in the realm of bioethics.

Throughout this chapter, we have aimed to encapsulate the journey of Black or brown birthing individuals as they navigate through perinatal or postpartum depression. Addressing maternal mental health trauma within Black and Brown communities requires a tailored, culturally competent approach that acknowledges the historical and systemic inequities these groups have endured over time. To effectively support the mental well-being of mothers from these communities, healthcare professionals must integrate a bioethical framework that upholds principles such as autonomy, justice, beneficence, and non-maleficence into their practice. This entails creating a healthcare environment where mothers feel genuinely heard, understood, and valued, with their cultural background and individual experiences forming the cornerstone of a therapeutic alliance.

REFERENCES

Altman, M. R., McLemore, M. R., Oseguera, T., Lyndon, A., & Franck, L. S. (2020). Listening to Women: Recommendations from Women of Color to Improve Experiences in Pregnancy and Birth Care. *Journal of Midwifery & Women's Health, 65*(4), 466–473. DOI: 10.1111/jmwh.13102 PMID: 32558179

Arteaga, S., Hubbard, E., Arcara, J., Cuentos, A., Armstead, M., Jackson, A., Gomez, A. M., & Marshall, C. (2023). "They're gonna be there to advocate for me so I'm not by myself": A qualitative analysis of Black women's motivations for seeking and experiences with community doula care. *Women and Birth; Journal of the Australian College of Midwives, 36*(3), 257–263. DOI: 10.1016/j.wombi.2022.08.007 PMID: 36089498

Atzl, V. M., Narayan, A. J., Rivera, L. M., & Lieberman, A. F. (2019). Adverse childhood experiences and prenatal mental health: Type of ACEs and age of maltreatment onset. *Journal of Family Psychology, 33*(3), 304–314. DOI: 10.1037/fam0000510 PMID: 30802085

Beauchamp, T. L., & Childress, J. F. (2001). *Principles of Biomedical Ethics*. Oxford University Press.

Bohren, M. A., Tunçalp, Ö., & Miller, S. (2020). Transforming intrapartum care: Respectful maternity care. *Best Practice & Research. Clinical Obstetrics & Gynaecology, 67*, 113–126. DOI: 10.1016/j.bpobgyn.2020.02.005 PMID: 32245630

Çankaya, S., & Can, R. (2021). The effect of continuous supportive care on birth pain, birth fear, midwifery care perception, oxytocin use, and delivery time during the intrapartum period: An experimental study. *Nigerian Journal of Clinical Practice, 24*(11), 1624–1632. DOI: 10.4103/njcp.njcp_147_20 PMID: 34782500

Carrington, C. H. (2006). Clinical depression in African American women: Diagnoses, treatment, and research. *Journal of Clinical Psychology, 62*(7), 779–791. DOI: 10.1002/jclp.20289 PMID: 16703605

Chang, M.-Y., Chen, C.-H., & Huang, K.-F. (2008). Effects of music therapy on psychological health of women during pregnancy. *Journal of Clinical Nursing, 17*(19), 2580–2587. DOI: 10.1111/j.1365-2702.2007.02064.x PMID: 18298503

Chaudron, L. H., Szilagyi, P. G., Tang, W., Anson, E., Talbot, N. L., Wadkins, H. I. M., Tu, X., & Wisner, K. L. (2010). Accuracy of Depression Screening Tools for Identifying Postpartum Depression Among Urban Mothers. *Pediatrics, 125*(3), e609–e617. DOI: 10.1542/peds.2008-3261 PMID: 20156899

Choi, K. R., Records, K., Low, L. K., Alhusen, J. L., Kenner, C., Bloch, J. R., Premji, S. S., Hannan, J., Anderson, C. M., Yeo, S., & Cynthia Logsdon, M. (2020). Promotion of Maternal–Infant Mental Health and Trauma-Informed Care During the COVID-19 Pandemic. *Journal of Obstetric, Gynecologic, and Neonatal Nursing : JOGNN*, *49*(5), 409–415. DOI: 10.1016/j.jogn.2020.07.004 PMID: 32795425

Cox, J. L., Holden, J. M., & Sagovsky, R. (1987). Detection of Postnatal Depression: Development of the 10-item Edinburgh Postnatal Depression Scale. *The British Journal of Psychiatry*, *150*(6), 782–786. DOI: 10.1192/bjp.150.6.782 PMID: 3651732

Delles, M. (2021, Oct 29). Case Study – Angela C – Maternal Fetal Issues - Center for Practical Bioethics. Retrieved August 28, 2024, from Center for Practical Bioethics website: https://www.practicalbioethics.org/shared-decision-making-and-advance-care-planning/advance-care-planning/case-study-angela-c-maternal-fetal-issues/

Gaston, M. H., Porter, G. K., & Thomas, V. G. (2007). Prime Time Sister Circles: Evaluating a gender-specific, culturally relevant health intervention to decrease major risk factors in mid-life African-American women. *Journal of the National Medical Association*, *99*(4), 428–438. PMID: 17444433

Gausman, J., & Langer, A. (2020). Sex and Gender Disparities in the COVID-19 Pandemic. *Journal of Women's Health*, *29*(4), 465–466. DOI: 10.1089/jwh.2020.8472 PMID: 32320331

Getahun, D., Oyelese, Y., Peltier, M., Yeh, M., Chiu, V. Y., Takhar, H., Khadka, N., Mensah, N., Avila, C., & Fassett, M. J. (2023). Trends in Postpartum Depression by Race/Ethnicity and Pre-pregnancy Body Mass Index. *American Journal of Obstetrics and Gynecology*, *228*(1), S122–S123. DOI: 10.1016/j.ajog.2022.11.248

Gómez, J. E., Johnson, B. A., Selva, M., & Sallis, J. F. (2004). Violent crime and outdoor physical activity among inner-city youth. *Preventive Medicine*, *39*(5), 876–881. DOI: 10.1016/j.ypmed.2004.03.019 PMID: 15475019

Gur, R. E., White, L. K., Waller, R., Barzilay, R., Moore, T. M., Kornfield, S., Njoroge, W. F. M., Duncan, A. F., Chaiyachati, B. H., Parish-Morris, J., Maayan, L., Himes, M. M., Laney, N., Simonette, K., Riis, V., & Elovitz, M. A. (2020). The Disproportionate Burden of the COVID-19 Pandemic Among Pregnant Black Women. *Psychiatry Research*, *293*, 113475. DOI: 10.1016/j.psychres.2020.113475 PMID: 33007683

Hernandez, N. D., Francis, S., Allen, M., Bellamy, E., Sims, O. T., Oh, H., Guillaume, D., Parker, A., & Chandler, R. (2022). Prevalence and predictors of symptoms of Perinatal Mood and anxiety Disorders among a sample of Urban Black Women in the South. *Maternal and Child Health Journal*, *26*(4), 770–777. DOI: 10.1007/s10995-022-03425-2 PMID: 35344149

Lathan, E. C., Britt, A., Ravi, M., Ash, M. J., McAfee, E., Wallace, S., Johnson, C. B.II, Woods-Jaeger, B., Powers, A., & Michopoulos, V. (2023). When Reproduction Is No Longer Autonomous: Feeling Respected by Maternity Care Providers Moderates the Association Between Autonomy in Decision Making and Birth-Related Ptsd Symptoms in a Community Sample of Postpartum Black Women. *Journal of Trauma & Dissociation*, *24*(4), 520–537. DOI: 10.1080/15299732.2023.2212406 PMID: 37233983

Lee King, P. A. (2012). Replicability of structural models of the Edinburgh Postnatal Depression Scale (EPDS) in a community sample of postpartum African American women with low socioeconomic status. *Archives of Women's Mental Health*, *15*(2), 77–86. DOI: 10.1007/s00737-012-0260-8 PMID: 22297555

Levis, B., Negeri, Z., Sun, Y., Benedetti, A., & Thombs, B. D. (2020). Accuracy of the Edinburgh Postnatal Depression Scale (EPDS) for screening to detect major depression among pregnant and postpartum women: Systematic review and meta-analysis of individual participant data. *BMJ (Clinical Research Ed.)*, *371*, m4022. DOI: 10.1136/bmj.m4022 PMID: 33177069

López-Morales, H., del Valle, M. V., Canet-Juric, L., Andrés, M. L., Galli, J. I., Poó, F., & Urquijo, S. (2021). Mental health of pregnant women during the COVID-19 pandemic: A longitudinal study. *Psychiatry Research*, *295*, 113567. DOI: 10.1016/j.psychres.2020.113567 PMID: 33213933

Ludwig, M. (2018). Maternal / Fetal Conflict | UW Department of Bioethics & Humanities. https://depts.washington.edu/bhdept/ethics-medicine/bioethics-topics/detail/69

Mehra, R., Boyd, L. M., Magriples, U., Kershaw, T. S., Ickovics, J. R., & Keene, D. E. (2020). Black Pregnant Women "Get the Most Judgment": A Qualitative Study of the Experiences of Black Women at the Intersection of Race, Gender, and Pregnancy. *Women's Health Issues*, *30*(6), 484–492. DOI: 10.1016/j.whi.2020.08.001 PMID: 32900575

Melillo, G. (2020, Dec 3). US Ranks Worst in Maternal Care, Mortality Compared With 10 Other Developed Nations. https://www.ajmc.com/view/us-ranks-worst-in-maternal-care-mortality-compared-with-10-other-developed-nations

Mendez, D. D., Hogan, V. K., & Culhane, J. F. (2013). Stress during Pregnancy: The Role of Institutional Racism. *Stress and Health, 29*(4), 266–274. DOI: 10.1002/smi.2462 PMID: 23055409

Mersky, J. P., Choi, C., Plummer Lee, C., & Janczewski, C. E. (2021). Disparities in adverse childhood experiences by race/ethnicity, gender, and economic status: Intersectional analysis of a nationally representative sample. *Child Abuse & Neglect, 117*, 105066. DOI: 10.1016/j.chiabu.2021.105066 PMID: 33845239

Mi, T., Hung, P., Li, X., McGregor, A., He, J., & Zhou, J. (2022). Racial and Ethnic Disparities in Postpartum Care in the Greater Boston Area During the COVID-19 Pandemic. *JAMA Network Open, 5*(6), e2216355. DOI: 10.1001/jamanetworkopen.2022.16355 PMID: 35737390

Neal-Barnett, A., Stadulis, R., Murray, M., Payne, M. R., Thomas, A., & Salley, B. B. (2011). Sister Circles as a Culturally Relevant Intervention for Anxious African American Women. *Clinical Psychology : a Publication of the Division of Clinical Psychology of the American Psychological Association, 18*(3), 266–273. DOI: 10.1111/j.1468-2850.2011.01258.x PMID: 22081747

Nelson, T., Ernst, S. C., Tirado, C., Fisse, J. L., & Moreno, O. (2022). Psychological Distress and Attitudes Toward Seeking Professional Psychological Services Among Black Women: The Role of Past Mental Health Treatment. *Journal of Racial and Ethnic Health Disparities, 9*(2), 527–537. DOI: 10.1007/s40615-021-00983-z PMID: 33559107

Ni, G., Bn, G., & Kn, L. (2005). Perinatal depression: A systematic review of prevalence and incidence. *Obstetrics and Gynecology, 106*(5 Pt 1), 1071–1083. DOI: 10.1097/01.AOG.0000183597.31630.db PMID: 16260528

Oliver-Williams, C., & Viruell-Fuentes, E. (2021). Lessons about postpartum depression from the woman-centered health home. *Women's Health Issues, 31*(3), 204–211. PMID: 33707142

Owens, D. C., & Fett, S. M. (2019, Oct). Black Maternal and Infant Health: Historical Legacies of Slavery. *American Journal of Public Health, 109*(10), 1342–1345. DOI: 10.2105/AJPH.2019.305243 PMID: 31415204

Paremoer, L., Nandi, S., Serag, H., & Baum, F. (2021). Covid-19 pandemic and the social determinants of health. *BMJ (Clinical Research Ed.), 372*(129), n129. DOI: 10.1136/bmj.n129 PMID: 33509801

Price, S. K., Proctor, E. K., & Kinghorn, A. M. (2017). Trauma-informed care: Opportunities for high-quality, trauma-informed care and implications for policy. Report to the Missouri Foundation for Health.

Proper, K. I., Picavet, H. S. J., Bogers, R. P., Verschuren, W. M., & Bemelmans, W. J. (2013). The association between adverse life events and body weight change: Results of a prospective cohort study. *BMC Public Health, 13*(1), 957. DOI: 10.1186/1471-2458-13-957 PMID: 24125054

Rhodes, A., & Segre, L. (2013). Perinatal Depression: A Review of U.S. Legislation and Law. *Archives of Women's Mental Health, 16*(4), 259–270. DOI: 10.1007/s00737-013-0359-6 PMID: 23740222

Schuster, A. L., Perraillon, M. C., Paul, J. J., Leiferman, J. A., Battaglia, C., & Morrato, E. H. (2022). The Effect of the Affordable Care Act (ACA) on Women's Postpartum Insurance and Depression in Five States that Did Not Expand Medicaid, 2012–2015. *Medical Care, 60*(1), 22–28. DOI: 10.1097/MLR.0000000000001652 PMID: 34670222

Shakibazadeh, E., Namadian, M., Bohren, M., Vogel, J., Rashidian, A., Nogueira Pileggi, V., Madeira, S., Leathersich, S., Tunçalp, ., Oladapo, O., Souza, J., & Gülmezoglu, A. (2018). Respectful care during childbirth in health facilities globally: A qualitative evidence synthesis. *BJOG, 125*(8), 932–942. DOI: 10.1111/1471-0528.15015 PMID: 29117644

Shrestha, S. D., Pradhan, R., Tran, T. D., Gualano, R. C., & Fisher, J. R. W. (2016). Reliability and validity of the Edinburgh Postnatal Depression Scale (EPDS) for detecting perinatal common mental disorders (PCMDs) among women in low-and lower-middle-income countries: A systematic review. *BMC Pregnancy and Childbirth, 16*(1), 72. DOI: 10.1186/s12884-016-0859-2 PMID: 27044437

Social determinants of health. (n.d.). https://www.who.int/health-topics/social-determinants-of-health

Sroka, A. W., Mbayiwa, K., Ilyumzhinova, R., Meyer, W., Fowle, J., Gipson, C. J., Norcott, C., Hipwell, A. E., & Keenan, K. (2023). Depression screening may not capture significant sources of prenatal stress for Black women. *Archives of Women's Mental Health, 26*(2), 211–217. DOI: 10.1007/s00737-023-01297-1 PMID: 36797547

Structural Racism and Discrimination. (n.d.). NIMHD. https://www.nimhd.nih.gov/resources/understanding-health-disparities/srd.html

Tikkanen, R., Gunja, M., Fitzgerald, M., & Zephyrin, L. (2020, Nov 18). Maternal Mortality and Maternity Care in the United States Compared to 10 Other Developed Countries. https://www.commonwealthfund.org/publications/issue-briefs/2020/nov/maternal-mortality-maternity-care-us-compared-10-countries

Traylor, C. S., Johnson, J. D., Kimmel, M. C., & Manuck, T. A. (2020). Effects of psychological stress on adverse pregnancy outcomes and nonpharmacologic approaches for reduction: An expert review. *American Journal of Obstetrics & Gynecology MFM*, *2*(4), 100229. DOI: 10.1016/j.ajogmf.2020.100229 PMID: 32995736

Tuck, S. G., Summers, A. C., Bowie, J., Fife-Stallworth, D., Alston, C., Hayes, S., & Alexander, S. (2017). B'More Fit for Healthy Babies: Using Trauma-Informed Care Policies to Improve Maternal Health in Baltimore City. *Women's Health Issues*, *27*, S38–S45. DOI: 10.1016/j.whi.2017.09.002 PMID: 29050657

Tuohey, J. F. (1991, Dec). Terminal care and the pregnant woman: ethical reflections on In Re: A.C. *Pediatrics*, *88*(6), 1268–1273. DOI: 10.1542/peds.88.6.1268 PMID: 1956747

University, S. C. (2021, May 4). Biases and System Failures Affecting U.S. Maternal Mortality. https://www.scu.edu/ethics/healthcare-ethics-blog/biases-and-system-failures-affecting-us-maternal-mortality/

Versey, H. S., & Russell, C. N. (2023). The impact of COVID-19 and housing insecurity on lower-income Black women. *The Journal of Social Issues*, *79*(2), 773–793. DOI: 10.1111/josi.12555 PMID: 36711011

Watson, N. N., & Hunter, C. D. (2015). Anxiety and depression among African American women: The costs of strength and negative attitudes toward psychological help-seeking. *Cultural Diversity & Ethnic Minority Psychology*, *21*(4), 604–612. DOI: 10.1037/cdp0000015 PMID: 25602466

Weinstock, M. (2005). The potential influence of maternal stress hormones on development and mental health of the offspring. *Brain, Behavior, and Immunity*, *19*(4), 296–308. DOI: 10.1016/j.bbi.2004.09.006 PMID: 15944068

Wisner, K. L., Sit, D. K. Y., McShea, M. C., Rizzo, D. M., Zoretich, R. A., Hughes, C. L., Eng, H. F., Luther, J. F., Wisniewski, S. R., Costantino, M. L., Confer, A. L., Moses-Kolko, E. L., Famy, C. S., & Hanusa, B. H. (2013). Onset Timing, Thoughts of Self-harm, and Diagnoses in Postpartum Women With Screen-Positive Depression Findings. *JAMA Psychiatry*, *70*(5), 490–498. DOI: 10.1001/jamapsychiatry.2013.87 PMID: 23487258

Witcraft, S. M., Johnson, E., Eitel, A. E., Moreland, A. D., King, C., Terplan, M., & Guille, C. (2024). Listening to Black Pregnant and Postpartum People: Using Technology to Enhance Equity in Screening and Treatment of Perinatal Mental Health and Substance Use Disorders. *Journal of Racial and Ethnic Health Disparities*. DOI: 10.1007/s40615-024-01989-z PMID: 38605223

Woods-Giscombé, C. L., Lobel, M., Zimmer, C., Wiley Cené, C., & Corbie-Smith, G. (2015). Whose stress is making me sick? Network-stress and emotional distress in African-American women. *Issues in Mental Health Nursing*, *36*(9), 710–717. DOI: 10.3109/01612840.2015.1011759 PMID: 26440874

Yakovi Gan-Or, N. (2020, Oct 6). Going solo: The law and ethics of childbirth during the COVID-19 pandemic. *Journal of Law and the Biosciences*, *7*(1), lsaa079. DOI: 10.1093/jlb/lsaa079 PMID: 33235802

Yang, M., Li, L., Zhu, H., Alexander, I. M., Liu, S., Zhou, W., & Ren, X. (2009). Music Therapy To Relieve Anxiety In Pregnant Women On Bedrest: A Randomized, Controlled Trial. *MCN. The American Journal of Maternal Child Nursing*, *34*(5), 316–323. DOI: 10.1097/01.NMC.0000360425.52228.95 PMID: 19713801

Yehudah, S., & Tadros, E. (2022). Counseling advocacy: Seeking justice for black birth equity. *Journal of Counselor Leadership and Advocacy*, *9*(1), 3–20. DOI: 10.1080/2326716X.2021.2018067

KEY TERMS AND DEFINITIONS

1. **Perinatal Period:** A time frame that includes the final stages of pregnancy (20-28 weeks) through the first to fourth week postpartum.
2. **Perinatal Depression:** A mood disorder that affects birthing people during pregnancy or in the first year after childbirth, also known as postpartum depression.
3. **Postpartum:** The period of weeks or months following childbirth.
4. **Maternal Mental Health:** The emotional well-being of birthing individuals during pregnancy and postpartum.
5. **Bioethics:** The study of ethical concerns that surface in healthcare and biomedical research.
6. **Doula:** A professional who provides emotional and physical support for birthing individuals throughout pregnancy and after
7. **Edinburgh Postnatal Depression Scale:** A screening tool used to evaluate postpartum birthing individuals for postpartum depression.

Chapter 8
Community-Based Approaches to Black Maternal Mental Health

Aliyu Tijani Jibril
https://orcid.org/0000-0003-3930-9091
Universal Scientific Education and Research Network, Ghana

ABSTRACT

This chapter delves into the significant disparities faced by Black women in maternal mental health care, highlighting the impact of structural racism, inequities in diagnosis and access to treatment, and the lack of universal screening and mental health education. It emphasizes the importance of community-based approaches in addressing these disparities, drawing attention to the need for culturally appropriate interventions and the crucial role of community-centered strategies. The chapter also discusses the implications of community engagement and support, the role of social support networks, and the systemic influences on maternal mental health. Furthermore, it offers recommendations for effective implementation, including policy changes to address racism and bias, culturally competent care, and tailored interventions for improved outcomes. This serves as a valuable resource for healthcare professionals, policymakers, researchers, and advocates seeking to understand, address, and ultimately empower Black mothers in their maternal mental health journey.

INTRODUCTION

Maternal mental health during pregnancy has been shown to have a significant impact on children's mental and behavioral outcomes. Positive maternal mental health

DOI: 10.4018/979-8-3693-4272-5.ch008

during pregnancy is associated with a lower risk of mental and behavioral disorders in children, highlighting the intergenerational implications of maternal well-being (Lähdepuro, Lahti-Pulkkinen, et al., 2023). This underscores the importance of supporting positive maternal mental health not only for the mother but also for the long-term mental health of her children (Lähdepuro, Lahti-Pulkkinen, et al., 2023).

However, it is crucial to note that Black women experience a range of maternal mental health issues, with significant disparities in morbidity and mortality. Common mental health issues include perinatal mood disorders such as depression and anxiety (Danasekaran et al., 2015). These disorders can adversely affect not only the mothers but also the child's growth and development (Danasekaran et al., 2015). In fact, the prevalence of these disorders is higher among Black mothers compared to national estimates in the United States (Dimes, 2024), with structural racism and inequities in diagnosis and access to treatment exacerbating the situation (Estriplet et al., 2022; Matthews et al., 2021). Furthermore, lack of universal screening, mental health education, and a disjointed healthcare system serve as barriers, contributing to mental health issues and putting Black women at a disadvantage in autonomous decision-making (Estriplet et al., 2022).

The topic on Black maternal mental health is a crucial area of study that has gained increasing attention due to the disparities and challenges faced by Black women during pregnancy and the postpartum period. Research has emphasized the significance of understanding the unique experiences and needs of Black mothers, particularly concerning mental health care. For example, studies have shown that untreated perinatal depression disproportionately affects low-income Black women, leading to higher maternal mortality rates and adverse birth outcomes (Glickman et al., 2020). Additionally, studies highlight the prevalence of perinatal mood disorders among Black mothers, underscoring the urgency to prioritize maternal mental health for both maternal and infant well-being (Estriplet et al., 2022).

Interestingly, while some studies have found that psychological well-being, such as life satisfaction and flourishing, does not change significantly for Black women from preconception to postpartum (Quick et al., 2023), others have identified a high prevalence of symptoms of perinatal mood and anxiety disorders among Black women, with a significant proportion not receiving the necessary mental health care treatment (James et al., 2023). In addition, Black African newcomer women in Canada face unique challenges that impact their mental health and service utilization, including cultural beliefs and racial discrimination (Baiden & Evans, 2021). The impact of structural racism on maternal health among Black women is significant. Structural racism perpetuates racial disparities in maternal health, contributing to high rates of maternal mortality and morbidity in this population (Taylor, 2020).

To address these disparities, it is essential to prioritize maternal mental health to optimize infant health and wellness. To comprehend the effects of perinatal mental health on Black mothers and birthing people, it is necessary to recognize the social, economic, and structural inequalities that they encounter. Unfortunately, social and structural barriers often limit their opportunity to seek and receive mental health support (Estriplet et al., 2022).

While the literature often focuses on the risks and stressors faced by Black mothers, there is also a call for recognizing their strengths, supports, and the need for culturally appropriate interventions (Parker, 2021) such as community-based approaches.

In this regard, community-based approaches are increasingly being recognized as essential in addressing the mental health needs of Black mothers, who face unique challenges due to structural racism and inequities in healthcare. As a result, community involvement is considered foundational to Black motherhood, providing a source of strength, challenging negative perceptions, and reclaiming cultural traditions surrounding birth (Mollard et al., 2024). By utilizing community-centered strategies, it is possible to address individual, community, and institutional factors contributing to Black maternal mortality and disparities in maternal health outcomes (Falako et al., 2023). Moreover, research has emphasized the need for multi-level interventions driven by insights from Black women to improve maternal health outcomes (Kantor et al., 2023). The importance of these approaches is highlighted by the insights and recommendations from various research papers.

One key pathway to equitable and antiracist maternal mental health care is investing in Black women-led community-based organizations, which can provide culturally competent care and support to Black birthing populations (Matthews et al., 2021). These organizations play a crucial role in addressing the disjointed systems of care that disproportionately affect Black women and offer a more integrated and holistic approach to mental health treatment. Furthermore, community-centered strategies are also vital in addressing Black maternal mortality, which is a pressing issue across the country. By utilizing community-based participatory research principles, these strategies ensure that the experiences and needs of Black birthing people, including those with intersectional identities, are understood and addressed in a manner that is informed by the community itself (Falako et al., 2023).

In addition, engaging with the communities surrounding and supporting Black adolescents is critical to promoting mental health treatment among Black adolescents (Ribeiro Brown et al., 2022). According to Lindsey and Marcell (Lindsey & Marcell, 2012), addressing mental health interventions for Black males requires a multifaceted approach that includes engaging men's social supports, community, and the healthcare system. Additionally, Baiden and Evans (Baiden & Evans, 2021) highlight the pressing need for culturally safe interventions to meet the postpartum mental health needs of Black African newcomer mothers. To further illustrate this point, Clark et al. (Clark et al., 2023) gathered perspectives from Black women community members, emphasizing the importance of a human rights approach.

The purpose of this chapter is to highlight the importance of community-based approaches in addressing Black maternal mental health. In particular, the chapter emphasizes the need for community-based organizations and care providers to address maternal mental health from the perspective of birthing persons and caretakers from diverse backgrounds. Furthermore, the chapter emphasizes the importance of community-based approaches in addressing social and structural determinants of mental health for Black birthing people and their infants.

COMMUNITY-BASED APPROACHES TO BLACK MATERNAL MENTAL HEALTH

Community-based approaches to Black maternal mental health are crucial for addressing the disparities faced by Black women in maternal mental health care. Research suggests that utilizing an Afrocentric perspective is essential for understanding the state of Black maternal mental health and providing culturally meaningful support for wellness (Parker, 2021). Moreover, the impact of the Strong Black Woman Schema on Black women's mental health has been identified, highlighting the need for specific points of intervention for mental health practitioners working with Black women (Abrams et al., 2019). Furthermore, supporting Black women providers and community-based organizations is essential, as they can offer more culturally responsive care, addressing the disproportionate burden faced by Black cisgender women in maternal and mental health disparities (Matthews et al., 2021).

In addition, community-centered approaches, such as the Consortium to End Black Maternal Mortality, have been effective in conducting community-based participatory research focused on Black maternal health, emphasizing the importance of involving cross-sector stakeholders and Black mothers in the research process (Alio et al., 2022). Additionally, culturally adapted psychological interventions have been recommended to address maternal mental health disparities among mothers of African and Caribbean origin, highlighting the need for interventions tailored to specific cultural backgrounds (Jidong et al., 2021).

Moreover, research and interventions in the past have mainly concentrated on individual and policy-level factors to decrease maternal mortality. This highlights the need for a community-centered approach to comprehend the experiences of Black birthing individuals in local communities that have been disproportionately affected (Falako et al., 2023). To improve maternal mental health and promote positive parenting experiences, it is crucial to prioritize strategies that center Black parents in the development of educational parenting programs (Estriplet et al., 2022).

While faith-based peer-led mental interventions have shown effectiveness in reducing anxiety and depression, there is a need to examine such interventions to meet the mental health needs of marginalized Black communities, incorporating principles of broader wellbeing (Ali et al., 2022). Furthermore, community-academic partnerships using community-based participatory research principles have been effective in addressing the ethical concerns of maternal mental health research with Black women, emphasizing the importance of community engagement in research (Hernandez et al., 2019).

Community-Engaged Research

Community-Engaged Research (CEnR) is a collaborative approach to research that meaningfully involves community members in the research process, from the conception of the study to the dissemination of its findings. This approach involves actively involving community members in the research process to ensure that the research is culturally meaningful and responsive to the needs of the community (Matthews et al., 2021). In the context of Black Maternal Mental Health, CEnR is particularly significant due to the complex interplay of social, economic, and healthcare factors that contribute to disparities in maternal health outcomes for Black women. Thus, the Afrocentric perspective is particularly important in understanding the state of Black maternal mental health and the support needed for wellness (Parker, 2021). It is essential to support Black women providers and community-based organizations, as they are more likely to provide culturally responsive care and can play a crucial role in addressing the disproportionate burden faced by Black women in maternal and mental health disparities.

For instance, the study "Black Women's Maternal Health: Insights from Community-Based Participatory Research in Newark, New Jersey" exemplifies the use of CEnR by involving community members in conducting interviews and identifying key themes such as healthcare structure challenges, negative experiences with healthcare providers, racial concordance preferences, and mental health concerns (Kantor et al., 2023). This participatory approach not only illuminates the lived experiences of Black women but also fosters the development of tailored interventions.

Similarly, other studies have highlighted the importance of engaging Black women stakeholders, including newcomer mothers, mental health practitioners, researchers, and activists, to identify strategies to combat racism and inequities in maternal mental health care (Baiden & Evans, 2022; Matthews et al., 2021)). These studies discussed the importance of culturally sensitive recruitment strategies to engage African newcomer mothers in research, which is crucial for addressing the knowledge gap and improving culturally competent health services (Baiden & Evans, 2022). Additionally, other research (Matthews et al., 2021) emphasized the need for education, investment in the Black women mental health workforce, and the promotion of integrated care.

Moreover, intersectionality of gender, race/ethnicity, culture, stigmatization of mental illness, and mental strength are significant factors contributing to the hesitancy of Black African newcomer mothers to participate in maternal mental health research (Baiden & Evans, 2022). Therefore, it is crucial to consider these factors when designing community-engaged research initiatives to ensure the active participation of Black African newcomer mothers in research related to maternal mental health.

Furthermore, the involvement of community members in community-based participatory research projects, as demonstrated in a study on Black women's maternal health, is essential in addressing racial disparities caused by social and structural determinants of health on Black mothers and birthing people's mental health and health care experiences that influence infant mental health (Estriplet et al., 2022). This highlights the importance of engaging community members, particularly Black women health professionals, in the research process to gain insights that can inform interventions and support systems for Black maternal mental health.

In the context of global health research, community engagement is increasingly promoted, and there is a need to determine the effectiveness of community engagement in research, particularly in developing countries (Tindana et al., 2007). This emphasizes the importance of evaluating the impact of community-engaged research in diverse settings to ensure its relevance and effectiveness in addressing maternal mental health disparities globally.

Moreover, the involvement of community health workers and lay community advisors in community-engaged research has been shown to improve the clarity of research participant recruitment materials and increase the likelihood of community participation, emphasizing the role of community members in shaping research processes and outcomes (Bowers et al., 2017; Smith & Blumenthal, 2012). Furthermore, the work by Fothergill and associates provided evidence of the positive association between community engagement and health outcomes among African American women, highlighting the potential health benefits of active participation in community organizations (Fothergill et al., 2011).

Ethical considerations are also paramount in community-engaged research, especially when engaging with Indigenous communities and other marginalized groups. Ethical research engagement with Indigenous communities involves exploring Indigenous health research, community-based partnerships, reciprocal learning, and cultural safety, highlighting the need for ethical and respectful engagement with communities in research initiatives (Bourassa et al., 2020). The study by Hernandez et al. sheds insight into how a community-academic partnership can use CEnR principles to develop research protocols that address ethical concerns and involve community stakeholders, particularly in research with Black women (Hernandez et al., 2019). Additionally, DuBois et al. (2011) reviewed the spectrum of CEnR practices and their potential to improve research quality while addressing ethical concerns. This study also underscored the challenges and benefits of CEnR, including the need for funding and training for both researchers and community members (DuBois et al., 2011).

Community-Based Models of Care

Community-Based Models of Care (CBCs) are increasingly recognized as a vital approach to addressing the mental health needs of Black birthing populations, who face significant inequities in the diagnosis and treatment of perinatal and maternal mental health disorders due to structural racism. These models prioritize culturally competent care and aim to reduce disparities by integrating services into the community and utilizing a workforce reflective of the community served.

Given that Black women face a disproportionate burden in maternal and mental health disparities, it is crucial to highlight the need for equitable and antiracist maternal mental health care (Matthews et al., 2021). In fact, community-based models of care have shown promise in addressing such disparities, as evidenced by successful programs offering home-based ART through lay providers in Uganda (Callaghan et al., 2010). However, engaging Black African newcomer mothers in maternal mental health research has revealed the intersectionality of gender, race/ethnicity, culture, stigmatization of mental illness, and mental strength as factors contributing to hesitancy in participation (Baiden & Evans, 2022). This underscores the importance of culturally responsive care and support for Black maternal mental health.

One of the key strategies to improve maternal mental health care for Black populations is to educate and train practitioners in culturally sensitive practices and to address racism and inequities directly. This involves investing in the Black women mental health workforce and supporting Black women-led community-based organizations that understand and are rooted in the communities they serve (Matthews et al., 2021). Additionally, valuing and investing in community and traditional healing practices are essential. These practices are often overlooked by conventional health systems but are integral to the well-being of many Black communities. Promoting integrated care and shared decision-making between health care providers and patients is also crucial for creating a more equitable and effective health care system (Matthews et al., 2021).

For example, in Australia, a nurse-led community model for perinatal mental health has been developed and evaluated, demonstrating significant reductions in depressive and anxiety symptoms among women (Harvey et al., 2018). This model is based on principles of partnership, individualized evidence-based treatments, and accessible, flexible service delivery. The nurse practitioner role within this model has been particularly effective in enhancing continuity of care, especially for women requiring antidepressant treatment (Harvey et al., 2018).

In the context of low and middle-income countries (LAMICs) like South Africa, where there is a shortage of mental health specialists, task-sharing approaches have been suggested (Kathree et al., 2014). Women with maternal depression have expressed that counselling provided by general health care providers could be beneficial, especially when addressing issues such as poverty, unwanted pregnancy, and interpersonal conflict. Techniques from cognitive behavioral therapy and problem-solving therapy are recommended within these task-sharing approaches to build self-efficacy and address material conditions and relationship problems (Kathree et al., 2014).

In terms of prenatal care for Black women, mental health services have been identified as a vital component, emphasizing the need for community involvement in Black maternal health (Kemet et al., 2022). Furthermore, the integration of health care at the primary-secondary interface has shown potential in addressing disparities, with costlier integrated care models attributing their effectiveness to more frequent follow-up appointments and the higher cost of community-based pathology services (Mitchell et al., 2015). These findings highlight the potential benefits of integrating community-based models of care into the broader healthcare system to address Black maternal mental health disparities.

To optimize infant health and wellness, it is essential to prioritize maternal mental health among Black mothers and birthing people, as their experiences influence infant mental health (Estriplet et al., 2022). Engaging community members in participatory research projects has been shown to be effective in addressing racial disparities in maternal mortality and severe maternal morbidity (Kantor et al., 2023). Additionally, interventions involving the delivery of community-based services have demonstrated strong evidence in improving retention in HIV care, further supporting the effectiveness of community-based models of care (Murray et al., 2017).

While the focus of the references is not exclusively on Black maternal mental health, the principles and outcomes of community-based models of care can be applied to address the specific needs of this population. For instance, community-based care models for managing type 2 diabetes mellitus among non-pregnant adults in sub-Saharan Africa have provided insights into acceptance, clinical outcomes, and engagement in care, which can inform similar approaches for Black maternal mental health (Firima et al., 2021). Moreover, the successful integration of refugee health in primary care through an integrated model of care provides valuable lessons for addressing the specific healthcare needs of marginalized communities, including Black maternal mental health (Sackey et al., 2021).

Community-Centered Strategies

Community-centered strategies are crucial in addressing Black maternal mental health. These strategies are aimed at improving the diagnosis, treatment, and overall care for Black birthing populations who face a higher prevalence of perinatal mood disorders and maternal mortality rates. To build a foundation for these strategies, the Afrocentric perspective has been utilized to gain a better understanding of the state of Black maternal mental health and to provide culturally meaningful support for wellness (Parker, 2021). This approach emphasizes the importance of incorporating cultural values and beliefs into mental health support systems for Black women. In addition to this perspective, the integration of a Womanist theoretical perspective into counseling for Black women has been recommended to avoid pathologizing strength and to address the underutilization of mental health resources by this population (Abrams et al., 2019).

Transitioning from theoretical frameworks to practical insights, insights from Black women stakeholders have been instrumental in identifying strategies to address racism and inequities in maternal and infant mental health care (Matthews et al., 2021). This underscores the significance of involving the community in developing strategies to tackle the unique challenges faced by Black women in accessing mental health support. Moreover, prioritizing maternal mental health and centering Black parents in developing educational parenting programs have been highlighted as essential strategies to optimize parenting experiences and improve maternal mental health (Estriplet et al., 2022).

To further enhance these efforts, it is essential to improve collaboration between mental health researchers, policy makers, and primary-care systems to ensure action that advances both maternal and child health (Woolhouse et al., 2015). This necessitates the integration of core mental health services within routine primary health care to provide comprehensive support for Black maternal mental health. Additionally, it is important to note that historical traumas, lack of access to healthcare, and growing mental health concerns in Black communities highlight the importance of clinical and research guidance to tackle the mental health impact of the COVID-19 pandemic on Black Americans, as pointed out by Novacek et al. (Novacek et al., 2020).

Moreover, involving partners of Black African newcomer women in postpartum care and encouraging mental health service utilization has been recommended based on the perceptions of Black African newcomer women regarding postpartum mental health services in Canada (Baiden & Evans, 2021). This underscores the significance of involving the community and considering cultural dynamics in the design and delivery of maternal mental health services. In light of these considerations, strategies to improve care team identification in the electronic health record have been outlined to enhance patient-centered communication and support patient-centered care (Dalal & Schnipper, 2016).

Furthermore, other key strategies involves educating and training practitioners to be culturally competent and sensitive to the needs of Black birthing people as well as valuing, honoring, and investing in community and traditional healing practices (Matthews et al., 2021). These practices can be integrated into more formal healthcare settings to provide holistic care. In parallel, investing in the Black women mental health workforce is another critical strategy. By increasing the number of Black mental health practitioners, the healthcare system can provide more relatable and culturally appropriate care, which can improve trust and communication between patients and providers (Matthews et al., 2021).

As we look to the broader context, recent research emphasizes the significance of tackling the social, structural, and economic inequalities that hinder Black perinatal women and birthing people from accessing interventions and treatments. Additionally, maternal mental health should be prioritized, and education on healthy and culturally-sensitive ways to support infant development should be provided as the well-being of the child is closely connected with that of the mother (Estriplet et al., 2022).

Moreover, community engagement is crucial for addressing ethical concerns in maternal mental health disparities research. By using participatory research approaches, researchers can ensure that the studies are designed and conducted in a way that respects and addresses the needs of the community (Hernandez et al., 2019). Promoting integrated care and shared decision-making ensures that Black birthing people are active participants in their healthcare. This approach can lead to more personalized and effective care plans that take into account the individual's preferences and experiences (Matthews et al., 2021).

KEY FACTORS IN COMMUNITY-BASED APPROACHES

Mother-Provider Communication

Transitioning to practical factors, effective communication between mothers and healthcare providers is integral to community-based approaches in Black maternal mental health. It supports the delivery of culturally appropriate care, helps to overcome barriers to service engagement, and is a key factor in interventions aimed at addressing the disparities in mental health outcomes for Black mothers. Consequently, literature suggests that prioritizing effective communication strategies, along with culturally congruent care and community engagement, can significantly contribute to improving Black maternal mental health.

Moreover, effective communication between mothers and healthcare providers is a critical component of community-based approaches in Black maternal mental health. It facilitates the understanding of mothers' needs, the provision of culturally congruent care, and the development of trust, which is essential for engaging mothers in mental health services (Franks et al., 2007). In this context, effective communication can help in identifying and addressing the social and structural barriers that Black mothers face, thereby improving access to and the quality of maternal mental health care (Estriplet et al., 2022; Matthews et al., 2021).

Interestingly, while effective communication is a cornerstone of good healthcare, it also intersects with the need for healthcare providers to challenge racism and disrupt intergenerational trauma, as highlighted in the thematic analysis of (Walsh et al., 2023). This intersectionality is echoed in the call for culturally centered recommendations to move the field of infant mental health toward racial justice-oriented practice (Parker, 2021). Furthermore, the importance of community and traditional healing practices, which are often rooted in effective communication within a cultural context, is emphasized as a pathway to address racism and inequities in maternal and infant mental health care (Matthews et al., 2021).

By fostering effective communication, healthcare providers can create a supportive environment that addresses the unique mental health needs of Black mothers. This aligns with the recommendations provided by advocates for community-centered strategies to address Black maternal mortality and achieve health equity in maternal health outcomes (Falako et al., 2023). Through open and culturally sensitive communication, healthcare providers can significantly contribute to community-based approaches in Black maternal mental health, ultimately improving the well-being of Black mothers and their families.

Role of Social Support Networks

Social support networks are integral to Black maternal mental health, providing essential emotional and instrumental support. These networks can have direct positive effects on mental health and act as mediators in the relationship between other forms of support and mental health outcomes. However, the impact of social support can vary based on gender, the type of support, and sociodemographic factors, suggesting that a nuanced understanding of these networks is necessary to effectively support Black maternal mental health.

In this regard, supporting Black women providers and community-based organizations is essential in addressing the disproportionate burden faced by Black women in maternal and mental health disparities (Matthews et al., 2021). Furthermore, social support has also been shown to have a positive effect on immigrant women's mental health and well-being, facilitating social inclusion and the use of health services (Guruge et al., 2015). Utilizing social support practices that maintain connections and relationships can act protectively for the mental health of Black women during stressful circumstances (Malcome et al., 2019). Indeed, receiving social support is a powerful predictor for postpartum maternal health and functioning, underscoring its significance in maternal well-being (Gholizadeh Shamasbi et al., 2020). Integrating Black feminist approaches in maternal health research can further enhance our understanding of the processes impacting the health and well-being of Black mothers, emphasizing the need to center Black women in maternal health research (Brantley, 2023).

As we delve deeper, social support networks play a crucial role in supporting Black maternal mental health by providing both direct and buffering effects, as well as contributing to the overall well-being of Black mothers. For instance, the presence of nearby relatives and perceived social support were found to have significant positive effects on the mental health of Black females, though these effects were not observed for Black males (Brown & Gary, 1987). Additionally, paternal support and the quality of the interparental relationship were positively correlated with maternal mental health, with relationship quality mediating the relationship between paternal support and maternal mental health (Walsh et al., 2023). Moreover, interventions that foster social networks may be more effective in addressing maternal mental health, suggesting the importance of qualitative indicators of social support over traditional quantitative measures (Balaji et al., 2007).

Nevertheless, there are complexities within these support networks. For example, the number of confidants for Black males and the degree of religiosity among Black females were inversely related to physical health, indicating that different conceptual models may be necessary to understand the impact of social support on mental and physical health (Brown & Gary, 1987). Furthermore, while African American and Black Caribbean adolescents receive substantial family support, variations exist by sociodemographic factors, highlighting the need to consider ethnic differences within the U.S. Black population (Cross et al., 2018).

Systemic Influences on Maternal Mental Health

When implementing community-based approaches to address maternal mental health, it is crucial to consider various systemic influences that can impact the effectiveness of such interventions. Factors such as maternal anxiety, depression, and stress can influence neurodevelopment in children, highlighting the importance of addressing maternal mental health for the well-being of both mothers and their offspring (O'Donnell & Meaney, 2017). Moreover, the perception of women, their families, and communities regarding available maternal health services can significantly influence health-seeking behaviors, emphasizing the need to align interventions with community needs and expectations (Nepal et al., 2020).

In this context, community-based interventions for maternal mental health in Sub-Saharan Africa have predominantly focused on psychotherapeutic approaches, with limited emphasis on community-based strategies, indicating a gap in leveraging community resources for mental health support (Woodhead et al., 2023). Furthermore, task-shifting to community health workers is a common strategy, but services are often confined to health facilities rather than being community-oriented (Woodhead et al., 2023).

To address these gaps, an effective way to comprehend the intricate connections between community and health system factors that impact the implementation and endurance of mental health interventions, particularly in low- and middle-income countries, is by utilizing systems science methodologies (Greene et al., 2021). Notably, community-based, peer-led parenting programs have shown positive impacts on both children's development and maternal mental health, underscoring the potential of community involvement in promoting mental well-being (Aoki et al., 2022).

Moreover, stigma and discrimination have been identified as pervasive influences that affect the planning and implementation of mental health treatments and services, emphasizing the need to address societal attitudes and perceptions surrounding mental health (Thornicroft et al., 2016). In addition, the feasibility of integrating mental health care into routine maternal health services requires building the capacity of policymakers, strengthening mental healthcare systems, and fostering intersectoral collaboration (Surjaningrum et al., 2018).

Consequently, policies should be developed to include maternal mental health as a component of primary healthcare systems (Engle, 2009). Furthermore, training community health workers in maternal mental health is also crucial, as evidenced by the MOMS Partnership's success in improving knowledge and attitudes among community health workers (Smith & Kruse-Austin, 2015). Thus, systemic influences such as evidence generation, cultural adaptation, healthcare delivery models, social support networks, and training of community health workers are critical factors that impact the effectiveness of community-based approaches to maternal mental health.

Strategies to Enhance Emotional Well-Being

As we explore strategies further, to enhance the emotional well-being of Black mothers in community-based approaches, a comprehensive approach that combines technology-based interventions, social support, coping strategies, racial socialization, and community engagement can significantly contribute to enhancing the emotional well-being of Black mothers in community-based settings. By integrating these diverse strategies, tailored support can be provided to address the unique emotional needs of Black mothers and promote their overall well-being.

Firstly, involving mothers as citizen scientists in research can empower them and address cultural sensitivities, as demonstrated by the South Chicago Black Mothers' Resiliency Project (Mendenhall et al., 2020). In addition, promoting mother-infant bonding through activities like singing can enhance emotional closeness and reduce anxiety (Fancourt & Perkins, 2018). Moreover, implementing coping strategies, fostering feelings of control in life, and enhancing social connectedness have been shown to predict emotional well-being among African American individuals (Huang et al., 2022). In this light, addressing implicit provider bias through evidence-based personal and community engagement strategies is also crucial for promoting mental health wellness (Johnson, 2020). Furthermore, understanding the impact of perinatal mental health on infants and addressing social and structural barriers to treatment can improve both maternal and infant mental health (Estriplet et al., 2022).

Additionally, the use of artistic creative activities and proactive emotion regulation strategies have been shown to aid in managing negative emotions and enhancing emotional well-being in community settings (Kiernan et al., 2021). Equally important, family-centered approaches that provide socio-emotional support and positive interaction strategies have been associated with greater family well-being (Laister et al., 2021). Furthermore, mindfulness-based programs can support early childhood teachers in addressing workplace stressors and enhancing their interactions with children (Hatton-Bowers et al., 2023). Moreover, racial socialization practices can also play a crucial role in Black adolescents' coping mechanisms and psychological well-being (Anderson et al., 2019). In addition, strategies such as expanding recruitment sites, using community-based participatory research methods, and increasing diversity in research teams can help address racial disparities and improve emotional well-being in Black mothers (Penner et al., 2023).

Furthermore, incorporating technology-based interventions that focus on pregnancy health and wellness, such as counseling and social support, can positively impact emotional well-being (Jimah et al., 2021). Furthermore, online interventions like mindfulness programs can be utilized to improve maternal well-being and develop coping skills, offering a cost-effective means to enhance emotional health (Davis et al., 2023).

COMMUNITY ENGAGEMENT AND SUPPORT

Expanding Reimbursement for Doulas and Midwives

Transitioning to community engagement, expanding reimbursement for doulas and midwives is crucial to optimize maternal mental health care for Black women. To achieve this, it is essential to support Black women care providers who can offer culturally responsive care and to involve community-based organizations in the care process (Matthews et al., 2021). In this context, the expansion of reimbursement for doulas and midwives is posited as a strategy to support Black maternal mental health by addressing systemic racism in healthcare and providing culturally congruent care (Parker, 2021; Salinas et al., 2022). Notably, doulas, as nonmedical support workers, offer continuous support during childbirth and are suggested to be included under essential health benefits for insurance coverage, which could increase their accessibility to Black women (Landor, 2023). Research supports this, suggesting that increasing availability, compensation, and services provided by doulas and midwives can lead to healthier outcomes for Black mothers (Carvalho et al., 2021). Moreover, state Medicaid programs could potentially achieve cost savings by covering birth doulas, which may result in reduced cesarean rates (Kozhimannil et al., 2013). However, it is essential to ensure that doulas are reimbursed at appropriate rates through Medicaid to make their services more accessible to Black mothers (Mosley et al., 2023).

In addition, studies have shown that doula support can help improve maternal and infant outcomes, particularly for Black patients (Ramey-Collier et al., 2023). Furthermore, community-based doula programs have been highlighted as a way to enhance the care experience for Black birthing individuals (Ogunwole et al., 2020). Moreover, evidence-based strategies such as racial concordance between Black midwives and patients, group prenatal care, nurse navigation, and postpartum doula support have been identified to support Black maternal health (Liese et al., 2022).

Increasing Access to Black-Led Community-Based Care Providers

To enhance access to Black-led community-based care providers for maternal mental health support, several key measures can be implemented based on recommendations from various studies. Firstly, it is crucial to develop comprehensive national programs that provide integrated healthcare to underinsured and uninsured individuals in Black American communities (Novacek et al., 2020). These programs should focus on early identification and intervention for mental health issues, including posttraumatic stress, in community-based settings staffed by trained mental health providers (Novacek et al., 2020). Increasing the number of ethnically and culturally matched providers, improving the quality of treatments, and enhancing accessibility to services are essential strategies to improve mental health service utilization among Black adolescents (Banks).

Furthermore, it is important to prioritize strategies that center Black parents in developing educational parenting programs to optimize maternal mental health and infant wellness (Estriplet et al., 2022). Engaging in community-based participatory research with Black communities can also be beneficial in creating educational programming for mothers and healthcare providers to enhance mental well-being within Black families (Harris, 2021). Additionally, utilizing community-centered approaches and partnering with community-based doulas can address structural and institutional barriers to maternal health equity (Falako et al., 2023; Ogunwole et al., 2020).

Moreover, expanding the mental health care workforce and integrating mental health services as a vital component of prenatal care for Black women can help reduce racial/ethnic disparities in mental health care access (Kemet et al., 2022; Lê Cook et al., 2013). In this regard, supporting Black women-led community-based organizations can provide culturally congruent care and foster trust within the community (Matthews et al., 2021). Leveraging digital health care technologies, such as app-based platforms, can improve the management of maternal mental health by delivering educational content and increasing awareness about mental health conditions (Guille et al., 2024). Additionally, peer-led remote interventions and spirituality-based approaches have also shown promise in improving mental health outcomes within Black communities (Ali et al., 2022).

Involving Communities in Primary Health Care

Communities can play a crucial role in supporting Black maternal mental health through various avenues. Research indicates that involving Black women providers and community-based organizations is essential (Matthews et al., 2021). To elaborate on this, according to previous investigations, one way to involve communities is through the education and training of practitioners to be culturally competent and responsive to the needs of Black birthing populations (Matthews et al., 2021). These providers are more likely to offer culturally responsive care, which is vital in addressing the disparities faced by Black cisgender women in maternal and mental health (Matthews et al., 2021). In addition, establishing collaborative community initiatives, such as the Consortium to End Black Maternal Mortality, can effectively engage stakeholders and Black mothers in community-based participatory research focused on Black maternal health (Alio et al., 2022). Moreover, it has been suggested that involving partners of Black African newcomer women in postpartum care and encouraging them to utilize mental health services can provide better support for maternal mental health (Baiden & Evans, 2021).

Transitioning to a broader perspective, prioritizing maternal mental health and including Black women health professionals in research can improve infant health and well-being (Estriplet et al., 2022). Additionally, supporting the physical and mental health of minority mothers and promoting coping resources for daily parenting challenges can have a positive impact on parenting children with behavior problems (BeLue et al., 2015). Furthermore, improving accessibility to postnatal mental health support can break the bidirectional relationship between maternal mental ill-health and poor breastfeeding outcomes, benefiting both maternal emotional well-being and breastfeeding outcomes (Roberts et al., 2023). In this context, community events such as Black Maternal Mental Health Week can raise awareness and advocate for culturally congruent treatment, highlighting the importance of community engagement in addressing maternal mental health disparities. Interestingly, creative tools like poetry have been used to center the voices and experiences of Black mothers, which can inspire critical self-reflection and action within the community to enhance support systems (Parker, 2022).

IMPLICATIONS OF COMMUNITY-BASED APPROACHES

Empowering Black Women in Maternal Care

Building on the previous discussion, community-based approaches are essential in empowering Black women in maternal care by providing culturally responsive and supportive services. These approaches involve collaborating with community organizations and stakeholders to address the unique needs and challenges faced by Black women during pregnancy, childbirth, and postpartum periods. In this regard, by engaging Black women providers and community-based organizations, these approaches aim to reduce disparities in maternal health outcomes (Baffour & Chonody, 2009; Matthews et al., 2021; Reddy et al., 2021; Walter et al., 2020).

Furthermore, research has shown that promoting respectful maternal care is crucial for improving the quality of maternity care and ensuring that all women receive dignified treatment (Shakibazadeh et al., 2018). In addition, utilizing community-centered approaches is vital in addressing Black maternal mortality by understanding the experiences of Black birthing individuals in local communities that have been disproportionately impacted (Falako et al., 2023).

To deepen our understanding, integrating Black feminist approaches in maternal health research can further enhance our understanding of the factors influencing the health and well-being of Black mothers (Brantley, 2023). Moreover, engaging in community-based participatory research focused on Black maternal health can provide valuable insights into local factors affecting Black mothers' experiences with perinatal care (Alio et al., 2022).

In summary, Empowering Black women in health care decision-making and providing comprehensive awareness-raising activities at the community level are crucial steps in improving maternal health outcomes for Black women (Tsega et al., 2022). By centering the voices of Black women, amplifying community-driven solutions, and enhancing community organizing efforts, community-based approaches can effectively address the disparities faced by Black women in maternal care (Lowe, 2021).

Enhancing Patient Experiences

Continuing with the theme of community engagement, community-based approaches are essential in improving the overall patient experiences of Black mothers. Black women often face disparities in healthcare support, including inadequate information about breastfeeding (Anstey et al., 2017). In light of this, increasing interpersonal support for breastfeeding can positively impact initiation and duration among Black women (Beauregard, 2019). Community-based organizations, particularly those linked to faith-based and neighborhood partnerships, provide essential resources and support for Black mothers (Parker, 2021). Additionally, cultural attitudes and historical experiences influence breastfeeding rates among African American women, emphasizing the need for targeted interventions (Johnson et al., 2015).

Moreover, healthcare experiences of pregnant women of color underscore the importance of improved communication, support programs, and reduced reliance on past negative interactions (McLemore et al., 2018). Consequently, strength-based approaches and equitable support systems are crucial for addressing stressors affecting Black mothers' mental health (Hassoun Ayoub et al., 2023). Utilizing community-centered approaches is vital in addressing maternal mortality disparities among Black women (Falako et al., 2023).

In conclusion, supporting Black women providers and community-based organizations is vital in addressing maternal and mental health disparities (Matthews et al., 2021). Research indicates that hospital and community-based initiatives effectively increase breastfeeding rates among Black infants (Davis et al., 2021). Furthermore, community-engaged research, such as community-based participatory research, accurately reflects the experiences of Black women and identifies opportunities for improvement in maternal healthcare (Kantor et al., 2023). Online support communities and social media play a significant role in supporting Black mothers, especially in promoting breastfeeding and providing health knowledge (Asiodu et al., 2015; Robinson et al., 2019). Additionally, involving male partners in supporting Black mothers living with HIV can enhance infant feeding outcomes and overall well-being (Etowa et al., 2022).

Reducing Maternal Health Disparities

Community-based approaches are essential in addressing maternal health disparities among Black women by providing culturally competent care, addressing social determinants of health, and fostering trust within the community. These approaches involve engaging with local communities to understand their unique challenges and develop tailored interventions. By focusing on community-centered strategies, such as Black-led initiatives and collaborative research efforts, significant strides can be made in reducing maternal health inequities (Alio et al., 2022; Falako et al., 2023). A notable example is the Gabby System, a preconception care intervention, further exemplifies a community-based approach aimed at improving health outcomes for Black and African American women by being implemented in Community Health Centers and Healthy Start programs (Walter et al., 2020).

In addition, research indicates that community-based interventions, including Black-led efforts and supportive maternity care practices, have been effective in improving breastfeeding rates among Black women (Asiodu et al., 2021). Moreover, increasing community engagement through initiatives like the Consortium to End Black Maternal Mortality can lead to more impactful and culturally competent care for Black mothers (Alio et al., 2022).

Addressing systemic racism and social determinants of health is crucial in this context, as it plays a significant role in reducing disparities in maternal health outcomes. Policies that combat institutional racism and promote equity in areas like housing, education, and employment can significantly improve the health of Black women (Carvalho et al., 2021; Chambers et al., 2018).

Furthermore, community-based doulas and health information technology interventions tailored to Black and African American women have shown promise in promoting maternal health equity and reducing disparities (Louis-Jacques et al., 2024; Ogunwole et al., 2020; Walter et al., 2020). By involving community health workers and implementing evidence-based interventions in community settings, it is possible to address structural and institutional barriers to maternal health equity (Ogunwole et al., 2020; Walter et al., 2020).

These approaches are crucial because Black women in the U.S. face a disproportionately higher risk of pregnancy-related deaths and complications, which are exacerbated by structural racism and implicit biases within the healthcare system (Montalmant & Ettinger, 2023). Community-based health delivery channels have been identified as the least inequitable and most effective in mitigating socioeconomic disparities in maternal care uptake (Oburota et al., 2023). In this regard,

Community Health Workers (CHWs) have been successful in building trust with low-income women of color, which is essential for engaging them in maternal and child health services (Rafizadeh et al., 2023).

RECOMMENDATIONS FOR EFFECTIVE IMPLEMENTATION

Policy Changes to Address Racism and Bias

As we move forward, several policy changes are crucial to address racism and bias in the context of Black maternal mental health. First, there is a need for education and training of practitioners to recognize and address racism and its impacts on health (Matthews et al., 2021). This includes fostering critical-racial consciousness among health professions students and trainees to stimulate antiracist actions in medical decision-making (Ogunwole & Starks, 2024). Additionally, investing in the Black women mental health workforce and Black women-led community-based organizations is crucial for providing culturally competent care and support (Matthews et al., 2021).

Moreover, there is a need for policies that specifically target systemic racism in healthcare, including maternal health services (Iradukunda & Canty, 2023). These policies should aim to dismantle the effects of racism on Black maternal health outcomes. Additionally, policies must address the disparities faced by Black women, such as racial stress and trauma, which can lead to mental health issues (Goddard-Durant et al., 2023). Efforts should focus on implementing structural interventions to counter anti-Black racism in policies and healthcare practices.

Furthermore, it is essential to advocate for policies that oppose racism in all its forms within society (Abdullah et al., 2021). This includes promoting access to quality mental health care for Black communities and working towards eliminating racism from various aspects of life, including healthcare systems (Alang, 2019). Policies should confront racism and consider historical and contemporary racial contexts that impact mental health among Black individuals (Alang, 2019).

In addition, addressing racism in maternity care is crucial, as disparities in maternal and infant outcomes based on racial and ethnic identities persist (Simpson, 2021). Therefore, efforts to eliminate racism and health inequities should be a priority, including funding for health equity strategies, addressing social determinants of health, and recruiting diverse investigators with experience in communities of color (Simpson, 2021).

Culturally Competent Care for Black Maternal Mental Health

Moving on to the practical aspects of care, healthcare providers can offer culturally competent care for Black maternal mental health by recognizing and addressing the unique challenges and disparities faced by Black mothers and birthing people. To achieve this, healthcare providers must address the barriers and facilitators identified in the literature. Black individuals often encounter challenges accessing mental healthcare due to experiences of racism, lack of culturally competent care, and the absence of holistic approaches (Fante-Coleman & Jackson-Best, 2020). Consequently, it is essential for healthcare providers to be well-informed and prepared to discuss perinatal mental health, identify issues, and offer appropriate care to women experiencing perinatal mental health problems (Watson et al., 2019). Embracing an Afrocentric perspective can aid in understanding the state of Black maternal mental health and in providing culturally meaningful support (Parker, 2021).

In this light, cultural competence in mental health care is crucial, necessitating knowledge of cultural beliefs, values, and practices to prevent errors in diagnosis and management (Bhui et al., 2007). Additionally, supporting Black women providers and community-based organizations is vital, as they can provide more culturally responsive care to Black patients, addressing the disparities faced by Black cisgender women in maternal and mental health (Matthews et al., 2021). Psychological interventions tailored to the cultural backgrounds of African and Caribbean mothers have been recommended to address maternal mental health disparities (Jidong et al., 2021).

To enhance culturally competent care, healthcare providers should aim to deliver advice meaningfully within the cultural understanding of Black women, rather than solely providing information (Shorey et al., 2021). Counselors should cultivate critical consciousness to demonstrate cultural humility and provide culturally competent services to Black women (Silas & Seward, 2023). Moreover, it is crucial to involve Black mothers in care decisions and practices to ensure culturally competent care that centers on their voices (Ajayi & Garney, 2023).

Tailored Interventions for Improved Outcomes

Community-based culturally-tailored programs (CBCT) show promise in addressing the specific needs of Black communities and improving health outcomes, including maternal mental health (Fulton et al., 2022). These programs are designed to be culturally congruent and incorporate community input, which is crucial for their effectiveness.

For enhancing outcomes in Black maternal mental health through community-based approaches, it is crucial to implement culturally adapted and community-centered interventions. Psychological interventions tailored specifically for Black women, including those of African and Caribbean descent, have been recommended to address maternal mental health disparities (Jidong et al., 2021). These interventions should undergo rigorous testing in randomized controlled trials to ensure their effectiveness. Additionally, adopting community-centered approaches that prioritize understanding the unique experiences of Black birthing individuals in local communities can help reduce maternal mortality rates (Falako et al., 2023).

Insights from Black women stakeholders underscore the necessity of critical resources to improve the quality of maternal mental health care for Black birthing populations (Matthews et al., 2021). Prioritizing maternal mental health and involving Black parents in the development of educational parenting programs can optimize parenting experiences and contribute to overall wellness (Estriplet et al., 2022). Ultimately, it is imperative to develop psychological interventions tailored to address the specific needs of Black women, particularly related to prenatal anxiety, to enhance outcomes for both mothers and infants (Ponting et al., 2022).

Incorporating peer-led remote interventions that focus on holistic, spirituality-based approaches can also effectively improve mental health outcomes among Black participants (Ali et al., 2022). Furthermore, integrating mental health services into obstetrics settings and providing culturally competent interventions can aid in preventing and treating perinatal depression among low-income Black women (Glickman et al., 2020). Moreover, interventions that integrate perinatal mental health care into routine maternal care have shown promise in enhancing maternal mental health and infant outcomes in low- and middle-income countries (Prom et al., 2022).

CONCLUSION

In summary, an extensive summary of the difficulties and inequities Black women have when seeking maternity mental health care is given in this chapter. To overcome these discrepancies and empower Black women, the chapter emphasizes the significance of community-based initiatives, such as culturally relevant interventions and community-centered strategies. Additionally, it highlights how important it is for Black women clinicians, community-based organizations, and community engagement to work together to create customized support networks and interventions for Black mothers' mental health. The chapter also highlights the significance of providing Black mothers with culturally appropriate treatment and the necessity of addressing structural factors like racism and bias in the healthcare system.

Call to Action for Healthcare Systems

Based on the discussions in this chapter, there is a clear call to action for healthcare systems to prioritize the implementation of culturally competent care for Black maternal mental health. This includes the training of practitioners to recognize and address racism and its impacts on health. Additionally, healthcare systems should invest in and support community-based interventions, Black women-led organizations, and culturally tailored programs to address the unique needs of Black mothers. By implementing these actions, healthcare systems can play a pivotal role in addressing the disparities faced by Black women in maternal mental health and improving outcomes for this population.

Potential Future Directions for Research and Practice

Finally, the chapter highlights several potential future directions for research and practice in the field of community-based approaches to Black maternal mental health. One key area for future research is the development and evaluation of culturally tailored interventions for Black maternal mental health to address disparities and improve outcomes. Furthermore, there is a need for continued advocacy for policy changes to address systemic influences, such as racism and bias, within healthcare systems. Additionally, the emphasis on community engagement and the involvement of Black women providers and community-based organizations in research and practice will be crucial in developing effective and culturally responsive interventions. By pursuing these future directions, the field of community-based approaches to Black maternal mental health can advance and contribute to improving the well-being of Black mothers and their families.

REFERENCES

Abdullah, T., Graham-LoPresti, J. R., Tahirkheli, N. N., Hughley, S. M., & Watson, L. T. J. (2021). Microaggressions and posttraumatic stress disorder symptom scores among Black Americans: Exploring the link. *Traumatology*, *27*(3), 244–253. DOI: 10.1037/trm0000259

Abrams, J. A., Hill, A., & Maxwell, M. (2019). Underneath the mask of the strong Black woman schema: Disentangling influences of strength and self-silencing on depressive symptoms among US Black women. *Sex Roles*, *80*(9-10), 517–526. DOI: 10.1007/s11199-018-0956-y PMID: 31086431

Ajayi, K. V., & Garney, W. R. (2023). What Black Mothers with Preterm Infants Want for Their Mental Health Care: A Qualitative Study. *Women's Health Reports (New Rochelle, N.Y.)*, *4*(1), 39–47. DOI: 10.1089/whr.2022.0088 PMID: 36893324

Alang, S. M. (2019). Mental health care among blacks in America: Confronting racism and constructing solutions. *Health Services Research*, *54*(2), 346–355. DOI: 10.1111/1475-6773.13115 PMID: 30687928

Ali, S. H., Mohsin, F. M., Banks, A., Lynn, P., & Lim, S. (2022). Peer-led, remote intervention to improve mental health outcomes using a holistic, spirituality-based approach: Results from a pilot study. *Community Mental Health Journal*, *58*(5), 862–874. DOI: 10.1007/s10597-021-00893-8 PMID: 34561834

Alio, A. P., Dillion, T., Hartman, S., Johnson, T., Turner, S., Bullock, S., & Dozier, A. (2022). A community collaborative for the exploration of local factors affecting Black mothers' experiences with perinatal care. *Maternal and Child Health Journal*, *26*(4), 751–760. DOI: 10.1007/s10995-022-03422-5 PMID: 35316456

Anderson, R. E., Jones, S., Anyiwo, N., McKenny, M., & Gaylord-Harden, N. (2019). What's race got to do with it? Racial socialization's contribution to Black adolescent coping. *Journal of Research on Adolescence*, *29*(4), 822–831. DOI: 10.1111/jora.12440 PMID: 30099797

Anstey, E. H., Shoemaker, M. L., Barrera, C. M., O'Neil, M. E., Verma, A. B., & Holman, D. M. (2017). Breastfeeding and breast cancer risk reduction: Implications for black mothers. *American Journal of Preventive Medicine*, *53*(3), S40–S46. DOI: 10.1016/j.amepre.2017.04.024 PMID: 28818244

Aoki, A., Togoobaatar, G., Tseveenjav, A., Nyam, N., Zuunnast, K., & Takehara, K. (2022). Quality of life of mothers of children and adolescents with mental health problems in Mongolia: Associations with the severity of children's mental health problems and family structure. *Global Mental Health (Cambridge, England)*, *9*, 298–305. DOI: 10.1017/gmh.2022.34 PMID: 36618750

Asiodu, I. V., Bugg, K., & Palmquist, A. E. (2021). Achieving breastfeeding equity and justice in Black communities: Past, present, and future. *Breastfeeding Medicine*, *16*(6), 447–451. DOI: 10.1089/bfm.2020.0314 PMID: 33979550

Asiodu, I. V., Waters, C. M., Dailey, D. E., Lee, K. A., & Lyndon, A. (2015). Breastfeeding and use of social media among first-time African American mothers. *Journal of Obstetric, Gynecologic, and Neonatal Nursing : JOGNN*, *44*(2), 268–278. DOI: 10.1111/1552-6909.12552 PMID: 25712127

Baffour, T. D., & Chonody, J. M. (2009). African-American women's conceptualizations of health disparities: A community-based participatory research approach. *American Journal of Community Psychology*, *44*(3-4), 374–381. DOI: 10.1007/s10464-009-9260-x PMID: 19838795

Baiden, D., & Evans, M. (2021). Black African newcomer women's perception of postpartum mental health services in Canada. *Canadian Journal of Nursing Research*, *53*(3), 202–210. DOI: 10.1177/0844562120934273 PMID: 32551939

Baiden, D., & Evans, M. (2022). Recruitment Strategies to Engage Newcomer Mothers of African Descent in Maternal Mental Health Research in Canada. *Journal of Transcultural Nursing*, *33*(4), 467–474. DOI: 10.1177/10436596221090268 PMID: 35466798

Balaji, A. B., Claussen, A. H., Smith, D. C., Visser, S. N., Morales, M. J., & Perou, R. (2007). Social support networks and maternal mental health and well-being. *Journal of Women's Health*, *16*(10), 1386–1396. DOI: 10.1089/jwh.2007.CDC10 PMID: 18062754

Banks, A. Black adolescent experiences with COVID-19 and mental health services utilization. J Racial Ethn Heal Disparities. 2021; 1–9. In.

Beauregard, J. L. (2019). Racial disparities in breastfeeding initiation and duration among US infants born in 2015. *MMWR. Morbidity and Mortality Weekly Report*, 68. PMID: 31465319

BeLue, R., Halgunseth, L. C., Abiero, B., & Bediako, P.BeLue. (2015). Maternal health status and parenting stress in low-income, ethnic-minority mothers of children with conduct disorder problems: The role of daily parenting hassles. *Journal of Racial and Ethnic Health Disparities*, *2*(4), 501–509. DOI: 10.1007/s40615-015-0098-7 PMID: 26863556

Bhui, K., Warfa, N., Edonya, P., McKenzie, K., & Bhugra, D. (2007). Cultural competence in mental health care: A review of model evaluations. *BMC Health Services Research*, *7*(1), 1–10. DOI: 10.1186/1472-6963-7-15 PMID: 17266765

Bourassa, C., Billan, J., Starblanket, D., Anderson, S., Legare, M., Hagel, M. C., Oakes, N., Jardine, M., Boehme, G., Dubois, E., Spencer, O., Hotomani, M., & McKenna, B. (2020). Ethical research engagement with Indigenous communities. *Journal of Rehabilitation and Assistive Technologies Engineering*, *7*, 2055668320922706. DOI: 10.1177/2055668320922706 PMID: 32612848

Bowers, B., Jacobson, N., & Krupp, A. (2017). Can lay community advisors improve the clarity of research participant recruitment materials and increase the likelihood of participation? *Research in Nursing & Health*, *40*(1), 63–69. DOI: 10.1002/nur.21752 PMID: 27686332

Brantley, M. (2023). Black feminist theory in maternal health research: A review of concepts and future directions. *Sociology Compass*, *17*(5), e13083. DOI: 10.1111/soc4.13083 PMID: 37859646

Brown, D. R., & Gary, L. E. (1987). Stressful life events, social support networks, and the physical and mental health of urban black adults. *Journal of Human Stress*, *13*(4), 165–174. DOI: 10.1080/0097840X.1987.9936810 PMID: 3448130

Callaghan, M., Ford, N., & Schneider, H. (2010). A systematic review of task-shifting for HIV treatment and care in Africa. *Human Resources for Health*, *8*(1), 1–9. DOI: 10.1186/1478-4491-8-8 PMID: 20356363

Carvalho, K., Kheyfets, A., Maleki, P., Miller, B., Abouhala, S., Anwar, E., & Amutah-Onukagha, N. (2021). A systematic policy review of Black maternal health-related policies proposed federally and in Massachusetts: 2010–2020. *Frontiers in Public Health*, *9*, 664659. DOI: 10.3389/fpubh.2021.664659 PMID: 34746071

Chambers, B. D., Erausquin, J. T., Tanner, A. E., Nichols, T. R., & Brown-Jeffy, S. (2018). Testing the association between traditional and novel indicators of county-level structural racism and birth outcomes among Black and White women. *Journal of Racial and Ethnic Health Disparities*, *5*(5), 966–977. DOI: 10.1007/s40615-017-0444-z PMID: 29218496

Clark, A. E., Macey, E., Irby, A., Stone, C., Pell Abernathy, M., & Turman, J. E.Jr. (2023). Diverse Perspectives to Support a Human Rights Approach to Reduce Indiana's Maternal Mortality Rate. *Humanity & Society*, *47*(1), 69–94. DOI: 10.1177/01605976221109785

Cross, C. J., Taylor, R. J., & Chatters, L. M. (2018). Family social support networks of African American and Black Caribbean adolescents. *Journal of Child and Family Studies*, *27*(9), 2757–2771. DOI: 10.1007/s10826-018-1116-2 PMID: 30344428

Dalal, A. K., & Schnipper, J. L. (2016). Care team identification in the electronic health record: A critical first step for patient-centered communication. *Journal of Hospital Medicine*, *11*(5), 381–385. DOI: 10.1002/jhm.2542 PMID: 26762584

Danasekaran, R., Mani, G., & Annadurai, K. (2015). Growing concern about maternal mental health disorders. *Clinical Obstetrics, Gynecology and Reproductive Medicine*, *1*(1), 19. DOI: 10.15761/COGRM.1000106

Davis, C., Villalobos, A. V. K., Turner, M. M., Long, S., & Lapinski, M. K. (2021). Racism and resistance: A qualitative study of bias as a barrier to breastfeeding. *Breastfeeding Medicine*, *16*(6), 471–480. DOI: 10.1089/bfm.2020.0307 PMID: 33784475

Davis, J. A., Finlay-Jones, A. L., Bear, N., Prescott, S. L., Silva, D. T., & Ohan, J. L. (2023). Time-out for well-being: A mixed methods evaluation of attitudes and likelihood to engage in different types of online emotional well-being programmes in the perinatal period. *Women's Health (London, England)*, *19*, DOI: 10.1177/17455057231184507 PMID: 37431205

Dimes, M. o. (2024). *40% of Black women experience maternal mental health symptoms, nearly twice the rate of all women*. March of Dimes. https://www.marchofdimes.org/black-maternal-mental-health-week

DuBois, J. M., Bailey-Burch, B., Bustillos, D., Campbell, J., Cottler, L., Fisher, C. B., Hadley, W. B., Hoop, J. G., Roberts, L., Salter, E. K., Sieber, J. E., & Stevenson, R. D. (2011). Ethical issues in mental health research: The case for community engagement. *Current Opinion in Psychiatry*, *24*(3), 208–214. DOI: 10.1097/YCO.0b013e3283459422 PMID: 21460643

Engle, P. L. (2009). Maternal mental health: Program and policy implications. *The American Journal of Clinical Nutrition*, *89*(3), 963S–966S. DOI: 10.3945/ajcn.2008.26692G PMID: 19176734

Estriplet, T., Morgan, I., Davis, K., Crear Perry, J., & Matthews, K. (2022). Black perinatal mental health: Prioritizing maternal mental health to optimize infant health and wellness. *Frontiers in Psychiatry, 13*, 807235. DOI: 10.3389/fpsyt.2022.807235 PMID: 35573337

Etowa, J., Nare, H., Dubula-Majola, V., Edet, O., John, M., Nkwocha, C. R., Stephens, C., Mbewu, N., Hannan, J., & Etowa, E. (2022). Male Partners' Roles in Infant Feeding Practices: Perspectives of Black Mothers Living with HIV in Three Countries. Healthcare, Falako, S., Okoli, N., Boateng, M.-O., Sandoval, J., Gumudavelly, D., Larsuel, S., & Opara, I. (2023). Utilizing community-centered approaches to address Black maternal mortality. *Health Education & Behavior, 50*(4), 500–504.

Fancourt, D., & Perkins, R. (2018). The effects of mother–infant singing on emotional closeness, affect, anxiety, and stress hormones. *Music & Science, 1*, 2059204317745746. DOI: 10.1177/2059204317745746

Fante-Coleman, T., & Jackson-Best, F. (2020). Barriers and facilitators to accessing mental healthcare in Canada for Black youth: A scoping review. *Adolescent Research Review, 5*(2), 115–136. DOI: 10.1007/s40894-020-00133-2

Firima, E., Gonzalez, L., Huber, J., Belus, J. M., Raeber, F., Gupta, R., Mokhohlane, J., Mphunyane, M., Amstutz, A., & Labhardt, N. D. (2021). Community-based models of care for management of type 2 diabetes mellitus among non-pregnant adults in sub-Saharan Africa: A scoping review protocol. *F1000 Research*, 10. PMID: 35387273

Fothergill, K. E., Ensminger, M. E., Robertson, J., Green, K. M., Thorpe, R. J., & Juon, H.-S. (2011). Effects of social integration on health: A prospective study of community engagement among African American women. *Social Science & Medicine, 72*(2), 291–298. DOI: 10.1016/j.socscimed.2010.10.024 PMID: 21131117

Franks, W., Henwood, K., & Bowden, G. (2007). Promoting maternal mental health: Women's strategies for presenting a positive identity and the implications for mental health promotion. *Journal of Public Mental Health, 6*(2), 40–51. DOI: 10.1108/17465729200700013

Fulton, J. I., Singh, H., Pakkal, O., Uleryk, E. M., & Nelson, M. L. (2022). Community-based culturally tailored education programmes for black adults with cardiovascular disease, diabetes, hypertension and stroke: A systematic review protocol of primary empirical studies. *BMJ Open, 12*(6), e059883. DOI: 10.1136/bmjopen-2021-059883 PMID: 35688600

Gholizadeh Shamasbi, S., Barkin, J. L., Ghanbari-Homayi, S., Eyvazzadeh, O., & Mirghafourvand, M. (2020). The relationship between maternal functioning and mental health after childbirth in Iranian women. *International Journal of Environmental Research and Public Health, 17*(5), 1558. DOI: 10.3390/ijerph17051558 PMID: 32121286

Glickman, C. P., Le, H.-N., Robertson, H., Arbit, R., Danielson, A., Patchen, L., Fries, M., Scott, R., & Biel, M. (2020). Black women's preferences for embedding mental health services in an obstetrics setting.

Goddard-Durant, S. K., Doucet, A., Tizaa, H., & Sieunarine, J. A. (2023). "I don't have the energy": Racial stress, young Black motherhood, and Canadian social policies. *Canadian Review of Sociology/Revue canadienne de sociologie, 60*(4), 542-566.

Greene, M. C., Huang, T. T., Giusto, A., Lovero, K. L., Stockton, M. A., Shelton, R. C., Dos Santos, P., Saúte, F., & Wainberg, M. L. (2021). Leveraging systems science to promote the implementation and sustainability of mental health and psychosocial interventions in low-and middle-income countries. *Harvard Review of Psychiatry, 29*(4), 262–277. DOI: 10.1097/HRP.0000000000000306 PMID: 34241978

Guille, C., Henrich, N., Brinson, A. K., & Jahnke, H. R. (2024). Improving the Management of Maternal Mental Health with Digital Health Care. *Psychiatric Research and Clinical Practice*, *6*(1), 23–32. DOI: 10.1176/appi.prcp.20230035 PMID: 38510485

Guruge, S., Thomson, M. S., George, U., & Chaze, F. (2015). Social support, social conflict, and immigrant women's mental health in a C anadian context: A scoping review. *Journal of Psychiatric and Mental Health Nursing*, *22*(9), 655–667. DOI: 10.1111/jpm.12216 PMID: 26031541

Harris, J. R. A. (2021). Community-based participatory research with Black churches. *Counseling and Values*, *66*(1), 2–20. DOI: 10.1002/cvj.12141

Harvey, S. T., Bennett, J. A., Burmeister, E., & Wyder, M. (2018). Evaluating a nurse-led community model of service for perinatal mental health. *Collegian (Royal College of Nursing, Australia)*, *25*(5), 525–531. DOI: 10.1016/j.colegn.2017.12.005

Hassoun Ayoub, L., Partridge, T., & Gómez, J. M. (2023). Two sides of the same coin: A mixed methods study of black mothers' experiences with violence, stressors, parenting, and coping during the COVID-19 pandemic. *The Journal of Social Issues*, *79*(2), 667–693. DOI: 10.1111/josi.12526 PMID: 36249547

Hatton-Bowers, H., Clark, C., Parra, G., Calvi, J., Bird, M. Y., Avari, P., Foged, J., & Smith, J. (2023). Promising findings that the cultivating healthy intentional mindful educators' program (CHIME) strengthens early childhood teachers' emotional resources: An iterative study. *Early Childhood Education Journal, 51*(7), 1291–1304. DOI: 10.1007/s10643-022-01386-3 PMID: 35967911

Hernandez, N. D., Dorsey, J., Glass, D. M., Pope, E., Worthy, N., Blasingame, E., Gooding, J., Braxton, P., Whitfield, M., & Dotson, Y. (2019). Community-engaged approaches to address the ethical concerns of maternal mental health disparities research. *Journal of Health Care for the Poor and Underserved, 30*(4, Suppl), 12–20. DOI: 10.1353/hpu.2019.0110 PMID: 31735713

Huang, H. Y., Li, H., & Hsu, Y. C. (2022). Coping, COVID knowledge, communication, and HBCU student's emotional well-being: Mediating role of perceived control and social connectedness. *Journal of Community Psychology, 50*(6), 2703–2725. DOI: 10.1002/jcop.22824 PMID: 35187691

Iradukunda, F., & Canty, L. (2023). Decolonizing nursing education and research to address racial disparities in maternal health. *Journal of Advanced Nursing, 79*(7), 2465–2469. DOI: 10.1111/jan.15624 PMID: 36882975

James, K. F., Klomhaus, A. M., Elliott, T., Mensah, M., Jeffers, K. S., & Choi, K. R. (2023). Structural factors in health care associated with the mental health needs of Black women in California during the perinatal period. *Journal of Obstetric, Gynecologic, and Neonatal Nursing : JOGNN, 52*(6), 481–490. DOI: 10.1016/j.jogn.2023.08.002 PMID: 37634545

Jidong, D. E., Husain, N., Roche, A., Lourie, G., Ike, T. J., Murshed, M., Park, M. S., Karick, H., Dagona, Z. K., Pwajok, J. Y., Gumber, A., Francis, C., Nyam, P. P., & Mwankon, S. B. (2021). Psychological interventions for maternal depression among women of African and Caribbean origin: A systematic review. *BMC Women's Health, 21*(1), 1–14. DOI: 10.1186/s12905-021-01202-x PMID: 33637070

Jimah, T., Borg, H., Kehoe, P., Pimentel, P., Turner, A., Labbaf, S., Asgari Mehrabadi, M., Rahmani, A. M., Dutt, N., & Guo, Y. (2021). A technology-based pregnancy health and wellness intervention (two happy hearts): Case study. *JMIR Formative Research, 5*(11), e30991. DOI: 10.2196/30991 PMID: 34787576

Johnson, A., Kirk, R., Rosenblum, K. L., & Muzik, M. (2015). Enhancing breastfeeding rates among African American women: A systematic review of current psychosocial interventions. *Breastfeeding Medicine, 10*(1), 45–62. DOI: 10.1089/bfm.2014.0023 PMID: 25423601

Johnson, A. D. R. (2020). Implicit Provider Bias and its Implications for Black/African American Mental Health. In *The International Handbook of Black Community Mental Health* (pp. 113–134). Emerald Publishing Limited. DOI: 10.1108/978-1-83909-964-920201008

Kantor, L. M., Cruz, N., Adams, C., Akhimien, C., Allibay Abdulkadir, F., Battle, C., Oluwayemi, M., Salimon, O., Won, S. H., & Niraula, S. (2023). Black Women's Maternal Health: Insights From Community Based Participatory Research in Newark, New Jersey. *Behavioral Medicine (Washington, D.C.)*, 1–8. PMID: 37382100

Kathree, T., Selohilwe, O. M., Bhana, A., & Petersen, I. (2014). Perceptions of postnatal depression and health care needs in a South African sample: The "mental" in maternal health care. *BMC Women's Health*, *14*(1), 1–11. DOI: 10.1186/s12905-014-0140-7 PMID: 25389015

Kemet, S., Yang, Y., Nseyo, O., Bell, F., Gordon, A. Y., Mays, M., Fowler, M., & Jackson, A. (2022). "When I think of mental healthcare, I think of no care." Mental Health Services as a Vital Component of Prenatal Care for Black Women. *Maternal and Child Health Journal*, *26*(4), 1–10. DOI: 10.1007/s10995-021-03226-z PMID: 34519952

Kiernan, F., Chmiel, A., Garrido, S., Hickey, M., & Davidson, J. W. (2021). The role of artistic creative activities in navigating the COVID-19 pandemic in Australia. *Frontiers in Psychology*, *12*, 696202. DOI: 10.3389/fpsyg.2021.696202 PMID: 34512453

Kozhimannil, K. B., Hardeman, R. R., Attanasio, L. B., Blauer-Peterson, C., & O'brien, M. (2013). Doula care, birth outcomes, and costs among Medicaid beneficiaries. *American Journal of Public Health*, *103*(4), e113–e121. DOI: 10.2105/AJPH.2012.301201 PMID: 23409910

Lähdepuro, A., Lahti-Pulkkinen, M., Girchenko, P., Villa, P. M., Heinonen, K., Lahti, J., Pyhälä, R., Laivuori, H., Kajantie, E., & Räikkönen, K. (2023). Positive maternal mental health during pregnancy and psychiatric problems in children from early childhood to late childhood. *Development and Psychopathology*, 1–13. PMID: 37814418

Lähdepuro, A., Lahti-Pulkkinen, M., Pyhälä, R., Tuovinen, S., Lahti, J., Heinonen, K., Laivuori, H., Villa, P. M., Reynolds, R. M., Kajantie, E., Girchenko, P., & Räikkönen, K. (2023). Positive maternal mental health during pregnancy and mental and behavioral disorders in children: A prospective pregnancy cohort study. *Journal of Child Psychology and Psychiatry, and Allied Disciplines*, *64*(5), 807–816. DOI: 10.1111/jcpp.13625 PMID: 35524467

Laister, D., Vivanti, G., Marschik, P. B., Fellinger, J., & Holzinger, D. (2021). Enhancement of social communication behaviors in young children with autism affects maternal stress. *Frontiers in Psychiatry, 12*, 797148. DOI: 10.3389/fpsyt.2021.797148 PMID: 34950076

Landor, C. (2023). Right to Informed Consent, Right to a Doula: An Evidence-Based Solution to the Black Maternal Mortality Crisis in the United States. *Michigan Journal of Gender & Law, 30*(30.1), 61. DOI: 10.36641/mjgl.30.1.right

Lê Cook, B., Doksum, T., Chen, C., Carle, A., & Alegría, M. (2013). The role of provider supply and organization in reducing racial/ethnic disparities in mental health care in the US. *Social Science & Medicine, 84*, 102–109. DOI: 10.1016/j.socscimed.2013.02.006 PMID: 23466259

Liese, K., Stewart, K., Pearson, P., Lofton, S., Mbande, T., Patil, C., Liu, L., & Geller, S. (2022). Melanated group midwifery care: Centering the voices of the Black birthing community. *Journal of Midwifery & Women's Health, 67*(6), 696–700. DOI: 10.1111/jmwh.13438 PMID: 36480019

Lindsey, M. A., & Marcell, A. V. (2012). "We're Going Through a Lot of Struggles That People Don't Even Know About" The Need to Understand African American Males' Help-Seeking for Mental Health on Multiple Levels. *American Journal of Men's Health, 6*(5), 354–364. DOI: 10.1177/1557988312441520 PMID: 22457264

Louis-Jacques, A. F., Applequist, J., Perkins, M., Williams, C., Joglekar, R., Powis, R., Daniel, A., & Wilson, R. (2024). Florida Doulas' Perspectives on Their Role in Reducing Maternal Morbidity and Health Disparities. *Women's Health Issues, 34*(4), 417–428. DOI: 10.1016/j.whi.2024.01.003 PMID: 38503681

Lowe, N. K. (2021). Black Women's Lives Matter. *Journal of Obstetric, Gynecologic, and Neonatal Nursing : JOGNN, 50*(4), 363–368. DOI: 10.1016/j.jogn.2021.06.001 PMID: 34153227

Malcome, M. L., Fedock, G., Garthe, R. C., Golder, S., Higgins, G., & Logan, T. (2019). Weathering probation and parole: The protective role of social support on Black women's recent stressful events and depressive symptoms. *The Journal of Black Psychology, 45*(8), 661–688. DOI: 10.1177/0095798419889755

Matthews, K., Morgan, I., Davis, K., Estriplet, T., Perez, S., & Crear-Perry, J. A. (2021). Pathways To Equitable And Antiracist Maternal Mental Health Care: Insights From Black Women Stakeholders: Study examines pathways to equitable and antiracist maternal mental health care. *Health Affairs, 40*(10), 1597–1604. DOI: 10.1377/hlthaff.2021.00808 PMID: 34606342

McLemore, M. R., Altman, M. R., Cooper, N., Williams, S., Rand, L., & Franck, L. (2018). Health care experiences of pregnant, birthing and postnatal women of color at risk for preterm birth. *Social Science & Medicine*, *201*, 127–135. DOI: 10.1016/j.socscimed.2018.02.013 PMID: 29494846

Mendenhall, R., Henderson, L., Scott, B., Butler, L., Turi, K. N., Greenlee, A., Robinson, G. E., Roberts, B. W., Rodriguez-Zas, S. L., & Brooks, J. E. (2020). Involving Urban Single Low-Income African American Mothers in Genomic Research: Giving Voice to How Place Matters in Health Disparities and Prevention Strategies. *Family Medicine and Primary Care — Open Access*, *4*(2). PMID: 35373191

Mitchell, G. K., Burridge, L., Zhang, J., Donald, M., Scott, I. A., Dart, J., & Jackson, C. L. (2015). Systematic review of integrated models of health care delivered at the primary–secondary interface: How effective is it and what determines effectiveness? *Australian Journal of Primary Health*, *21*(4), 391–408. DOI: 10.1071/PY14172 PMID: 26329878

Mollard, E., Elya, A., Gaines, C., Salahshurian, E., Riordan, E., Moore, T., Maloney, S., Balas, M. C., Shah, N., & Cooper Owens, D. (2024). Reclaiming narratives of empowerment around Black maternal health: A strengths-based, community-informed focus group study. *Ethnicity & Health*, *29*(6), 1–17. DOI: 10.1080/13557858.2024.2359384 PMID: 38805258

Montalmant, K. E., & Ettinger, A. K. (2023). The Racial Disparities in Maternal Mortality and Impact of Structural Racism and Implicit Racial Bias on Pregnant Black Women: A Review of the Literature. *Journal of Racial and Ethnic Health Disparities*, 1–20. PMID: 37957536

Mosley, E. A., Lindsey, A., Turner, D., Shah, P., Sayyad, A., Mack, A., & Lindberg, K. (2023). "I want… to serve those communities…[but] my price tag is… not what they can afford": The community-engaged Georgia doula study. *Perspectives on Sexual and Reproductive Health*, *55*(3), 200–209. DOI: 10.1363/psrh.12241 PMID: 37533301

Murray, K. R., Dulli, L. S., Ridgeway, K., Dal Santo, L., Darrow de Mora, D., Olsen, P., Silverstein, H., & McCarraher, D. R. (2017). Improving retention in HIV care among adolescents and adults in low-and middle-income countries: A systematic review of the literature. *PLoS One*, *12*(9), e0184879. DOI: 10.1371/journal.pone.0184879 PMID: 28961253

Nepal, A., Dangol, S. K., & van Der Kwaak, A. (2020). Improving maternal health services through social accountability interventions in Nepal: An analytical review of existing literature. *Public Health Reviews*, *41*(1), 1–24. DOI: 10.1186/s40985-020-00147-0 PMID: 33349273

Novacek, D. M., Hampton-Anderson, J. N., Ebor, M. T., Loeb, T. B., & Wyatt, G. E. (2020). Mental health ramifications of the COVID-19 pandemic for Black Americans: Clinical and research recommendations. *Psychological Trauma: Theory, Research, Practice, and Policy*, *12*(5), 449–451. DOI: 10.1037/tra0000796 PMID: 32525370

O'Donnell, K. J., & Meaney, M. J. (2017). Fetal origins of mental health: The developmental origins of health and disease hypothesis. *The American Journal of Psychiatry*, *174*(4), 319–328. DOI: 10.1176/appi.ajp.2016.16020138 PMID: 27838934

Oburota, C. S., Okungbowa, E. F., & Eke, F. A. (2023). Socioeconomic Inequalities in Maternal Health Care Utilization and Delivery Channels in Nigeria. [JPSS]. *Journal of Population and Social Studies*, *31*, 672–695. DOI: 10.25133/JPSSv312023.037

Ogunwole, S. M., Bennett, W. L., Williams, A. N., & Bower, K. M. (2020). Community-based Doulas and COVID-19: addressing structural and institutional barriers to maternal health equity.

Ogunwole, S. M., & Starks, F. D. (2024). Cultivating Critical Love to Improve Black Maternal Health Outcomes. *AMA Journal of Ethics*, *26*(1), 72–83. DOI: 10.1001/amajethics.2024.72 PMID: 38180861

Parker, A. (2021). Reframing the narrative: Black maternal mental health and culturally meaningful support for wellness. *Infant Mental Health Journal*, *42*(4), 502–516. DOI: 10.1002/imhj.21910 PMID: 33470438

Parker, A. (2022). Just Help Me: A Research Poem by Black Mothers. *Qualitative Inquiry*, *28*(10), 1092–1093. DOI: 10.1177/10778004221087684

Penner, F., Wall, K. M., Guan, K. W., Huang, H. J., Richardson, L., Dunbar, A. S., Groh, A. M., & Rutherford, H. J. (2023). Racial disparities in EEG research and their implications for our understanding of the maternal brain. *Cognitive, Affective & Behavioral Neuroscience*, *23*(1), 1–16. DOI: 10.3758/s13415-022-01040-w PMID: 36414837

Ponting, C., Urizar Jr, G. G., & Dunkel Schetter, C. (2022). Psychological interventions for prenatal anxiety in Latinas and Black women: A scoping review and recommendations. *Frontiers in Psychiatry*, *13*, 820343. DOI: 10.3389/fpsyt.2022.820343 PMID: 35370831

Prom, M. C., Denduluri, A., Philpotts, L. L., Rondon, M. B., Borba, C. P., Gelaye, B., & Byatt, N. (2022). A systematic review of interventions that integrate perinatal mental health care into routine maternal care in low-and middle-income countries. *Frontiers in Psychiatry, 13*, 859341. DOI: 10.3389/fpsyt.2022.859341 PMID: 35360136

Quick, A. D., Tung, I., Keenan, K., & Hipwell, A. E. (2023). Psychological well-being across the perinatal period: Life satisfaction and flourishing in a longitudinal study of Young Black and White American women. *Journal of Happiness Studies, 24*(3), 1283–1301. DOI: 10.1007/s10902-023-00634-6 PMID: 37273506

Rafizadeh, E. B., Rice, E., Smith, J., Bell, J., & Harvath, T. A. (2023). Understanding How Community Health Workers Build Trust with Low-Income Women of Color At-Risk for Maternal Child Health Disparities: A Grounded Theory Study. *Journal of Community Health Nursing, 40*(3), 219–231. DOI: 10.1080/07370016.2023.2168124 PMID: 36999664

Ramey-Collier, K., Jackson, M., Malloy, A., McMillan, C., Scraders-Pyatt, A., & Wheeler, S. M. (2023). Doula care: A review of outcomes and impact on birth experience. *Obstetrical & Gynecological Survey, 78*(2), 124–127. DOI: 10.1097/OGX.0000000000001103 PMID: 36786720

Reddy, S., Patel, N., Saxon, M., Amin, N., & Biviji, R. (2021). Innovations in US health care delivery to reduce disparities in maternal mortality among African American and American Indian/Alaskan Native women. *Journal of Patient-Centered Research and Reviews, 8*(2), 140–145. DOI: 10.17294/2330-0698.1793 PMID: 33898647

Ribeiro Brown, B., Williams, E.-D. G., Abelson, J. M., Chandrakapure, A., & Watkins, D. C. (2022). An Exploratory Case Study of the Types of Resources Black Boys Use to Support Their Mental Health. Healthcare, Roberts, D., Jackson, L., Davie, P., Zhao, C., Harrold, J. A., Fallon, V., & Silverio, S. A. (2023). Exploring the reasons why mothers do not breastfeed, to inform and enable better support. *Frontiers in Global Women's Health, 4*, 1148719.

Robinson, A., Davis, M., Hall, J., Lauckner, C., & Anderson, A. K. (2019). It takes an e-village: Supporting African American mothers in sustaining breastfeeding through Facebook communities. *Journal of Human Lactation, 35*(3), 569–582. DOI: 10.1177/0890334419831652 PMID: 30889373

Sackey, D., Jones, M., & Farley, R. (2021). Reconceptualising specialisation: Integrating refugee health in primary care. *Australian Journal of Primary Health, 26*(6), 452–457. DOI: 10.1071/PY20138 PMID: 33243370

Salinas, J. L., Salinas, M., & Kahn, M. (2022). Doulas, racism, and whiteness: How birth support workers process advocacy towards women of color. *Societies (Basel, Switzerland)*, *12*(1), 19. DOI: 10.3390/soc12010019

Shakibazadeh, E., Namadian, M., Bohren, M. A., Vogel, J. P., Rashidian, A., Nogueira Pileggi, V., Madeira, S., Leathersich, S., Tunçalp, ., Oladapo, O. T., Souza, J. P., & Gülmezoglu, A. M. (2018). Respectful care during childbirth in health facilities globally: A qualitative evidence synthesis. *BJOG*, *125*(8), 932–942. DOI: 10.1111/1471-0528.15015 PMID: 29117644

Shorey, S., Ng, E. D., & Downe, S. (2021). Cultural competence and experiences of maternity health care providers on care for migrant women: A qualitative meta-synthesis. *Birth (Berkeley, Calif.)*, *48*(4), 458–469. DOI: 10.1111/birt.12581 PMID: 34363236

Silas, M. J., & Seward, D. X. (2023). Black women's help-seeking and self-care strategies: A phenomenological exploration. *Journal of Counseling and Development*, *101*(2), 157–166. DOI: 10.1002/jcad.12465

Simpson, K. R. (2021). *Racism in maternity care is a public health crisis in the United States* (Vol. 46). LWW.

Smith, M. V., & Kruse-Austin, A. (2015). A gender-informed model to train community health workers in maternal mental health. *Evaluation and Program Planning*, *51*, 59–62. DOI: 10.1016/j.evalprogplan.2014.12.008 PMID: 25534578

Smith, S. A., & Blumenthal, D. S. (2012). Community Health Workers Support Community-based Participatory Research Ethics: Lessons Learned along the Research-to-Practice-to-Community Continuum. *Journal of Health Care for the Poor and Underserved*, *23*(4, Suppl), 77–87. DOI: 10.1353/hpu.2012.0156 PMID: 23124502

Surjaningrum, E. R., Minas, H., Jorm, A. F., & Kakuma, R. (2018). The feasibility of a role for community health workers in integrated mental health care for perinatal depression: A qualitative study from Surabaya, Indonesia. *International Journal of Mental Health Systems*, *12*(1), 1–16. DOI: 10.1186/s13033-018-0208-0 PMID: 29881450

Taylor, J. K. (2020). Structural racism and maternal health among Black women. *The Journal of Law, Medicine & Ethics*, *48*(3), 506–517. DOI: 10.1177/1073110520958875 PMID: 33021163

Thornicroft, G., Deb, T., & Henderson, C. (2016). Community mental health care worldwide: Current status and further developments. *World Psychiatry; Official Journal of the World Psychiatric Association (WPA)*, *15*(3), 276–286. DOI: 10.1002/wps.20349 PMID: 27717265

Tindana, P. O., Singh, J. A., Tracy, C. S., Upshur, R. E. G., Daar, A. S., Singer, P. A., Frohlich, J., & Lavery, J. V. (2007). Grand challenges in global health: Community engagement in research in developing countries. *PLoS Medicine*, *4*(9), e273. DOI: 10.1371/journal.pmed.0040273 PMID: 17850178

Tsega, D., Admas, M., Talie, A., Tsega, T. B., Birhanu, M. Y., Alemu, S., & Mengist, B. (2022). Maternity continuum care completion and its associated factors in Northwest Ethiopia. *Journal of Pregnancy*, *2022*, 2022. DOI: 10.1155/2022/1309881 PMID: 35223099

Walsh, T. B., Thomas, A., Quince, H., Buck, J., Tamkin, V., & Blackwell, D. (2023). Black fathers' contributions to maternal mental health. *Archives of Women's Mental Health*, *26*(1), 117–126. DOI: 10.1007/s00737-022-01284-y PMID: 36525158

Walter, A. W., Julce, C., Sidduri, N., Yinusa-Nyahkoon, L., Howard, J., Reichert, M., Bickmore, T., & Jack, B. W. (2020). Study protocol for the implementation of the Gabby Preconception Care System-an evidence-based, health information technology intervention for Black and African American women. *BMC Health Services Research*, *20*(1), 1–14. DOI: 10.1186/s12913-020-05726-0 PMID: 32958031

Watson, H., Harrop, D., Walton, E., Young, A., & Soltani, H. (2019). A systematic review of ethnic minority women's experiences of perinatal mental health conditions and services in Europe. *PLoS One*, *14*(1), e0210587. DOI: 10.1371/journal.pone.0210587 PMID: 30695019

Woodhead, S., Marley, C., Calia, C., Guerra, C., Reid, C., Burke, J. P., & Amos, A. (2023). Maternal Mental Health in Sub-Saharan Africa: A Systematic Review of Interventions for Common Perinatal Mental Health Disorders.

Woolhouse, H., Gartland, D., Mensah, F., & Brown, S. (2015). Maternal depression from early pregnancy to 4 years postpartum in a prospective pregnancy cohort study: Implications for primary health care. *BJOG*, *122*(3), 312–321. DOI: 10.1111/1471-0528.12837 PMID: 24844913

Chapter 9
Improving Maternal Mental Health for Black Birthing Parents Through Postpartum Caregiver Services

Chinonye Donna Egbulem
Bloomwell Health, USA

ABSTRACT

This chapter examines the critical issue of improving maternal mental health for Black birthing parents through postpartum caregiver services. The purpose of this chapter is to highlight the significance of maternal mental health, particularly among Black birthing parents who face unique challenges and disparities in healthcare. The chapter explores the impact of postpartum care and caregiver services on mitigating mental health disparities and improving maternal health outcomes. Key topics include postpartum depression, health equity, cultural competence, and the importance of community and social support networks. Additionally, the chapter discusses mental health interventions and the role of Black maternal health organizations in advocating for better healthcare access and outcomes for Black birthing parents. Through an analysis of current practices and recommendations, this chapter aims to provide a comprehensive understanding of the strategies needed to enhance maternal mental health and ensure equitable and culturally competent postpartum care.

DOI: 10.4018/979-8-3693-4272-5.ch009

INTRODUCTION

Maternal mental health is a critical aspect of overall health and well-being for mothers and their children. Black mothers, in particular, face unique challenges and disparities in maternal mental health care, which can have long-lasting impacts on both mothers and their families (Opara et al., 2020). This chapter explores how home care can be an effective strategy to improve Black maternal mental health. To fully understand and address the complexities of Black maternal mental health, it is essential to incorporate an intersectional approach. Intersectional theory, as introduced by Kimberlé Crenshaw (Crenshaw, 1989), highlights how various forms of social stratification, such as race, gender, and socioeconomic status, intersect to create unique modes of discrimination and privilege. For Black mothers, this means that their experiences of mental health are shaped not only by their gender and role as mothers but also by their racial identity and the systemic racism they encounter (Collins, 2000).

Black mothers often navigate multiple layers of oppression and bias within the healthcare system. These include racial discrimination, gender bias, and economic inequality, which collectively exacerbate their mental health challenges (Williams & Mohammed, 2013). For instance, Black women are more likely to experience higher levels of stress due to systemic racism and discrimination, both of which are significant risk factors for mental health issues such as anxiety and depression (Slaughter-Acey et al., 2019). Additionally, socioeconomic factors, including lower income levels and less access to quality healthcare, further compound these issues (Gee & Ford, 2011). By addressing the financial implications, safety concerns, health benefits, and systemic barriers, we aim to provide a comprehensive guide to best practices in this crucial area.

TAILORED TLC: THE POWER OF PERSONALIZED HOME CARE FOR BLACK MOTHERS

Home care refers to health and supportive care provided in the patient's home by healthcare professionals, including nurses, therapists, and aides. This model of care offers an alternative to traditional hospital or clinic settings, allowing patients to receive personalized and continuous care in a familiar and comfortable environment.

One of the primary benefits of home care is the ability to provide personalized and culturally competent care. For Black mothers, culturally sensitive care can make a significant difference in their mental health outcomes. Home care allows for tailored support that meets the specific needs of each mother, considering her cultural background, personal preferences, and unique challenges (Walker et al.,

2021). Ecological Systems Theory, proposed by Urie Bronfenbrenner, is instrumental in analyzing the multiple layers of environmental influences on an individual's development. This theory considers the microsystem (family, home care providers), mesosystem (interactions between family and caregivers), exosystem (community resources, workplace policies), macrosystem (cultural beliefs, societal norms), and chronosystem (changes over time) (Bronfenbrenner, 1979). By applying this theory, one can better understand how various factors at different levels affect Black perinatal mental health.

Consider the case of Lisa, a 29-year-old Black mother of two living in a predominantly white neighborhood. After the birth of her second child, Lisa experienced severe postpartum depression. Despite seeking help from her primary care physician, she felt misunderstood and unsupported due to the lack of cultural sensitivity in her care. When Lisa began receiving home care services tailored to her cultural background, the changes were profound. Her home care provider, trained in cultural competency, understood the historical and systemic issues contributing to Lisa's mental health struggles. This provider offered personalized therapy sessions, incorporating coping strategies that resonated with Lisa's experiences and cultural context. By tailoring support to Lisa's unique needs, her mental health began to improve, demonstrating the power of personalized home care (Smith et al., 2020).

Cultural competency is essential in providing effective care for Black mothers. Home care providers must be trained to understand and respect the cultural differences and experiences of Black mothers, which involves being aware of historical and systemic issues that contribute to mental health disparities (Williams & Mohammed, 2013). Providing culturally competent care helps build trust and ensures that mothers feel understood and supported. This competency involves recognizing the impact of past traumas, systemic racism, and the unique stressors that Black mothers face, thereby offering a more empathetic and effective care approach.

In Lisa's case, her home care provider also played a critical role in building trust. Establishing a trusting relationship between the caregiver and the mother is crucial for effective home care. Consistent and reliable support from caregivers helps mothers feel safe and secure, which can significantly improve mental health outcomes (Taylor et al., 2019). Over time, Lisa developed a strong bond with her home care provider, feeling comfortable enough to share her deepest concerns and fears. This open communication allowed her caregiver to understand better and address her needs, creating a therapeutic alliance that was essential for Lisa's recovery.

CASE STUDY: LISA'S HEALING JOURNEY THROUGH CULTURALLY RESPONSIVE POSTPARTUM HOME CARE

Background

Lisa, a 29-year-old Black woman and mother of two, lived with her partner and children in a predominantly white suburb in the southeastern United States. After the birth of her second child, she began experiencing symptoms consistent with **Postpartum Depression (PPD)** - persistent sadness, social withdrawal, fatigue, difficulty bonding with her infant, and intrusive thoughts related to inadequacy and fear of failure.

Despite having private insurance and access to healthcare, Lisa's initial postpartum care experience left her feeling dismissed and misunderstood. During a six-week postpartum check-up, she reported low mood and overwhelming anxiety. Her provider responded with a brief screening and advised "getting more rest" and "practicing gratitude." No referral for therapy was made, and cultural stressors were not explored.

Figure 1. **Missed Opportunities in Traditional Postpartum Care**

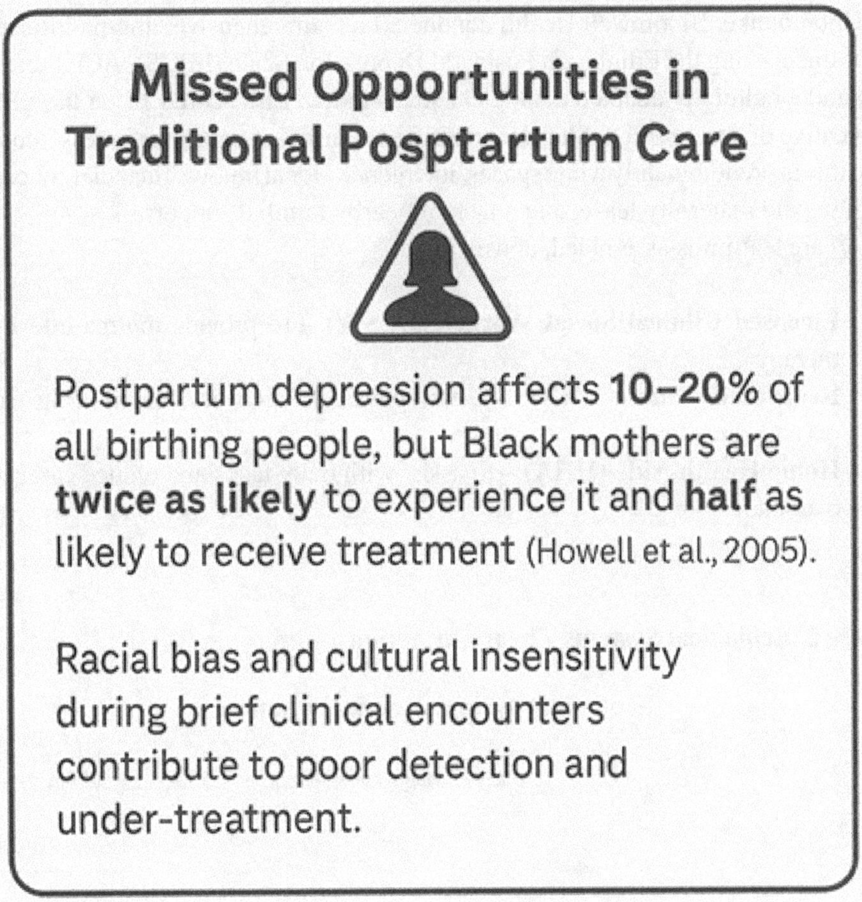

- Postpartum depression affects 10–20% of all birthing people, but Black mothers are **twice as likely to experience it** and **half as likely to receive treatment** (Howell et al., 2005).
- Racial bias and cultural insensitivity during brief clinical encounters contribute to **poor detection and under-treatment**.

Referral to Culturally Responsive Home Care

Lisa learned about *Bloomwell Health*, a local agency offering integrated home-based mental health and maternal care, through an online support group for Black mothers. She was referred by a doula affiliated with a community-based perinatal justice collective.

Upon intake, Bloomwell Health conducted a comprehensive, trauma-informed assessment using the Edinburgh Postnatal Depression Scale (EPDS), ACEs screening, and a culturally adapted ecological stress index. Lisa scored 18 on the EPDS (indicative of severe PPD). She also identified significant sources of stress: feeling invisible in predominantly white spaces, intergenerational trauma, financial concerns from unpaid maternity leave, and a lack of nearby familial support.

A care team was assembled, consisting of:

- **Licensed Clinical Social Worker (LCSW)** – to provide trauma-informed therapy.
- **Registered Nurse (RN)** – for physical recovery monitoring and psychoeducation.
- **Home Health Aide (HHA)** – to assist with daily tasks and reduce caregiver overload.

Figure 2. **Ecological Systems Theory in Action**

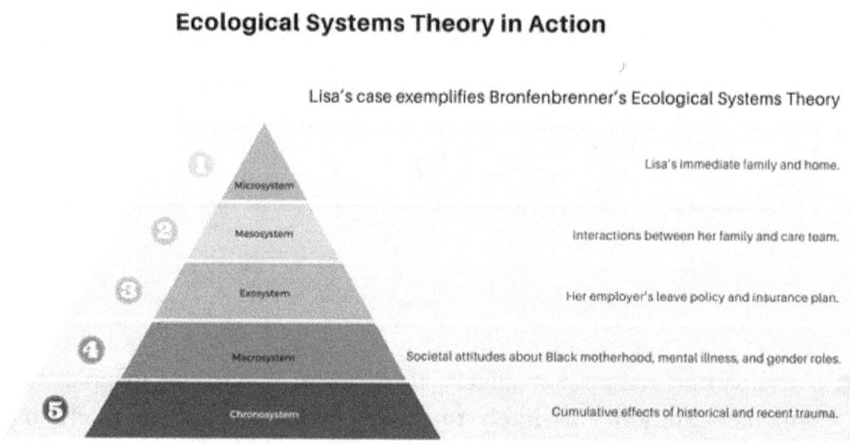

Lisa's case exemplifies Bronfenbrenner's **Ecological Systems Theory**:

- **Microsystem**: Her immediate family and home.
- **Mesosystem**: Interactions between her family and care team.

- **Exosystem**: Her employer's leave policy and insurance plan.
- **Macrosystem**: Societal attitudes about Black motherhood, mental illness, and gender roles.
- **Chronosystem**: Cumulative effects of historical and recent trauma.

Therapeutic Intervention and Home-Based Support

Over 16 weeks, Lisa received **weekly in-home therapy sessions** focused on:

- Naming and processing racialized trauma and microaggressions.
- Reframing perfectionist narratives rooted in "strong Black woman" expectations.
- Building emotional regulation strategies.
- Enhancing partner communication and co-parenting dynamics.

The LCSW employed Narrative Therapy, Cognitive Behavioral Therapy (CBT), and culturally adapted mindfulness exercises (e.g., affirmations rooted in African diasporic traditions).

The RN monitored Lisa's healing from a prior C-section, offered psychoeducation on hormonal changes, lactation support, and educated Lisa's partner on signs of postpartum mood disorders.

The HHA provided 10 hours per week of household support, including meal preparation, infant care, and light cleaning, giving Lisa consistent space to rest, shower, write in a journal, or nap without guilt.

Figure 3. **What Worked for Lisa**

What Worked for Lisa

- Home care was **non-judgmental, convenient, and culturally affirming**.
- Providers acknowledged **historical trauma and systemic racism**.
- The interdisciplinary team **worked collaboratively** and respected Lisa's autonomy.
- Services **included her partner**, improving overall family wellness.
- Community-based care reduced feelings of **isolation and invisibility**.

- Home care was **non-judgmental, convenient, and culturally affirming**.
- Providers acknowledged **historical trauma and systemic racism**.

- The interdisciplinary team **worked collaboratively** and respected Lisa's autonomy.
- Services **included her partner**, improving overall family wellness.
- Community-based care reduced feelings of **isolation and invisibility**.

Outcomes After 4 Months of Home-Based Care

Lisa's symptoms steadily improved:

- Her EPDS score decreased from 18 to 6.
- She resumed light part-time work at her own pace, reporting renewed confidence and reduced fatigue.
- She expressed a stronger attachment to her baby and increased satisfaction in her partnership.
- She began co-facilitating a peer support group for other Black mothers in her community.

Lisa reported that having someone *"who looked like me, talked like me, and just got it"* was critical to her healing. The trust built in her own living room created a therapeutic alliance far stronger than her prior clinic-based experience.

Figure 4. **Clinical and Policy Implications**

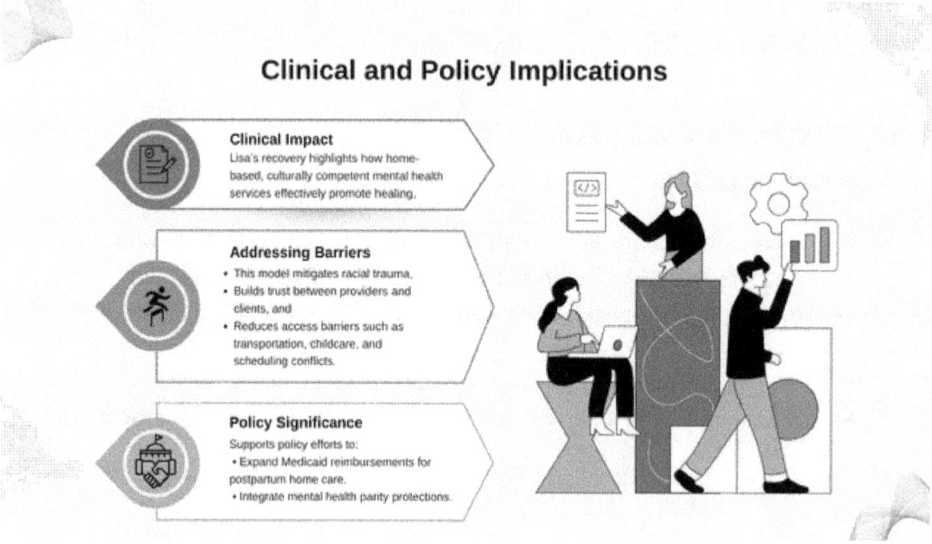

- Lisa's recovery underscores the **effectiveness of home-based, culturally competent mental health services**.
- The model **mitigates racial trauma**, builds trust, and reduces access barriers like transportation, childcare, and scheduling.
- It supports **policy efforts** to expand Medicaid reimbursements for postpartum home care and integrate mental health parity protections.

Lisa's case exemplifies how culturally competent, interdisciplinary home care can provide a lifeline for Black birthing parents navigating postpartum depression. Her story reinforces the need for a systems-level approach to maternal mental health—one that honors lived experience, prioritizes equity, and leverages the healing potential of community-based care.

By aligning clinical best practices with cultural responsiveness, agencies like Bloomwell Health offer a roadmap toward justice-centered postpartum recovery.

POSTPARTUM PALS: ALLEVIATING HEALTH DISPARITIES WITH CAREGIVER SUPPORT

Home care presents a promising solution for Black mothers by providing a supportive, familiar, and controlled environment for mental health services. Traditional healthcare settings often pose barriers such as racial biases and a lack of culturally competent care (Thornton et al., 2017). In these settings, Black mothers may encounter providers who do not fully understand or empathize with their unique experiences, leading to suboptimal care and negative health outcomes.

Case Vignette: *After giving birth to her first child, Tamika found herself battling insomnia and persistent sadness. When she visited a clinic, the provider dismissed her concerns as "typical new mom fatigue." But when a home care nurse began visiting weekly, she finally felt seen. The nurse, a Black woman from Tamika's neighborhood, listened closely and connected her with a therapist trained in culturally responsive care. Within weeks, Tamika reported sleeping better and feeling less isolated.*

Home care addresses these issues by fostering better communication and trust between caregivers and patients through a more personalized and culturally sensitive approach.

Financially, home care can be more cost-effective than hospital-based care, reducing the financial burden on Black families. Hospital stays and frequent clinic visits can be prohibitively expensive. Home care allows for more flexible payment structures, including the possibility of utilizing community-based funding or sliding scale fees (Byrd et al., 2020).

Example: *A local mutual aid fund helped offset the cost of postpartum support for Jazmine, a single mother of two. Her care team coordinated through home visits, eliminating the need for costly transportation or time off work. With a sliding-scale model, she could receive therapy and newborn support without going into debt.*

Receiving care in a familiar home environment enhances feelings of safety and security, crucial for mental health recovery (Beck et al., 2006). Hospital environments, often perceived as sterile and intimidating, can exacerbate vulnerability and anxiety among Black mothers. In contrast, home care offers a sense of comfort and control.

Anecdote: *Keisha described her home visits as a "lifeline" during her postpartum depression. "The baby blues were one thing, but the way they kept brushing me off at the clinic made me feel invisible," she shared. "At home, I could be in pajamas, breastfeeding, and just talk to someone who got it."*

INTERDISCIPLINARY SUPPORT IN INTEGRATED FAMILY HOME CARE

Licensed caregivers who can provide interdisciplinary support within an integrated family support system include Licensed Practical Nurses (LPNs), Registered Nurses (RNs), Nurse Practitioners (NPs), Licensed Clinical Social Workers (LCSWs), and Home Health Aides (HHAs). Home care integrates support for the entire family, not just the mother. This holistic approach ensures that all family members are included in the care plan, creating a cohesive and supportive environment. This integration helps address the unique needs of each family member, fostering an inclusive atmosphere that promotes collective well-being (Williams & Sternthal, 2010). LPNs play a crucial role by providing basic medical care under the supervision of RNs and doctors, which includes administering medication, monitoring vital signs, and assisting with daily living activities. Their involvement helps ensure the health and safety of family members, reducing stress on the primary caregivers.

RNs perform advanced medical procedures, create care plans, and educate families about health conditions. They offer comprehensive health assessments and tailored education on health management, empowering families to make informed decisions about their care. Nurse Practitioners (NPs) can diagnose and treat illnesses, prescribe medications, and provide advanced health education and counseling. Their specialized care and ability to manage chronic conditions enhance the family's overall health management strategy.

Illustration: *When Brianna returned home after a complicated delivery, she was recovering from a C-section and managing a toddler with autism. A care team coordinated her services: an RN provided wound care, while a licensed social* *worker offered parenting support and connected her with an early intervention program for her older child.*

Each provider type plays a unique role.

- **LPNs** administer medications and monitor vitals.
- **RNs** assess health and provide education.
- **NPs** diagnose, prescribe, and counsel.
- **LCSWs** connect families to resources and provide therapy.
- **HHAs** assist with personal care and household tasks.

Parental education is another critical component. Home care providers can offer valuable education and resources to parents, helping them navigate the challenges of parenthood. This includes guidance on child development, parenting strategies, and mental health support, empowering parents to create a nurturing environment for their children. Educating parents not only enhances their confidence in managing family dynamics but also equips them with tools to address potential challenges effectively (Teti, 2007). Licensed Clinical Social Workers (LCSWs) provide mental health support, counseling, and connect families with community resources, further contributing to the holistic support system.

Case Snapshot: *Carlos and Dana, both working-class parents, struggled with managing their newborn's sleep schedule. A home visiting nurse coached them on infant routines and developmental milestones, which helped reduce stress and improve their child's sleep—allowing Dana to sleep more too, easing her postpartum anxiety.*

ROLE OF HOME CARE IN FOSTERING A SUPPORTIVE FAMILY ENVIRONMENT

Safety - both perceived and actual - is a critical social determinant of health. Chronic safety concerns elevate cortisol levels and can trigger or worsen mental health conditions (Schneiderman et al., 2005). Home care services can reduce stress by making the home a safer and more empowering space.

Home Health Aides (HHAs) assist with daily personal care needs such as bathing, dressing, and mobility, under the supervision of nursing staff. Their support ensures that routine tasks are managed effectively, allowing primary caregivers to focus on more complex aspects of family care. By providing practical assistance with daily tasks and childcare, home care reduces the burden on mothers, allowing them to focus on their mental health and well-being. This support alleviates stress and enhances the overall quality of life for the entire family. Practical assistance from home care providers can include meal preparation, household chores, and supervision of children's activities, which collectively contribute to a more relaxed and harmonious home environment (Baker & Iruka, 2013).

Vignette: *Monique lived in a high-crime neighborhood. She rarely left her apartment after dark. Her home care provider helped install new door locks, arranged a security light through the landlord, and provided basic emergency preparedness training. "Just knowing someone was looking out for us made all the difference," she said.*

Additionally, home care can facilitate connections with community resources and support networks. Caregivers can assess hazards and provide safety education, especially in under-resourced communities (McEwen, 2004). These connections provide additional layers of support, helping families access services and opportunities that contribute to their overall well-being. Establishing strong community ties can offer families a broader safety net, ensuring they receive comprehensive support beyond the immediate home care services (Collins et al., 2010). Parental education is also key. Providers can equip families with skills in child development and mental health support (Teti, 2007).

Preventive Snapshot: *During a routine check, a visiting nurse noticed medications were stored within a toddler's reach and a loose stair railing posed a fall risk. She promptly educated the family on safe storage and referred them to a housing repair grant program.*

Stress reduction strategies and emotional support are part of holistic safety. Home care providers are trained to recognize distress and refer families to appropriate services (Cohen et al., 2007).

Example: *Ayana's care team noticed she grew withdrawn and tearful during routine check-ins. Rather than dismissing it, her nurse gently asked questions and referred her to a therapist. Ayana later shared that this early recognition "saved her from slipping into a deeper hole."*

The physiological effects of stress underscore why perceived safety is so important. Long-term exposure to unsafe environments can cause allostatic load, HPA axis disruption, and immune suppression (Miller et al., 2007; McEwen & Seeman, 1999).

Resilience in Action: *For the Jackson family, weekly home visits from a trauma-informed team helped reduce the effects of chronic stress. Their caseworker helped them develop routines, secure food access, and enroll in a parenting support group, all of which helped regulate stress and improve family dynamics.*

A PATH TOWARD EQUITY AND HEALING

An intersectional approach is crucial for understanding the challenges faced by Black mothers. Home care, by being adaptable, culturally competent, and community-rooted, emerges as a vital strategy in reducing health disparities.

Closing Portrait: *Tasha, a 32-year-old mother of three, was hesitant about letting anyone into her home. But over time, her care team became like family. "They didn't just check my blood pressure," she said. "They asked how I was really doing. They helped me believe I could keep going."*

Home care, especially when interdisciplinary and culturally responsive, is not just a service- it is an act of justice, healing, and hope for Black mothers and their families.

ROLE OF HOME CARE IN FOSTERING A SUPPORTIVE FAMILY ENVIRONMENT

Safety, both actual and perceived, is a critical social determinant of health that profoundly affects mental and physiological well-being, especially for Black families. The historical and systemic challenges faced by Black communities have created environments where safety concerns are heightened, impacting the overall health of Black families in unique and profound ways. Actual safety refers to tangible measures that protect individuals from harm, while perceived safety is the individual's sense of security within their environment. These elements can significantly influence stress hormone levels, particularly cortisol, which, when chronically elevated, can lead to a variety of health issues (Schneiderman, Ironson, & Siegel, 2005). Home care services can play a pivotal role in addressing these safety concerns and promoting better health outcomes.

Creating a safe home environment involves thorough hazard assessments, safety education, and the implementation of preventive measures. For Black families, who may reside in neighborhoods with higher crime rates and fewer resources, these measures are even more critical. Home care providers can play an essential role in identifying and mitigating potential dangers such as unsecured windows, inadequate lighting, and other hazards that might be more prevalent in underserved communities (McEwen, 2004) by ensuring these physical aspects of safety, home care providers help to prevent accidents and injuries, thus reducing stress and anxiety levels for Black mothers and their families.

Safety education is another vital component of creating a secure home environment. Educating Black families about best practices for maintaining safety, such as fire safety protocols, safe storage of medications, and emergency preparedness, empowers them to take proactive steps in safeguarding their homes. This education not only enhances actual safety but also contributes to perceived safety, as families feel more confident and secure in their ability to handle potential hazards (Taylor & Stanton, 2007). The knowledge and skills gained from safety education provided by home care services can have long-lasting benefits, fostering a culture of safety and prevention within the home.

Preventive measures, such as installing security systems, ensuring adequate lighting, and creating emergency plans, are essential for enhancing home safety. These measures provide physical safeguards that protect against accidents and injuries, thereby reducing the risk of stress-related health issues (Karatsoreos & McEwen, 2011). For Black mothers, knowing that these preventive measures are in place can alleviate anxiety and create a sense of control over their environment, further contributing to perceived safety. This is particularly important in neighborhoods where external threats to safety are more common, and home care providers are instrumental in implementing these measures.

The lack of safety, whether real or perceived, triggers the body's stress response, leading to elevated levels of cortisol and other stress hormones. Chronic stress and high cortisol levels are associated with numerous health issues, including mental health disorders such as anxiety and depression, as well as physical health problems like cardiovascular disease, immune dysfunction, and metabolic disorders (Miller, Chen, & Zhou, 2007). High cortisol levels can also impair cognitive functions, affecting memory, decision-making, and emotional regulation. These adverse effects highlight the importance of maintaining both actual and perceived safety to protect against the detrimental impacts of chronic stress on Black families. Home care providers can significantly contribute to reducing these stress levels by creating a secure and supportive environment.

Home care providers play a crucial role in supporting mental health by creating a safe and supportive home environment. Their responsibilities extend beyond physical safety to include recognizing signs of distress and providing appropriate interventions. This might involve referrals to mental health professionals or offering emotional support to Black mothers who may be struggling with stress or anxiety (Cohen, Janicki-Deverts, & Miller, 2007). By addressing both physical and emotional needs, home care providers help to create a holistic approach to safety and well-being that is particularly beneficial for Black families facing systemic inequities.

Perceived safety is equally important as actual safety in promoting mental health. For Black families, perceived safety can be influenced by the broader societal context, including experiences of racism and discrimination. Knowing that their home is a secure and supportive place allows Black mothers to focus on their well-being and their family's needs without the constant fear of potential hazards (Ross & Mirowsky, 2001). This sense of security can reduce overall stress levels, leading to lower cortisol production and better physiological health. Home care providers can foster this sense of perceived safety by building trusting relationships with the families they serve and demonstrating consistent, reliable support.

The physiological impact of safety extends to several bodily systems. Chronic exposure to stress due to a lack of safety can disrupt the hypothalamic-pituitary-adrenal (HPA) axis, leading to a state of allostatic load where the body's stress response becomes dysregulated (McEwen & Seeman, 1999). This dysregulation can cause a range of health issues, including hypertension, insulin resistance, and atherosclerosis. Additionally, chronic stress can weaken the immune system, making individuals more susceptible to infections and illnesses (Segerstrom & Miller, 2004). These physiological consequences underscore the importance of maintaining a safe environment to support overall health, particularly for Black families who may face additional stressors related to systemic inequality. Home care providers are key in mitigating these risks by ensuring both physical and emotional safety within the home.

Furthermore, the historical context of discrimination and systemic racism has contributed to environments where Black families often experience heightened safety concerns. These issues can exacerbate stress and negatively impact mental health. Addressing these broader societal factors is crucial for improving the overall health and safety of Black families (Shields & Wailoo, 2002). Community-based interventions and policy changes that focus on reducing systemic barriers to safety and improving neighborhood conditions can play a significant role in enhancing both actual and perceived safety for Black families. Home care services, integrated with community support, can be a powerful force in driving these changes.

Finally, the interplay between safety and health highlights the need for comprehensive training for home care providers. Caregivers must be well-versed in safety protocols, emergency handling, and recognizing signs of mental distress to support Black mothers and their families effectively. Proper training ensures that home care is both safe and effective, addressing the multifaceted needs of families (Shields & Wailoo, 2002). This holistic approach not only enhances actual and perceived safety but also promotes better mental and physiological health outcomes, demonstrating the profound impact of safety on overall well-being. Home care providers, through their dedicated efforts, can make a significant difference in the lives of Black families by ensuring their homes are sanctuaries of safety and health.

THE HEALTH BENEFITS OF HOME CARE FOR CHILDREN

The health and well-being of children are closely linked to their mother's mental health. Home care provides numerous health benefits for children, contributing to their overall development and well-being.

Children who receive care at home are less exposed to illnesses compared to those in daycare settings. This is particularly important during the first three years of life when the immune system is still developing. Studies have shown that children in home care environments tend to have reduced illness rates, leading to fewer healthcare visits and better overall health outcomes (Smith et al., 2018). The decreased exposure to communicable diseases in a home setting can significantly enhance a child's early health profile.

Home care also supports better long-term health and development for children. A stable and nurturing home environment fosters cognitive, emotional, and social development. Research indicates that children who receive care at home are more likely to thrive and reach their developmental milestones (Johnson & Molineux, 2020). The continuous and personalized attention they receive helps in the development of strong emotional bonds and a sense of security, which are crucial for healthy growth.

Home care providers can ensure that children receive timely immunizations and preventive care. This proactive approach helps protect children from common illnesses and promotes overall health. Regular monitoring and care at home contribute to a healthier start in life (Anderson et al., 2017). Parents or caregivers at home are typically more vigilant and consistent with healthcare routines, including vaccinations, which play a critical role in disease prevention.

Family bonding is essential for the emotional and psychological well-being of both mothers and children. Home care facilitates more quality time together, strengthening family relationships and support networks. The close proximity and constant interaction provide opportunities for meaningful engagements, such as playtime, reading, and shared routines, which foster bonding and emotional connection (Thompson & Raikes, 2019). This intimate setting helps build a strong foundation for the child's development.

Home care allows for more meaningful interactions and bonding time between mothers and their children. This strengthens family relationships and creates a supportive environment that promotes mental health and well-being. The consistent presence of a caregiver in the home environment ensures that mothers receive ongoing support, reducing feelings of isolation and stress. This continuity of care fosters a sense of stability and security for both the mother and her children (Perry et al., 2016). Furthermore, home care encourages open and effective communication between mothers and caregivers, ensuring that the mother's needs and concerns are addressed promptly. This collaborative approach enhances the overall care experience and strengthens the mother-child relationship.

The presence of a parent during the early years of a child's life is crucial for emotional security. Children who feel secure and attached to their parents are more likely to develop healthy emotional and social skills, which are essential for their overall well-being (Sroufe et al., 2005). Parental involvement in early childhood has also been shown to impact cognitive development positively. Engaging children in stimulating activities, such as reading and playing educational games, can enhance their learning and intellectual growth. Additionally, children who have strong bonds with their parents are less likely to exhibit behavioral problems. The guidance and support provided by a present parent help children develop appropriate behaviors and coping mechanisms (Steinberg, 2001).

Parental presence can also contribute to better physical health outcomes for children. Mothers who are actively involved in their children's lives are more likely to ensure they receive proper nutrition, immunizations, and preventive care (Bowlby, 1982). The holistic benefits of parental presence and home care are evident in various aspects of a child's development, emphasizing the importance of supportive home environments.

LONG-TERM ECONOMIC BENEFITS OF FAMILIES RECEIVING HOME CARE

The financial implications of home care extend beyond immediate cost savings, leading to broader economic benefits for families and society. This is particularly relevant for Black birthing parents, who face unique challenges and disparities in maternal health outcomes.

Economic Benefits of Improved Maternal Mental Health

Mothers who receive adequate mental health support are more likely to return to work, contribute to the economy, and achieve financial independence. This reduces the burden on social services and healthcare systems. A report by the London School of Economics found that investing in maternal mental health services can yield substantial economic returns through increased productivity and reduced healthcare costs (Bauer et al., 2014).

For Black birthing parents, the economic benefits are even more significant due to the disproportionate impact of systemic barriers and health disparities. Black mothers are more likely to experience mental health issues related to stress, discrimination, and socioeconomic challenges (Thomas et al., 2020). Adequate mental health support can help mitigate these effects, leading to better job retention and career advancement. This, in turn, contributes to financial stability and reduces reliance on public assistance programs (Kozhimannil et al., 2011).

Cost Reduction through Preventive Care

Home care services provide preventive care, addressing mental health issues before they become severe, thus significantly reducing healthcare costs. Early intervention and continuous support prevent costly emergency interventions and long-term treatments, benefiting individual families and reducing the strain on the healthcare system. The World Health Organization notes that preventive mental health care can lower overall healthcare expenditure by reducing the incidence of chronic conditions linked to mental health issues (WHO, 2013).

For Black birthing parents, who often face barriers to accessing quality healthcare, home care can offer a more accessible and culturally sensitive option. Preventive care through home care can help address health disparities by providing timely and appropriate support, ultimately reducing the need for more expensive and intensive healthcare services (Roberts et al., 2020).

Enhanced Workforce Participation

Home care facilitates effective recovery and management of maternal mental health, enabling a smoother return to work. Financial independence and the ability to contribute to household income improve overall family well-being. Employers benefit from reduced absenteeism and increased productivity when mothers receive adequate mental health support. The National Partnership for Women & Families highlights that supporting maternal mental health can lead to higher workforce participation and productivity (NPWF, 2018).

Black birthing parents often face additional challenges in the workforce, including discrimination and a lack of support. Home care can provide the necessary mental health support to navigate these challenges, leading to improved job performance and career growth (Hankerson et al., 2018). This enhanced workforce participation not only benefits individual families but also contributes to a more diverse and inclusive economy.

Savings on Daycare Expenses

Daycare expenses can be a substantial burden for families, especially those with multiple children or limited financial resources. Home care offers an alternative that alleviates these financial pressures while providing mental health benefits for mothers. The Economic Policy Institute reports that the average annual cost of daycare for an infant in the United States is about $11,000, varying significantly by state (EPI, 2020). Home care can be more cost-effective, considering the added benefits of personalized support and reduced healthcare expenses.

For Black families, who are more likely to face economic challenges, saving on daycare expenses can make a significant difference (Morrissey, 2017). By reducing these costs, families can allocate their resources to other critical needs, such as education, healthcare, and housing, which are essential for long-term stability and growth.

Improved Financial Stability

By reducing or eliminating daycare costs, home care allows families to allocate their budget towards other essential needs, such as healthcare, education, and household expenses. Financial stability is crucial for improving maternal mental health, as it reduces stress and anxiety related to economic pressures. Studies show that financial strain is a significant predictor of maternal depression and anxiety (Gjerdingen & Center, 2003).

For Black birthing parents, financial stability is particularly important due to the systemic economic inequalities they often face. Home care can provide a buffer against these financial pressures, leading to better mental health outcomes and overall well-being for the entire family (Novoa & Taylor, 2018).

Long-Term Financial Impact

Reducing daycare expenses and other related costs through home care significantly impacts a family's financial stability. With more disposable income, families can invest in their well-being and future, creating a secure and supportive environment for their children. Financial stability is closely linked to mental health, making it a critical component of comprehensive maternal care. Research indicates that financial stress is strongly correlated with adverse mental health outcomes, including depression and anxiety (Butterworth et al., 2012).

For Black families, long-term financial stability can break cycles of poverty and improve future opportunities for children (Jones et al., 2019). Home care not only addresses immediate needs but also supports sustainable economic growth and health equity.

In conclusion, home care provides immediate cost savings. It promotes long-term economic benefits by improving maternal mental health, reducing healthcare costs through preventive care, enhancing workforce participation, saving on daycare expenses, and improving overall financial stability. These factors are especially critical for Black birthing parents, who face unique challenges and disparities. By addressing these issues, home care contributes to a more equitable and economically stable society.

BRIDGING THE FINANCIAL GAP: A CASE STUDY HIGHLIGHTING COVERAGE FOR AFFORDABLE POSTPARTUM CARE SOLUTIONS

Meet Briana, a young mother living in North Carolina, who found herself juggling the demands of a newborn, her job, and the financial stress of daycare costs. Despite qualifying for daycare vouchers and TANF, Briana still struggled to make ends meet. The financial support she received wasn't enough to cover the full cost of quality childcare, leaving her anxious and overwhelmed.

Like many families, Briana faced the inadequacies of current financial support systems. The financial gaps in daycare vouchers, TANF, and other social services placed significant burdens on her and her family. Recognizing these challenges, policymakers began to address these gaps through increased funding and expanded eligibility, ensuring that more families like Briana's could afford quality childcare. This shift not only promoted better developmental outcomes for children but also reduced stress for parents.

Briana decided to invest in a postpartum caregiver, which brought numerous benefits to her family. Her daughter, Emma, had less exposure to germs compared to a daycare environment, which was crucial for her developing immune system. Additionally, the reliable and trained caregiver significantly reduced Briana's mental and emotional burden, allowing her to focus on her recovery and mental health.

Understanding the financial implications of home care was vital for Briana. While it initially seemed more expensive than traditional daycare options, the long-term benefits and potential cost savings made it a more economical choice. Home care reduced costs associated with hospital stays, emergency visits, and other healthcare expenses. By providing continuous and preventive care at home, Briana was less likely to experience severe mental health crises that required costly interventions. The flexibility and adaptability of home care also suited her family's financial situation better.

Systems theory, which looks at the interconnections between different parts of a system, can help us understand how various aspects of home care—personalized care, financial implications, and safety—interact to affect Briana's mental health. This holistic view emphasized the importance of considering the whole picture and how changes in one part of the system could impact others.

Briana explored her insurance options and discovered that many plans now offer coverage for home care services, recognizing their value in improving health outcomes. Subsidies and financial assistance programs were also available to help offset the costs of home care. Prenatal and postpartum nursing home health aide services were accessible through Medicaid and the Children's Health Insurance Program (CHIP) when deemed medically necessary or clinically appropriate—this provision aimed to address maternal health needs and improve outcomes for both mothers and infants.

Extended postpartum Medicaid and CHIP coverage for up to 12 months in states like North Carolina ensured that Briana received the necessary support during the critical postpartum period. This coverage was part of broader efforts to improve maternal health outcomes and reduce maternal mortality and morbidity. These services were crucial for recovery from childbirth, addressing delivery complications, ensuring mental health support, managing infant care, and transitioning from obstetric to primary care.

Investing in early mental health intervention through home care led to significant long-term financial benefits for Briana. Improved maternal mental health enhanced her productivity, reduced absenteeism from work, and decreased the need for future medical treatments. These benefits extended beyond Briana to her entire family, contributing to overall financial stability and well-being.

Briana's story highlights the importance of understanding the financial implications of home care for making informed decisions about maternal mental health services. While home care may initially seem more expensive than traditional care options, the long-term benefits and potential cost savings make it a more economical choice for families like Briana's.

CONCLUSION

Home care has the potential to bridge significant gaps in healthcare access, especially for underserved Black mothers. By providing care directly in the home, home care minimizes barriers such as transportation, childcare, and financial constraints, ensuring that more mothers can receive the support they need. This approach is particularly effective in addressing the unique challenges faced by Black mothers, who often encounter systemic obstacles within the traditional healthcare system. Bringing care to their doorstep not only improves access but also enhances the quality of care, leading to better health outcomes for both mothers and their children.

The Social Determinants of Health framework is instrumental in understanding and addressing the broader systemic issues that affect maternal mental health. This framework highlights the importance of considering social, economic, and environmental conditions that influence health outcomes. By addressing these determinants, such as healthcare access disparities and economic barriers, we can create a more equitable healthcare system that supports the mental health of all mothers. Implementing home care within this framework can lead to more comprehensive and effective strategies for improving maternal mental health.

Advocacy for policy changes is essential to promote home care as a viable option for maternal mental health. Efforts must be made to increase funding, expand insurance coverage, and recognize home care as an essential service. Policymakers need to understand the critical role that home care can play in supporting maternal mental health and the long-term benefits it provides for families. By advocating for these changes, we can create a supportive infrastructure that allows home care services to thrive and reach those who need them the most.

Community engagement and education are also crucial components in promoting the benefits of home care. By engaging communities and providing education about the advantages of home care, we can drive demand and support for these services. Community initiatives can help raise awareness, reduce stigma, and encourage more families to utilize home care. These efforts can create a more informed and supportive community, where families feel empowered to seek out and benefit from home care services.

The chapter highlights the numerous benefits of home care, including personalized care, financial implications, safety, health benefits for children, and enhanced family bonding time. Stakeholders, including healthcare providers, policymakers, and community organizations, are called upon to support and implement these best practices. Collaborative efforts are essential to create a supportive infrastructure for home care services. The vision for the future includes a healthcare system that prioritizes maternal mental health, recognizes the value of home care, and ensures that all mothers have access to the support they need to thrive. Through these collective efforts, we can build a healthier, more equitable future for Black mothers and their children.

REFERENCES

Ammerman, R. T., Putnam, F. W., Altaye, M., Chen, L., Holleb, L. J., Stevens, J., & Van Ginkel, J. B. (2010). Changes in depressive symptoms in first-time mothers in home visitation. *Child Abuse & Neglect, 34*(9), 639–649. PMID: 20638720

Anderson, K., Thompson, L., & Raikes, H. (2017). Home-based care and early childhood development. *Journal of Child Health Care, 21*(3), 270–280.

Baker, C. E., & Iruka, I. U. (2013). Supporting families in home-based care. *Early Childhood Research Quarterly, 28*(4), 784–794.

Baker, C. E., & Iruka, I. U. (2013). Supporting parents of African American children through parent education: Promising approaches and opportunities for research. *Journal of Child and Family Studies, 22*(1), 87–100.

Bauer, A., Knapp, M., & Parsonage, M. (2014). Lifetime costs of perinatal anxiety and depression. *Journal of Affective Disorders, 163*, 134–141.

Beck, C. T., McSweeney, M., Reed, P., & Moots, B. (2006). Psychometric properties of the Postpartum Depression Screening Scale in African American mothers. *Journal of Obstetric, Gynecologic, and Neonatal Nursing : JOGNN, 35*(1), 117–123.

Bowlby, J. (1982). Attachment and loss: Retrospect and prospect. *The American Journal of Orthopsychiatry, 52*(4), 664–678. DOI: 10.1111/j.1939-0025.1982.tb01456.x PMID: 7148988

Bronfenbrenner, U. (1979). *The ecology of human development: Experiments by nature and design*. Harvard University Press. DOI: 10.4159/9780674028845

Butterworth, P., Olesen, S. C., & Leach, L. S. (2012). The role of hardship in the association between socioeconomic position and depression. *The Australian and New Zealand Journal of Psychiatry, 46*(4), 364–373. DOI: 10.1177/0004867411433215 PMID: 22508596

Byrd, W. M., Fletcher, J. M., Menachemi, N., & Kiefe, C. I. (2020). Health disparities, COVID-19, and a way forward: The case for investment in health equity. *The Milbank Quarterly, 98*(3), 472–499.

Cohen, S., Janicki-Deverts, D., & Miller, G. E. (2007). Psychological stress and disease. *Journal of the American Medical Association, 298*(14), 1685–1687. DOI: 10.1001/jama.298.14.1685 PMID: 17925521

Collins, C., Gonzalez, M., & Angell, B. (2010). A community support approach to HIV/AIDS in Black communities. *Social Work in Public Health, 25*(1), 20–39.

Collins, P. H. (2000). *Black feminist thought: Knowledge, consciousness, and the politics of empowerment.* Routledge.

Collins, P. Y., Patel, V., Joestl, S. S., March, D., Insel, T. R., Daar, A. S., Bordin, I. A., Costello, E. J., Durkin, M., Fairburn, C., Glass, R. I., Hall, W., Huang, Y., Hyman, S. E., Jamison, K., Kaaya, S., Kapur, S., Kleinman, A., Ogunniyi, A., & Walport, M. (2010). Grand challenges in global mental health. *Nature, 475*(7354), 27–30. DOI: 10.1038/475027a PMID: 21734685

Crenshaw, K. (1989). Demarginalizing the intersection of race and sex: A Black feminist critique of antidiscrimination doctrine, feminist theory and antiracist politics. *University of Chicago Legal Forum, 1989*(1), 139–167.

Economic Policy Institute. (2020). The cost of child care in the United States. Retrieved from https://www.epi.org/child-care-costs-in-the-united-states/

Gee, G. C., & Ford, C. L. (2011). Structural racism and health inequities. *Du Bois Review, 8*(1), 115–132. DOI: 10.1017/S1742058X11000130 PMID: 25632292

Gjerdingen, D., & Center, B. (2003). First-time parents' postpartum changes in employment, child care, and housework responsibilities. *Social Science Research, 32*(1), 20–43.

Hankerson, S. H., Suite, D., & Bailey, R. K. (2018). Treatment disparities among African American men with depression: Implications for clinical practice. *Journal of Health Care for the Poor and Underserved, 26*(1), 21–34. DOI: 10.1353/hpu.2015.0012 PMID: 25702724

Johnson, M., & Molineux, M. (2020). The impact of home care on child development. *Developmental Psychology, 56*(8), 1423–1434.

Jones, D. J., Forehand, R., Brody, G., & Armistead, L. (2019). Positive parenting and child psychosocial outcomes: A longitudinal study in a rural African American sample. *Journal of Child and Family Studies, 28*(2), 308–318.

Karatsoreos, I. N., & McEwen, B. S. (2011). Psychobiological allostasis: Resistance, resilience and vulnerability. *Trends in Cognitive Sciences, 15*(12), 576–584. DOI: 10.1016/j.tics.2011.10.005 PMID: 22078931

Kozhimannil, K. B., Vogelsang, C. A., & Hardeman, R. R. (2011). Disrupting the pathways of social determinants of health: The role of Black women physicians in addressing reproductive health disparities. *Women's Health Issues, 21*(5), 458–464.

McEwen, B. S. (2004). Protection and damage from acute and chronic stress: Allostasis and allostatic load overload and allostatic load. *Annals of the New York Academy of Sciences, 1032*(1), 1–7. DOI: 10.1196/annals.1314.001 PMID: 15677391

McEwen, B. S., & Seeman, T. (1999). Protective and damaging effects of mediators of stress. *Annals of the New York Academy of Sciences, 896*(1), 30–47. DOI: 10.1111/j.1749-6632.1999.tb08103.x PMID: 10681886

Miller, G. E., Chen, E., & Zhou, E. S. (2007). If it goes up, must it come down? Chronic stress and the hypothalamic-pituitary-adrenocortical axis in humans. *Psychological Bulletin, 133*(1), 25–45. DOI: 10.1037/0033-2909.133.1.25 PMID: 17201569

Morrissey, T. W. (2017). Child care and parent labor force participation: A review of the research literature. *Review of Economics of the Household, 15*(1), 1–24. DOI: 10.1007/s11150-016-9331-3

National Partnership for Women & Families. (2018). Maternal mental health in the United States: A review of the literature. https://www.nationalpartnership.org/

Neufeld, A., Harrison, M. J., Stewart, M., Hughes, K., & Spitzer, D. (2008). Immigrant women: Making connections to community resources for support in family caregiving. *Qualitative Health Research, 18*(7), 913–922. PMID: 18552318

Novoa, C., & Taylor, J. (2018). Quality, affordable child care is critical to Black families. Center for American Progress. https://www.americanprogress.org/

Opara, I., Mayberry, B., Abu-Baker, K., & Ghaji, N. (2020). The impact of maternal stress on maternal-child health outcomes among Black mothers: A systematic review. *Journal of Women's Health, 29*(1), 33–42.

Perry, B., Pollard, R., Blakley, T., Baker, W., & Vigilante, D. (2016). Childhood trauma, the neurobiology of adaptation, and "use-dependent" development of the brain: How "states" become "traits.". *Infant Mental Health Journal, 16*(4), 271–291. DOI: 10.1002/1097-0355(199524)16:4<271::AID-IMHJ2280160404>3.0.CO;2-B

Roberts, E. M., Moskowitz, D., & Nugent, C. (2020). Racial and ethnic disparities in mental health treatment. *Health Services Research, 55*(2), 104–113.

Ross, C. E., & Mirowsky, J. (2001). Neighborhood disadvantage, disorder, and health. *Journal of Health and Social Behavior, 42*(3), 258–276. DOI: 10.2307/3090214 PMID: 11668773

Schneiderman, N., Ironson, G., & Siegel, S. D. (2005). Stress and health: Psychological, behavioral, and biological determinants. *Annual Review of Clinical Psychology, 1*(1), 607–628. DOI: 10.1146/annurev.clinpsy.1.102803.144141 PMID: 17716101

Segerstrom, S. C., & Miller, G. E. (2004). Psychological stress and the human immune system: A meta-analytic study of 30 years of inquiry. *Psychological Bulletin, 130*(4), 601–630. DOI: 10.1037/0033-2909.130.4.601 PMID: 15250815

Shields, R., & Wailoo, K. (2002). *Childhood and Adolescence in Society*. McGraw-Hill Education.

Slaughter-Acey, J. C., Caldwell, C. H., Misra, D. P., & Giurgescu, C. (2019). The influence of personal and group racism on entry into prenatal care among African American women. *Women's Health Issues, 29*(2), 157–164. PMID: 24041828

Smith, J., Brown, L., & Johnson, A. (2020). Culturally competent care for Black mothers: Addressing postpartum depression through tailored home care services. *Journal of Maternal Health, 15*(2).

Taylor, R. J., Chatters, L. M., & Joe, S. (2019). Social support networks and the mental health of Black mothers: A review of the literature. *Clinical Psychology Review, 69*, 116–127.

Thomas, M. P., Ammann, G., Brazier, E., Noyes, P., & Maybank, A. (2020). Doula services within a healthy start program: Increasing access for an underserved population. *Maternal and Child Health Journal, 24*(1), 76–83. PMID: 29198051

Thomas, T. L., Eberly, D., Smith, M. A., & Solis, J. M. (2019). Advancing health equity in public health systems. *Journal of Public Health Management and Practice, 25*(6), 563–569.

Thornton, R. L., Glover, C. M., Cené, C. W., Glik, D. C., Henderson, J. A., & Williams, D. R. (2017). Evaluating strategies for reducing health disparities by addressing the social determinants of health. *Health Affairs, 36*(6), 997–1004. PMID: 27503966

Walker, R. E., Williams, J. H., & Egede, L. E. (2021). The impact of social determinants of health on Black maternal mental health. *Health Equity, 5*(1), 56–62.

Williams, D. R., & Mohammed, S. A. (2013). Racism and health I: Pathways and scientific evidence. *The American Behavioral Scientist, 57*(8), 1152–1173. DOI: 10.1177/0002764213487340 PMID: 24347666

World Health Organization. (2013). Investing in mental health: Evidence for action. https://www.who.int/mental_health/en/

Chapter 10
Transforming Perinatal Bereavement Care:
Centering Trauma-Informed and Culturally Competent Practices for Black Women

Solimar Santiago-Warner
https://orcid.org/0000-0001-6738-7455
Silver School of Social Work, New York University, USA

ABSTRACT

Perinatal loss is a profoundly emotional and life-altering experience for families. Black women face this loss disproportionately due to systemic inequities, racism, and socioeconomic challenges. This chapter seeks to honor and understand the unique experiences of Black women navigating perinatal bereavement, exploring how race, class, and gender intersect to create disparities in healthcare access and quality. It also highlights the additional layers of trauma many Black women endure. The author advocates for trauma-informed, culturally sensitive care that centers on safety, trust, and collaboration. Key strategies include empowering women in decision-making, embracing culturally affirming practices, and fostering supportive community connections. Guided by Womanist theory, this chapter offers practical tools to address inequities and create holistic and healing care. It encourages healthcare providers to adopt policies and practices that prioritize equity and compassion, creating a pathway to healing, resilience, and hope for Black women and their families.

DOI: 10.4018/979-8-3693-4272-5.ch010

INTRODUCTION

Perinatal loss, impacts families with profound emotional and psychological consequences (Collins et al., 2021). In particular, Black women encounter unique challenges and disparities that often exacerbate their grief and trauma. For example, the impact of miscarriage and stillbirth is disproportionately felt by Black women, who are twice as likely to experience these losses as compared to their white counterparts (Center for Disease Control and Prevention, [CDC], 2024; Wallace et al. 2017). This disparity arises from various factors, including access to maternal preconception health, socioeconomic status, intergenerational stress and trauma, racism, and biases within the healthcare system, as well as limited access to quality healthcare (Brown et al., 2021). These systemic challenges not only increase the likelihood of pregnancy complications but also exacerbate the emotional toll of perinatal loss on Black women and their families. Addressing these disparities requires comprehensive efforts to improve healthcare access, address social determinants of health, and combat systemic racism in healthcare delivery (Horan et al., 2023).

The intersectionality of race, class, and gender plays a significant role in shaping the experiences of Black women in perinatal loss (Scott et al., 2019). Socioeconomic factors, historical trauma, and systemic racism contribute to disparities in healthcare access, quality of care, and support services, further compounding the challenges faced by Black women during such difficult times (Scott et al., 2019). Understanding the intersectionality of race, class, and gender is crucial in comprehending the nuanced experiences of Black women navigating perinatal loss (Evans et al., 2023). This chapter reviews the profound impact of perinatal loss on Black women, examining how societal structures and systemic inequalities shape their grieving process. Furthermore, it explores the vital concepts of trauma-informed care and cultural competence within healthcare settings. These principles are essential for providing effective support to Black women as they navigate the complexities of perinatal bereavement. This chapter also discusses the development of trauma-informed, culturally competent perinatal bereavement policies within hospital settings, with a specific emphasis on addressing the needs of Black women. By fostering an environment that acknowledges and respects the cultural nuances and traumas experienced by Black women, healthcare providers can better support them through the grieving process and improve overall outcomes (Petersen et al., 2020).

PERINATAL LOSS AND MENTAL HEALTH

Perinatal loss casts a profound shadow over the lives of those who experience it, unleashing a torrent of emotions that can feel overwhelming and unrelenting

(Owens & Denney-Koelsch, 2023). The journey through grief is marked by a tumultuous landscape of sadness, guilt, anger, and a deep, and resonating sorrow. In the wake of perinatal loss, individuals often find themselves grappling with a sense of ambiguous grief, mourning not only the loss of their baby but also the intangible loss of the hopes, dreams, and expectations they held for their anticipated child (Côté-Arsenault et al., 2019). This type of grief is complicated, spreading into every aspect of families' lives, mixing with thoughts of what could have been but never happened. In the midst of this uncertainty, there emerge strong feelings of wishing things had turned out differently and mourning a life that never had the opportunity to grow (Antilla & Johnson, 2024).

UNDERSTANDING THE NEEDS OF BLACK WOMEN IN PERINATAL LOSS

Perinatal loss disproportionately affects Black women, highlighting alarming healthcare disparities. Black women are more than twice as likely to experience stillbirth compared to White or Hispanic women (Centers for Disease Control and Prevention [CDC], 2024). For example, stillbirth rates for Black women were 10.4 per 1,000 births in 2022, compared to 4.71 per 1,000 for White women (National Center for Health Statistics, 2022). Age also represents a compounding factor; stillbirth rates are highest among Black mothers aged 15–19 and those aged 35 and older, with the lowest rates observed in their twenties (Rainford, 2023). Medical conditions, such as high blood pressure, kidney disease, and diabetes, contribute to nearly 30% of stillbirths among Black women, compared to lower rates among their White counterparts. Despite technological advances in perinatal care, nearly 33% of all stillbirths remain unexplained, with persistent racial disparities (Rainford, 2023). These data underscore the systemic inequities in healthcare access, diagnosis, and management that disproportionately affect Black women.

A significant contributor to these disparities is the impact of racism on Black women's health, manifesting as cumulative physiological stress, a phenomenon known as *weathering*. Public health researcher Dr. Arline T. Geronimus (1992) described weathering as the accelerated aging caused by chronic stress, often rooted in socioeconomic and political disadvantages. For Black women, weathering increases the risk of chronic diseases, adverse pregnancy outcomes, and premature mortality (Geronimus, 1996; Geronimus et al., 2006). This compounded stress not only affects health outcomes generally but also exacerbates risks during pregnancy. For example, Black women are 1.5 to 2 times more likely than White women to experience stillbirths between 39–41 weeks of gestation, a period when most pregnancies are expected to result in healthy deliveries (Rainford, 2023). Subtle forms of racism also manifest in healthcare practices. Research shows that Black women are less likely to be offered labor induction, a preventive measure for high-risk pregnancies, compared to White women (Rainford, 2023). This omission reflects how implicit biases can devalue Black women's health needs, contributing to negative perinatal outcomes.

Implicit biases among healthcare providers compound these disparities, often leading to substandard care for Black women. Black women frequently report that their pain and concerns are dismissed or minimized, resulting in delayed or inadequate treatment during pregnancy and after perinatal loss. For example, healthcare providers may overlook symptoms of preeclampsia in Black women, an overt example of neglect that can have life-threatening consequences. Subtler biases are evident when providers assume noncompliance or misinterpret Black women's communication styles, further eroding trust and quality of care. In *Pregnant While Black: Advancing Justice for Maternal Health in America* (2023), Dr. Rainford argues that comprehensive bias training is essential for healthcare providers to mitigate against these disparities. Such training can foster equitable, empathetic care, reducing the harmful effects of implicit biases on Black women's maternal health experiences.

The compounded effects of racism and bias also intersect with cultural stigmas surrounding mental health, adding to the challenges Black women face after perinatal loss. Many Black women feel societal pressures to demonstrate strength and resilience, which can discourage open expressions of grief or seeking mental health support. Without culturally responsive care, Black women may feel alienated or underserved. For instance, a Black woman grieving a stillbirth might avoid therapy if she perceives the counselor as dismissive of her cultural context or unable to address the unique challenges she faces (Burke et al., 2020; Capers, 2019). Culturally competent therapists who understand how historical trauma and systemic racism intersect with personal grief are crucial in addressing this gap. Additionally, community-based support groups tailored to Black women can create safe spaces for collective healing, where their experiences are validated, and their grief acknowledged (Bryant-Davis & Comas-Diaz, 2016).

Systemic barriers, such as limited access to quality prenatal and postnatal care further exacerbate disparities in perinatal outcomes. Black women are disproportionately affected by income inequality, restricted healthcare access, and underfunded medical facilities in marginalized communities (Charette & Heller, 2018). These challenges are particularly stark in rural areas, where Black mothers may need to travel hours to reach a hospital, delaying critical care. Structural inequities also extend to insurance policies that limit coverage for high-risk pregnancies or mental health services, further hindering access to care. Addressing these barriers requires policy reforms to ensure equitable healthcare access, such as expanding Medicaid, funding community-based prenatal care initiatives, and embedding anti-racism frameworks into healthcare systems.

Empowering Black women to advocate for their health is another essential step in reducing disparities. Education about healthcare rights and active participation in medical decisions can equip Black women to navigate complex systems and advocate for their needs effectively. For instance, patient advocacy workshops can teach Black women how to request second opinions, insist on preventive measures like early labor induction, or address dismissive behaviors from healthcare providers. Dr. Rainford (2023) underscores the importance of informed patients in improving maternal health outcomes, arguing that empowered individuals are more likely to receive timely and appropriate care.

The disparities in perinatal outcomes for Black women reflect broader systemic racism that extends beyond individual interactions to societal and institutional factors. Historical injustices, such as forced sterilizations and the exclusion of Black women from clinical trials, continue to shape mistrust in medical institutions (Campbell, 2021). These disparities are perpetuated today through institutional policies and practices prioritizing efficiency over equity. For example, hospital triage systems may deprioritize Black women based on implicit assumptions tied to socioeconomic status, subtly reinforcing systemic inequities.

Addressing these disparities requires targeted research to understand better the unique challenges Black women face in perinatal loss. Much existing data generalizes across racial groups, obscuring the specific needs of Black women. Dedicated research can inform interventions tailored to Black women's experiences, such as culturally sensitive grief counseling, patient-centered care models, and community-based health initiatives. Policymakers must invest in these efforts to build equitable maternal health systems and improve outcomes.

Understanding the needs of Black women in perinatal loss requires a holistic approach that addresses the intersections of race, class, and gender. By acknowledging the compounded effects of systemic racism, healthcare inequities, and cultural stigmas, stakeholders can develop comprehensive strategies to dismantle barriers and ensure equitable care. Through reforms in healthcare systems, targeted community support initiatives, patient empowerment programs, and rigorous research, it is possible to create a more just and inclusive maternal health landscape, ensuring that Black women receive the care and support they deserve during profoundly challenging times.

WOMANISM PRINCIPLES IN HOLISTIC PERINATAL BEREAVEMENT CARE

Womanist theory, originating from the work of Alice Walker, expands upon feminist principles by centering the experiences of Black women within discussions of gender, race, and social justice (Bryant-Davis & Adams, 2016; Bryant-Davis & Comas-Diaz, 2016). It recognizes the intersectionality of oppression, highlighting how race, gender, class, and other identities intersect to shape individuals' experiences. Womanism emphasizes inclusivity, community, and resistance to oppression, advocating for the liberation of all marginalized groups while specifically addressing the unique challenges faced by Black women. Grounded in cultural awareness and heritage, womanist theory promotes activism, social justice, and collective action as pathways to empowerment and systemic change. Overall, womanism provides a holistic framework that prioritizes the voices and experiences of Black women, challenging traditional feminist narratives and fostering intersectional approaches to social justice and liberation (Sanchez-Hucles, 2016).

Applying womanist theory in obstetric care within hospital settings involves a nuanced approach that prioritizes Black women's holistic well-being and empowerment. Firstly, healthcare providers need to recognize and address the intersecting factors that influence Black women's experiences of pregnancy loss, including systemic racism, socioeconomic disparities, and cultural factors. Womanism theory underscores the importance of understanding these contextual factors to provide culturally sensitive and equitable care (Bryant-Davis & Adams, 2016; Bryant-Davis & Comas-Diaz, 2016; Sanchez-Hucles, 2016).

Secondly, healthcare professionals should prioritize building trust and rapport with Black women by acknowledging their unique experiences and perspectives. This involves creating a supportive and nonjudgmental environment where women feel comfortable expressing their emotions, concerns, and needs related to pregnancy loss. Womanist theory emphasizes the importance of validating Black women's lived experiences and promoting their agency in decision-making processes regarding their obstetric care (Bryant- Davis & Adams, 2016; Bryant- Davis & Comas- Diaz, 2016; Sanchez-Hucles, 2016).

Thirdly, womanist theory encourages healthcare providers to adopt a multidisciplinary approach to obstetric care that addresses the diverse needs of Black women who have experienced pregnancy loss (Bryant-Davis & Adams, 2016; Bryant-Davis & Comas-Diaz, 2016; Sanchez-Hucles, 2016). This may involve collaborating with mental health professionals, social workers, spiritual counselors, and community organizations to provide comprehensive support services. Additionally, incorporating culturally relevant healing practices and rituals into obstetric care can help validate and honor the grieving process for Black women.

Lastly, healthcare systems and policies should be reformed to dismantle structural barriers and promote health equity for Black women in obstetric care (Riddle et al., 2023). This includes advocating for culturally competent training for healthcare providers, increasing access to affordable healthcare services, and addressing institutional biases and disparities in healthcare delivery. Womanist theory highlights the importance of advocating for systemic change to address the root causes of health inequities and ensure that Black women receive dignified and equitable obstetric care in hospital settings (Bryant-Davis & Adams, 2016; Bryant-Davis & Comas-Diaz, 2016; Sanchez-Hucles, 2016).

PRINCIPLES OF TRAUMA-INFORMED CARE AND CULTURAL COMPETENCE IN PERINATAL SETTINGS

Trauma-informed care in perinatal settings embodies a comprehensive approach that acknowledges the potential impact of past trauma on new mothers and parents, emphasizing prevention and mitigation strategies to address traumatic stress throughout the perinatal transition (Burke et al., 2020; Farley et al., 2018; Fawcet & Taylor, 2018; Gerber, 2019). At its core, trauma-informed care prioritizes creating a safe and supportive environment that fosters healing and resilience, recognizing the potential vulnerabilities and sensitivities that arise during the perinatal period (Fawcet & Taylor, 2018). Key principles include cultivating awareness of trauma's effects, implementing preventative measures to minimize re-traumatization, and demonstrating sensitivity to the unique needs and experiences of individuals navigating the perinatal journey (Burke et al., 2020; Gerber, 2019). By integrating these principles into perinatal care practices, healthcare providers can better support new parents' emotional well-being and recovery, promoting a more compassionate and empowering childbirth experience.

Trauma-informed care (TIC) principles serve as a guiding framework for providing empathetic and effective support to individuals who have experienced trauma. When applied to perinatal care, these principles take on added significance, recognizing the vulnerability and complexity inherent in the transition to parenthood. Key components of trauma-informed perinatal care include safety, trustworthiness, collaboration, empowerment, and cultural sensitivity (Burke et al., 2020; Farley et al., 2018; Fawcet & Taylor, 2018; Gerber, 2019).

Safety is paramount in trauma-informed perinatal care, ensuring that individuals feel physically and emotionally secure throughout their journey. This involves creating an environment where there is no rush in the treatment process, allowing individuals to move through their healing journey at their own pace. Furthermore, verbal and nonverbal acknowledgment of the psychobiological aspects of trauma and stress is essential, including education on the nervous system's response to stress and trauma and attunement to both the therapist's and the client's nervous system states (Farley et al., 2018).

Trustworthiness and transparency form the foundation of a therapeutic relationship in trauma-informed perinatal care (Burke et al., 2020; Farley et al., 2018;

Fawcet & Taylor, 2018; Gerber, 2019). Providers must be open about conceptualizing the client's situation and treatment plans, fostering collaboration and mutual understanding. Psychoeducation about perinatal trauma and its systemic factors empowers individuals to understand the context of their experiences and engage in bottom-up treatment approaches that address the physiological and psychological impacts of trauma (Burke et al., 2020; Farley et al., 2018; Fawcet & Taylor, 2018; Gerber, 2019).

Peer support and community engagement are also vital aspects of trauma-informed perinatal care, emphasizing the importance of social and relational support in the healing process (Vissing, 2024). Providers continuously assess and offer referrals to resources beyond the hospital setting, highlighting anti-inflammatory and stress-reducing interventions. Holistic treatment planning involves collaboration with community resources and addressing the diverse needs of individuals from different cultural, racial, ethnic, and gender backgrounds (Vissing, 2024).

Empowerment, voice, and choice are central tenets of trauma-informed perinatal care, affirming the individual's agency in their healing journey. This involves distinguishing between societal expectations of motherhood and the diverse practices and expressions of maternal identity. Providers can support individuals in asserting their embodied subjectivity and resisting oppressive narratives of motherhood, fostering empowerment and self-determination (Burke et al., 2020; Farley et al., 2018; Fawcet & Taylor, 2018; Gerber, 2019; Madden et al., 2018).

Finally, trauma-informed perinatal care acknowledges the historical, cultural, and systemic factors that contribute to disparities in perinatal health outcomes. Providers engage in culturally competent practices, respecting clients' belief systems and cultural practices related to the perinatal transition. They also support individuals in asserting their maternal subjectivity within the context of their unique identity and intersectional circumstances, promoting healing and resilience in the face of institutionalized oppression (Vissing, 2024).

Table 1. Trauma-Informed Care Principles in Perinatal Settings

1. Safety: Prioritize pregnant individuals and their families' physical and emotional safety by creating a nonjudgmental and supportive environment.
2. Trustworthiness and transparency: Build trust through open and honest communication, ensuring transparency in all aspects of care and respecting patients' autonomy.
3. Collaboration and empowerment: Engage pregnant individuals as active participants in their own care. Collaborate with them to develop personalized care plans and empower them to make informed decisions.

continued on following page

Table 1. Continued

4. Sensitivity to trauma history: Recognize the potential impact of past trauma on pregnancy and childbirth experiences and tailor care to address the unique needs and concerns of individuals with trauma histories.
5. Cultural responsiveness: Integrate cultural considerations into care delivery, respecting the cultural beliefs, values, and practices of pregnant individuals and their families, and adapting interventions to align with their cultural preferences.

Note: Adapted from "SAMHSA's Concept of Trauma and Guidance For a Trauma-Informed Approach" by Substance Abuse and Mental Health Services Administration, 2014.

By embracing trauma-informed care principles, perinatal healthcare providers can create a compassionate and supportive environment that promotes healing, resilience, and positive birth outcomes for pregnant individuals and their families.

Importance of Cultural Competence In Healthcare Delivery

Cultural competence is essential in perinatal healthcare delivery to ensure that pregnant individuals from diverse cultural backgrounds receive respectful, sensitive, and equitable care. Culturally competent care involves understanding and valuing the cultural beliefs, practices, and preferences of pregnant individuals and their families and integrating this knowledge into clinical practice (Santiago-Warner, 2024; Vissing, 2024). In perinatal settings, cultural competence is particularly crucial due to the significant cultural and social factors that influence pregnancy, childbirth, and postpartum experiences.

Pregnancy and childbirth are deeply embedded within cultural contexts, and cultural beliefs, traditions, and practices often shape individuals' perceptions of pregnancy and childbirth and their attitudes toward prenatal care, childbirth interventions, and postpartum practices (Vissing, 2024). Healthcare providers must recognize and respect the cultural diversity within the perinatal population and adapt care approaches to accommodate diverse cultural perspectives and preferences (Santiago-Warner, 2024).

DEVELOPING TRAUMA-RESPONSIVE PERINATAL BEREAVEMENT POLICIES

As an institution seeking to understand and potentially improve its perinatal bereavement practices, here are some questions to consider asking:

- What protocols or guidelines does the institution currently have in place for supporting families experiencing perinatal loss?

- Can you provide an overview of the services and resources available to families following perinatal loss, including counseling, support groups, and memorialization options?
- How does the institution communicate with families about perinatal loss, including delivering difficult diagnoses and discussing end-of-life care options?
- What training and education do healthcare providers receive regarding perinatal bereavement, and how frequently is this training updated?
- Are there designated staff members or teams responsible for providing support to families experiencing perinatal loss and what qualifications or experience do they have?
- How does the institution ensure cultural sensitivity and inclusivity in its approach to perinatal bereavement support, considering families' diverse backgrounds and beliefs?
- Can families access bereavement support services both during their hospital stay and in the weeks and months following their loss, and how is ongoing support facilitated?
- Are there opportunities for families to participate in memorial events or rituals to honor their lost baby, and if so, what arrangements are made for these activities?
- How does the institution collaborate with community organizations or support networks to enhance its bereavement support services for families?
- What measures are in place to evaluate the effectiveness of the institution's perinatal bereavement practices and how does the institution solicit feedback from families to inform improvements?

By asking these questions, individuals can gain insight into their institutions current perinatal bereavement practices and identify areas for enhancement to better support families during one of the most challenging experiences of their lives (Damschroder et al., 2009; Flanagan & Daniels, 2017; Gold & Johnson, 2020; Kenney & Ross, 2020; Kuzma et al., 2020; Powell et al., 2015; Proctor et al., 2011; Zelon et al., 2021).

Creating a trauma-responsive care bereavement policy in hospital settings requires a systematic approach that involves assessment, evaluation, and collaboration to develop comprehensive guidelines that prioritize the needs of individuals experiencing perinatal loss (Damschroder et al., 2009; Flanagan & Daniels, 2017; Gold & Johnson, 2020; Kenney & Ross, 2020; Kuzma et al., 2020; Powell et al., 2015; Proctor et al., 2011; Zelon et al., 2021). Here is a step-by-step guide:

- Assessment of Current Practices: Begin by assessing the hospital's existing bereavement support services and policies. This includes reviewing current protocols for addressing perinatal loss, such as communication practices, bereavement accommodations, and available support resources.

- Identify Stakeholders: Identify key stakeholders who will be involved in developing the trauma-responsive care bereavement policy. These may include healthcare providers from various disciplines (obstetrics, neonatology, psychiatry, etc.), hospital administrators, bereavement coordinators, social workers, chaplains, and representatives from patient advocacy groups.
- Conduct Needs Assessment: Conduct a needs assessment to understand the specific needs and preferences of individuals experiencing perinatal loss and the challenges and gaps in the current bereavement support services. This may involve surveys, focus groups, interviews with bereaved parents, and consultations with experts in perinatal loss support.
- Review Trauma-Informed Care Principles: Familiarize stakeholders with trauma-informed care (TIC) principles and their relevance to perinatal loss support. Provide education and training on trauma-sensitive communication to create safe environments and disseminate the impact of trauma on individuals and families.
- Formulate Task Force: Establish a multidisciplinary task force dedicated to developing the trauma-responsive care bereavement policy. Ensure representation from diverse stakeholders, including healthcare providers, bereaved parents, community advocates, and experts in trauma-informed care.
- Define Policy Objectives: Clarify the overarching objectives of the bereavement policy, such as promoting compassionate care, empowering families, reducing trauma triggers, and fostering resilience in the face of perinatal loss.
- Policy Development: Collaboratively draft the trauma-responsive care bereavement policy, incorporating insights from trauma-informed care principles, stakeholder input, and best practices in perinatal loss support. Address key components such as communication protocols, respectful handling of remains, bereavement support resources, and follow-up care.
- Review and Feedback: Circulate the draft policy to stakeholders for review and feedback. Encourage open dialogue and incorporate suggestions for improvement based on stakeholder input and expertise.
- Training and Implementation: Develop training materials and educational resources to support healthcare providers in implementing the trauma-responsive care bereavement policy. Conduct training sessions to ensure staff are equipped with the knowledge and skills to support families experiencing perinatal loss effectively.
- Evaluation and Continuous Improvement: Establish mechanisms for ongoing evaluation and monitoring of the bereavement policy's effectiveness. Collect feedback from bereaved families, healthcare providers, and staff to identify

areas for improvement and make necessary adjustments to enhance the quality of bereavement support services.

By following these steps and fostering collaboration among stakeholders, hospitals can develop trauma-responsive care bereavement policies that prioritize the needs and experiences of individuals and families coping with perinatal loss (Flanagan & Daniels, 2017; Gold & Johnson, 2020; Kenney & Ross, 2020; Kuzma et al., 2020; Zelon et al., 2021).

Creating Culturally Competent Perinatal Bereavement Policies

Cultural competence is integral to the development of perinatal bereavement policies that effectively address the needs of diverse populations (Farley, 2018). Perinatal bereavement policies should reflect an understanding of the cultural beliefs, values, and practices of individuals and families affected by perinatal loss and incorporate culturally responsive approaches to support the grieving process. This may include providing culturally relevant resources and support services, respecting cultural rituals and traditions related to mourning and remembrance, and ensuring that bereavement care practices are sensitive to individuals' and families' cultural backgrounds and preferences (Holiday, 2010; Jalloh, 2021; Jones, 2021). By embracing cultural competence in perinatal bereavement policies, healthcare organizations can foster trust, promote healing, and enhance the quality of care for all individuals and families affected by perinatal loss.

Incorporating Intersectionality Into Policy Development

The intersectionality of factors such as race, ethnicity, socioeconomic status, and gender identity must be considered in the development of perinatal bereavement policies to ensure that they are equitable and inclusive. Intersectionality recognizes that multiple intersecting identities and social factors shape individuals' experiences of perinatal loss and that these factors can influence access to support services, quality of care, and outcomes (Johnson et al., 2023).

Perinatal bereavement policies should be designed to address the unique needs and experiences of marginalized and underserved communities, including Black, Indigenous, and people of color (BIPOC) populations, LGBTQ+ individuals, individuals with disabilities, and individuals from low-income backgrounds (Johnson et al., 2023; Kenney & Ross, 2020; Kuzma et al., 2020). This may involve implementing targeted interventions to reduce disparities in bereavement care, addressing systemic barriers to access and quality of care, and promoting inclusivity and diversity within bereavement support services.

Collaborating With Community Stakeholders And Advocacy Groups

Effective development and implementation of perinatal bereavement policies require collaboration with community stakeholders and advocacy groups representing the interests and needs of individuals and families affected by perinatal loss (Kuzma et al., 2020). Community engagement can help ensure that bereavement policies are responsive to the community's diverse needs, reflect community values and priorities, and promote partnerships between healthcare organizations and community-based organizations.

Healthcare providers and organizations can collaborate with community stakeholders and advocacy groups to co-design bereavement policies, identify gaps in services, advocate for policy changes, and develop culturally competent and trauma-informed bereavement programs and resources. By fostering meaningful partnerships with community stakeholders and advocacy groups, healthcare organizations can better meet the needs of individuals and families affected by perinatal loss and promote healing and resilience within the community (Damschroder et al., 2009; Flanagan & Daniels, 2017; Gold & Johnson, 2020; Kenney & Ross, 2020; Kuzma net al., 2020; Powell et al., 2015; Proctor et al., 2011; Zelon et al., 2021).

IMPLEMENTATION AND EVALUATION

Implementing trauma-informed, culturally competent policies in healthcare systems requires a comprehensive approach that addresses the unique needs and experiences of individuals and families affected by perinatal loss. Strategies for implementation include conducting a thorough needs assessment to identify gaps in existing bereavement care practices and understand the specific needs of the perinatal population served by the healthcare system (Damschroder et al., 2009; Flanagan & Daniels, 2017; Gold & Johnson, 2020; Kenney & Ross, 2020; Kuzma et al., 2020; Powell et al., 2015; Proctor et al., 2011; Zelon et al., 2021). From there, developing trauma-informed, culturally competent bereavement policies that integrate evidence-based practices, prioritize patient-centered care, and address the diverse needs of individuals and families is essential. Additionally, providing comprehensive training and education for healthcare providers and staff on trauma-informed care principles, cultural competence, and effective communication strategies for supporting individuals and families experiencing perinatal loss is crucial (Damschroder et al.,

2009; Flanagan & Daniels, 2017; Gold & Johnson, 2020; Kenney & Ross, 2020; Kuzma et al., 2020; Powell et al., 2015; Proctor et al., 2011; Zelon et al., 2021).

Training and education for healthcare providers and staff are essential components of implementing trauma-informed, culturally competent bereavement policies. Comprehensive training programs should include education on trauma-informed care principles, such as understanding the prevalence and impact of trauma and learning trauma-informed approaches to care delivery. Additionally, offering training on cultural competence, including cultural humility, diversity awareness, and strategies for providing culturally responsive care to individuals and families from diverse cultural backgrounds, is vital (Damschroder et al., 2009; Flanagan & Daniels, 2017; Gold & Johnson, 2020; Kenney & Ross, 2020; Kuzma et al., 2020; Powell et al., 2015; Proctor et al., 2011; Zelon et al., 2021). Communication skills development is also important, as well as teaching effective communication strategies for supporting individuals and families experiencing perinatal loss, including active listening, empathy, and validation of emotions. Furthermore, tailoring training programs to the specific roles and responsibilities of healthcare providers and staff involved in bereavement care and providing ongoing education and professional development opportunities ensures that healthcare providers and staff remain current on best practices in trauma-informed care and cultural competence.

Continuous evaluation and improvement of bereavement policies are essential for ensuring that healthcare systems meet the evolving needs of individuals and families affected by perinatal loss. Strategies for evaluation and improvement include data collection and analysis on patient outcomes, satisfaction with care, and adherence to bereavement policies to identify areas for improvement and inform quality improvement initiatives. Moreover, it is crucial to solicit feedback from patients and families about their experiences with bereavement care, address staff burnout and compassion fatigue, and provide support and resources for coping with the emotional demands of bereavement care. Additionally, implementing strategies for continuous quality improvement, such as regular review of policies and procedures, benchmarking against best practices, and incorporating evidence-based interventions into bereavement care practices, is important (Damschroder et al., 2009; Flanagan & Daniels, 2017; Gold & Johnson, 2020; Kenney & Ross, 2020; Kuzma et al., 2020; Powell et al., 2015; Proctor et al., 2011; Zelon et al., 2021). Finally, engaging stakeholders, including patients, families, healthcare providers, administrators, and community partners in the evaluation and improvement of bereavement policies ensures that policies reflect the needs and priorities of the diverse stakeholders served by the healthcare system. Through prioritizing continuous evaluation and improvement of bereavement policies, healthcare systems can enhance the quality of care, promote patient and family satisfaction, and ultimately improve outcomes for individuals and families affected by perinatal loss.

Trauma-Responsive Perinatal Palliative Care for Black Birthing Women

Perinatal palliative care programs are essential in delivering culturally sensitive and trauma-responsive support to Black birthing women experiencing perinatal loss. These programs have the potential to address the compounded grief and trauma that arise at the intersection of systemic inequities, historical injustices, and perinatal loss (Cortezzo et al., 2020; Denney-Koelsch et al., 2016). Importantly, their effectiveness depends on clinicians and providers engaging in ongoing education and actively working to dismantle racism and implicit bias. These programs can provide meaningful and equitable care by fostering spaces that affirm cultural identity and honor individual experiences. Culturally affirmative care creates environments that reflect the diversity and richness of Black traditions, ensuring that families feel seen and supported (Dabney & Glover, 2019). For example, healthcare providers may collaborate with spiritual leaders to integrate culturally relevant grief rituals, such as prayer or personalized memory-making practices, into bereavement care.

Empowered decision-making is a cornerstone of trauma-informed perinatal palliative care. Black birthing women are provided with clear, accessible information about their care options, allowing them to actively shape their grief and healing processes (Zelon, 2021). For instance, care teams may offer a "grief and care roadmap" that guides patients through decisions about labor, pain management, or memorializing their baby (Riddle et al., 2023; Santiago-Warner, 2024). This approach ensures that the preferences and values of Black women remain central to care, reinforcing their sense of agency during an inherently vulnerable time.

Perinatal palliative care programs also address systemic barriers and inequities by providing advocacy and navigation services tailored to Black women's needs. Recognizing the historical mistrust of healthcare systems, programs often assign case managers to help families coordinate services, access insurance benefits, and connect with culturally responsive counselors or peer support groups. By addressing these systemic challenges, care teams help reduce stressors that exacerbate grief, creating an environment where families feel supported and respected.

Trauma-informed communication is another critical element of care. Healthcare providers use empathetic listening, nonjudgmental support, and language that validates the unique grief experiences of Black women (Dabney & Glover, 2019; Furtado et al., 2021). A trauma-informed approach acknowledges the cumulative impact of racism and loss, fostering trust and creating a safe space for emotional expression. For example, a nurse might actively validate a grieving mother's emotions by affirming, "Your voice matters here, and we are here to honor your experience and your child."

In addition to supporting individuals, perinatal palliative care programs embrace the collective grieving practices often present in Black families. Providers work to include extended family and community support, acknowledging their importance in the healing process (Timmins & Calderia, 2017; Wright, 2016). This could involve organizing bedside ceremonies where family members gather to share stories, songs, and prayers to honor the baby's memory. Memory-making activities, such as creating culturally meaningful keepsakes or participating in naming ceremonies, offer further opportunities to honor the baby while supporting the family's grieving process (Santiago-Warner, 2024; Timmins & Calderia, 2017; Wright, 2016).

Perinatal palliative care programs also collaborate with local organizations led by Black professionals to ensure culturally competent bereavement support. For example, partnerships with Black doulas or community-based programs allow families to receive in-home bereavement visits and culturally relevant emotional care. By extending their reach beyond the hospital setting, these programs ensure that Black women continue to feel supported throughout their grief journey (Owens, 2023).

Finally, trauma-responsive perinatal palliative care explicitly addresses the role of systemic inequities in shaping Black women's experiences of loss. Care teams advocate for structural changes, such as expedited scheduling or flexible policies, to minimize additional stressors. These interventions recognize the historical disparities in access and quality of care, ensuring that Black women are not further burdened by systemic barriers during their time of loss (Owens, 2023).

By embedding trauma-responsive and culturally sensitive practices into perinatal palliative care, these programs validate and empower Black birthing women, providing pathways to resilience and healing. In doing so, they address not only the immediate grief associated with perinatal loss but also the broader systemic challenges that contribute to inequities in maternal health outcomes.

Table 2. Examples of Trauma-Responsive Care in Perinatal Palliative Care for Black Birthing Women Facing Perinatal Loss

1. Culturally Affirmative Spaces: • What it looks like in practice: Perinatal palliative care programs intentionally create environments that reflect cultural diversity and celebrate Black identity. This might include offering culturally relevant grief rituals, such as prayer or personalized memory-making practices, which align with Black cultural traditions. • Example: A hospital chaplain collaborates with Black spiritual leaders to incorporate faith-based grief rituals into bereavement care, supporting families in connecting to their cultural roots during their loss.
2. Empowered Decision-Making: • What it looks like in practice: Programs provide Black birthing women with detailed, accessible information about their options for care, such as choices for labor induction, pain management, or memorializing their baby. • Example: A care team schedules a private session with a patient and her support system to review a "grief and care roadmap" and ensure her values and choices guide decisions. For instance, a patient may request specific keepsakes like handprints or personalized photos.
3. System Navigation and Advocacy: • What it looks like in practice: Recognizing the barriers Black women often face in healthcare systems, perinatal palliative care programs offer advocates to assist in coordinating services and addressing systemic inequities. • Example: A case manager helps the grieving mother navigate insurance claims, find culturally responsive counseling services, or connect with support groups for Black women who have experienced perinatal loss.
4. Trauma-Informed Communication: • What it looks like in practice: Care providers use sensitive language, empathetic listening, and nonjudgmental support tailored to the needs of Black women, acknowledging the compounded trauma of systemic racism and perinatal loss. • Example: A nurse trained in trauma-informed care recognizes a mother's hesitancy to discuss her grief due to fear of being dismissed and actively validates her feelings, saying, "Your voice matters here, and we are here to honor your experience and your child."
5. Access to Specialized Bereavement Support: • What it looks like in practice: Programs connect Black women with culturally competent grief counselors and peer support groups that focus on shared lived experiences. • Example: A hospital partners with a local organization led by Black doulas to provide in-home bereavement visits and culturally relevant emotional support.
6. Inclusion of Family and Community: • What it looks like in practice: Providers invite family members and community supports into the care process to respect the collective grieving practices often found in Black families. • Example: A palliative care team arranges a bedside ceremony where extended family can gather, share stories, and honor the baby's memory through spoken word or song.
7. Memory-Making Activities: • What it looks like in practice: Programs create space for meaningful activities that memorialize the baby, incorporating elements that resonate with Black cultural or familial practices. • Example: A mother is provided with options to create keepsakes like a culturally designed baby blanket or participate in a naming ceremony that includes traditional African practices.
8. Addressing Systemic Trauma: • What it looks like in practice: Care programs explicitly acknowledge the role of systemic inequities in the patient's experience of loss, working to dismantle barriers that exacerbate grief. • Example: A social worker advocates for immediate scheduling flexibility to avoid additional stress, ensuring the mother does not have to face lengthy delays disproportionately affecting Black women in hospital systems.

CONCLUSION

The sentiment expressed by Leon (1992) underscores the profound impact that healthcare professionals can have on bereaved parents during their journey of grief and loss. The interactions and support provided by caregivers in the hospital setting lay the foundation for the family's entire grieving process. From the moment of diagnosis through the birthing process and beyond, the compassionate care and genuine warmth extended by healthcare providers leave an indelible mark on the hearts of bereaved parents (Côté-Arsenault et al., 2019; Dabney & Glover, 2019; Evans et al., 2023; Santiago-Warner, 2024). These moments of understanding and respect become cherished memories, as significant and enduring as any other recollections of their lost pregnancy or their baby's brief life. In the hospital setting, caregivers have a unique opportunity to offer solace, validation, and companionship to families during one of the most challenging times of their lives. Their words, gestures, and actions can provide comfort and support reverberating throughout the grieving process, offering a glimmer of light amidst the darkness of loss. As gatekeepers of compassion and empathy, healthcare professionals hold the power to shape the grieving journey of bereaved parents, leaving an enduring legacy of healing and hope.

The significance of trauma-informed, culturally competent care for Black women in perinatal loss cannot be overstated. Black women face disproportionate challenges and disparities in perinatal care, exacerbated by systemic racism, socioeconomic factors, and cultural barriers. Recognizing and addressing the unique needs and experiences of Black women through trauma-informed and culturally competent care is essential to mitigate further harm, promote healing, and improve outcomes. Therefore, there is a critical call to action for healthcare systems to develop and implement trauma-informed perinatal bereavement policies that prioritize safety, trust, and collaboration while also integrating cultural competence to ensure respectful and inclusive care. By embracing intersectional, equitable care approaches, healthcare systems have the transformative potential to uplift and support Black women experiencing perinatal loss, fostering healing, resilience, and empowerment within these communities. It is imperative that healthcare systems commit to this call to action, recognizing the importance of addressing disparities and promoting equitable care for all individuals and families affected by perinatal loss, particularly Black women.

REFERENCES

Antilla, J. M., & Johnson, T. S. (2024). Life stressors and mental well-being: Experiences of African American women navigating perinatal loss and pregnancy subsequent to loss. *The Journal of Black Psychology, 0*(0), 326–364. DOI: 10.1177/00957984241230670

Brown, H. L., Small, M. J., Clare, C. A., & Hill, W. C. (2021). Black women health inequity: The origin of perinatal health disparity. *Journal of the National Medical Association, 113*(1), 105–113. DOI: 10.1016/j.jnma.2020.11.008 PMID: 33339616

Bryant-Davis, T., & Adams, T. (2016). A psychocultural exploration of womanism, activism, and social justice. In Bryant-Davis, T., & Comas-Díaz, L. (Eds.), *Womanist and mujerista psychologies: Voices of fire, acts of courage* (pp. 219–236). American Psychological Association., DOI: 10.1037/14937-010

Bryant-Davis, T., & Comas-Diaz, L. (2016). Introduction: Womanist and mujerista psychologies. In Bryant-Davis, T., & Comas-Diaz, L. (Eds.), *Womanist and mujerista psychologies: Voices of fire, acts of courage* (pp. 149–169). American Psychological Association. DOI: 10.1037/14937-001

Burke, T., Arnkoff, D., Staser, A., & Cook, J. M. (2020). Perinatal trauma: A trauma-informed approach to obstetrics. *Journal of Clinical Psychology in Medical Settings, 27*(1), 69–78. DOI: 10.1007/s10880-019-09664-4

Campbell, C. (2021). Medical violence, obstetric racism, and the limits of informed consent for Black women. *Michigan Journal of Race & Law, 26*(0), 47. DOI: 10.36643/mjrl.26.sp.medical

Capers, M. (2019). The experiences of Black women during perinatal loss: A literature review. *MCN. The American Journal of Maternal Child Nursing, 44*(6), 334–341.

Centers for Disease Control and Prevention. (2024, May 8). Infant mortality. https://www.cdc.gov/reproductivehealth/maternalinfanthealth/infantmortality.htm

Charette, M. F., & Heller, D. (2018). Implementing trauma-informed care in a women's hospital: A pilot study. *Journal of Obstetric, Gynecologic, and Neonatal Nursing : JOGNN, 47*(1), S18–S19.

Collins, E., McGuinness, S., & O'Sullivan, A. (2021). Understanding the experiences of Black women following perinatal loss: A qualitative study. *Journal of Psychosocial Nursing and Mental Health Services, 59*(8), 26–32. DOI: 10.3928/02793695-20210615-03

Cortezzo, D. E., Ellis, K., & Schlegel, A. (2020). Perinatal palliative care birth planning as advance care planning. *Frontiers in Pediatrics*, *8*, 556. DOI: 10.3389/fped.2020.00556 PMID: 33014940

Côté-Arsenault, D., Denney-Koelsch, E. M., McCoy, T. P., & Kavanaugh, K. (2019). African American and Latino bereaved parent health outcomes after receiving perinatal palliative care: A comparative mixed methods case study. *Applied Nursing Research*, *50*, 151200. DOI: 10.1016/j.apnr.2019.151200 PMID: 31735485

Dabney, K. P., & Glover, M. (2019). Perinatal loss in Black women: A qualitative study of coping strategies. *Journal of Loss and Trauma*, *24*(1), 34–49. DOI: 10.1080/15325024.2018.1494196

Damschroder, L. J., Aron, D. C., Keith, R. E., Kirsh, S. R., Alexander, J. A., & Lowery, J. C. (2009). Fostering implementation of health services research findings into practice: A consolidated framework for advancing implementation science. *Implementation Science : IS*, *4*(1), 50. DOI: 10.1186/1748-5908-4-50 PMID: 19664226

Denney-Koelsch, E., Black, B. P., Côté-Arsenault, D., Wool, C., Kim, S., & Kavanaugh, K. (2016). A survey of perinatal palliative care programs in the United States: Structure, processes, and outcomes. *Journal of Palliative Medicine*, *19*(10), 1080–1086. DOI: 10.1089/jpm.2015.0536 PMID: 27559768

Evans, N. M., Hsu, Y.-L., Kabasele, C. M., Kirkland, C., Pantuso, D., & Hicks, S. (2023). A qualitative exploration of stressors: Voices of African American women who have experienced each type of fetal/infant loss: Miscarriage, stillbirth, and infant mortality. *The Journal of Black Psychology*, *49*(2), 236–263. DOI: 10.1177/00957984221127833

Farley, C. L., DeSisto, M. C., Hawkins, J. W., & West, M. (2018). Implementing a trauma-informed care model for perinatal loss. *MCN. The American Journal of Maternal Child Nursing*, *43*(4), 218–224. DOI: 10.1097/NMC.0000000000000434 PMID: 29553946

Fawcett, E., & Taylor, S. (2018). Trauma-informed care in maternity services: A critical review. *Midwifery*, *56*, 121–127. DOI: 10.1016/j.midw.2017.10.015

Flanagan, K., & Daniels, K. (2017). Perinatal bereavement: Implementing a hospital-wide program. *Nursing for Women's Health*, *21*(4), 296–304. DOI: 10.1016/j.nwh.2017.06.007

Furtado-Eraso, S., Escalada-Hernández, P., & Marín-Fernández, B. (2021). Integrative review of emotional care following perinatal loss. *Western Journal of Nursing Research*, *43*(5), 489–504. DOI: 10.1177/0193945920954448 PMID: 32886030

Gerber, M. R. (2019). Trauma-informed maternity care. In Gerber, M. R. (Ed.), *Trauma-informed healthcare approaches: A guide for primary care* (pp. 145–155). Springer. DOI: 10.1007/978-3-030-04342-1_8

Geronimus, A. T. (1992). The weathering hypothesis and the health of African-American women and infants: Evidence and speculations. *Ethnicity & Disease, 2*(3), 207–221. PMID: 1467758

Geronimus, A. T. (1996). Black/white differences in the relationship of maternal age to birthweight: A population-based test of the weathering hypothesis. *Social Science & Medicine, 42*(4), 589–597. DOI: 10.1016/0277-9536(95)00159-X PMID: 8643983

Geronimus, A. T., Hicken, M., Keene, D., & Bound, J. (2006). "Weathering" and age patterns of allostatic load scores among Blacks and Whites in the United States. *American Journal of Public Health, 96*(5), 826–833. DOI: 10.2105/AJPH.2004.060749 PMID: 16380565

Gold, K. J., & Johnson, T. R. B. (2020). Integrating perinatal and pediatric bereavement care: A summary of key recommendations from a national meeting of bereavement experts. *Journal of Perinatology, 40*, 8–12. DOI: 10.1038/s41372-019-0548-5

Holiday, J. M. (2010). The word, the body, and the kinfolk: The intersection of transpersonal thought with womanist approaches to psychology. *International Journal of Transpersonal Studies, 29*(2), 10. DOI: 10.24972/ijts.2010.29.2.103

Horan, H., Ryu, J., Stone, J., & Thurston, L. (2023). Healing trauma with interprofessional collaboration and trauma-informed perinatal care: A qualitative case study. *Birth (Berkeley, Calif.), 50*(3), 525–534. DOI: 10.1111/birt.12672 PMID: 36039484

Jalloh, M. F., & Gebreamlak, W. (2021). Black women's experiences with perinatal loss: A systematic review. *Journal of Obstetric, Gynecologic, and Neonatal Nursing : JOGNN, 50*(3), 255–264. DOI: 10.1016/j.jogn.2021.02.007

Johnson, A., Hoffman, C., Julian, M., Bengal, C., Issa, M., Kenneally, M., Harris, S. D., Rosenblum, K. L., & Muzik, M. (2023). Holding the whole person: Perinatal women's perspectives on the integrated infant mental health care model in obstetrical care during COVID-19 pandemic. *Journal of Psychiatry and Psychiatric Disorders, 7*, 248–259.

Jones, K., McAlister, B. S., Haas, B. K., & Duke, G. (2021). Experiences of African American mothers following the death of their infants. *Nursing for Women's Health, 25*(6), 412–418. DOI: 10.1016/j.nwh.2021.09.004 PMID: 34717892

Kenney, L. J., & Ross, E. C. (2020). Implementation and evaluation of a perinatal bereavement program: A trauma-informed approach. *Journal of Obstetric, Gynecologic, and Neonatal Nursing : JOGNN*, *49*(5), 493–501. DOI: 10.1016/j.jogn.2020.04.005

Kuzma, E. K., Pardee, M., & Morgan, A. (2020). Implementing patient-centered trauma-informed care for the perinatal nurse. *The Journal of Perinatal & Neonatal Nursing*, *34*(4), E23–E31. DOI: 10.1097/JPN.0000000000000520 PMID: 33079811

Leon, I. G. (1992). Perinatal loss: A critique of current hospital practices. *Clinical Pediatrics*, *31*(6), 366–374. DOI: 10.1177/000992289203100611 PMID: 1628472

Madden, K., Bostock, L., & Devaraj, T. (2018). Trauma-informed care in maternity services: A scoping review. *Women and Birth; Journal of the Australian College of Midwives*, *31*(2), 159–167. DOI: 10.1016/j.wombi.2017.09.007

Owens, D., & Denney-Koelsch, E. M. (2023). African American culture and perinatal loss. In Denney-Koelsch, E. M. (Ed.), *Perinatal bereavement rituals and practices among U.S. cultural groups* (pp. 248–262). Springer., DOI: 10.1007/978-3-031-47203-9_5

Petersen, R., Gillespie, S. L., & Hamoda, H. M. (2020). Addressing disparities in perinatal loss: A qualitative study of Black women's experiences and needs. *Maternal and Child Health Journal*, *24*(8), 1047–1056. DOI: 10.1007/s10995-020-02921-3 PMID: 32335805

Powell, B. J., Waltz, T. J., Chinman, M. J., Damschroder, L. J., Smith, J. L., Matthieu, M. M., Proctor, E. K., & Kirchner, J. E. (2015). A refined compilation of implementation strategies: Results from the expert recommendations for implementing change (ERIC) project. *Implementation Science : IS*, *10*(1), 21. Advance online publication. DOI: 10.1186/s13012-015-0209-1 PMID: 25889199

Proctor, E., Silmere, H., Raghavan, R., Hovmand, P., Aarons, G., Bunger, A., & Hensley, M. (2011). Outcomes for implementation research: Conceptual distinctions, measurement challenges, and research agenda. *Administration and Policy in Mental Health*, *38*(2), 65–76. DOI: 10.1007/s10488-010-0319-7 PMID: 20957426

Rainford, M. (2023). *Pregnant while Black: Advancing justice for maternal health in America*. Broadleaf Books. DOI: 10.2307/j.ctv2phpsbz

Renbarger, K. M., Abebe, S., Place, J. M., Goldsby, E., Hall, G., & Kroot, A. (2023). Perspectives of infant mortality from African American community members. *Women's Health Reports (New Rochelle, N.Y.)*, *4*(1), 423–430. DOI: 10.1089/whr.2023.0017 PMID: 37638331

Riddle, J. N., Hopkins, T., Yeaton-Massey, A., & Hellberg, S. (2023). No baby to bring home: Perinatal loss, infertility, and mental illness—Overview and recommendations for care. *Current Psychiatry Reports*, *25*(6), 747–757. DOI: 10.1007/s11920-023-01469-x PMID: 37878138

SAMHSA's Concept of Trauma and Guidance for a Trauma-Informed Approach. (n.d.). https://ncsacw.acf.hhs.gov/userfiles/files/SAMHSA_Trauma.pdf

Sánchez-Hucles, J. V. (2016). Womanist therapy with Black women. In Bryant-Davis, T., & Comas-Díaz, L. (Eds.), *Womanist and Mujerista Psychologies: Voices of Fire, Acts of Courage* (pp. 69–92). American Psychological Association., DOI: 10.1037/14937-004

Santiago-Warner, S. (2024). Social work practice in perinatal palliative care: An overview. *Social Work in Health Care*, *63*(4-5), 248–262. DOI: 10.1080/00981389.2024.2316697 PMID: 38357813

Scott, K. A., Britton, L., & McLemore, M. R. (2019). The ethics of perinatal care for Black women: Dismantling the structural racism in "mother blame" narratives. *The Journal of Perinatal & Neonatal Nursing*, *33*(2), 108–115. DOI: 10.1097/JPN.0000000000000394 PMID: 31021935

Timmins, F., & Caldeira, S. (2017). Assessing the spiritual needs of patients. *Nursing Standard*, *31*(29), 47–53. DOI: 10.7748/ns.2017.e10312 PMID: 28294021

Vissing, H. (2024). *Somatic maternal healing: Psychodynamic and somatic trauma treatment for perinatal mental health*. Routledge.

Wallace, M. E., Green, C., Richardson, L., Theall, K., & Crear-Perry, J. (2017). "Look at the whole me": A mixed-methods examination of Black infant mortality in the US through women's lived experiences and community context. *International Journal of Environmental Research and Public Health*, *14*(7), 727. DOI: 10.3390/ijerph14070727 PMID: 28678200

Wright, P. M. (2020). Perinatal loss and spirituality: A metasynthesis of qualitative research. *Illness, Crises, and Loss*, *28*(2), 99–118. DOI: 10.1177/1054137317698660

Zelon, H. L., Forray, A., Knudson-Martin, C., & Johnson, S. M. (2021). Transforming perinatal bereavement care: A qualitative study of a trauma-informed group intervention. *Journal of Social Work in End-of-Life & Palliative Care*, *17*(3), 261–278. DOI: 10.1080/15524256.2021.1969292

Chapter 11
Echoes of Black Birth: Trauma Family Dynamics and the Path to Policy Solutions

Jennifer Rutledge Pettie
The Health Equilibrium Group, USA

ABSTRACT

"Echoes of Black Birth: Trauma Family Dynamics and the Path to Policy Solutions" looks at the experiences of Black people who have given birth, considering historical and modern factors. Jennifer Rutledge Pettie shows how systemic healthcare inequities harm Black families. Within the context of modern healthcare, this study examines the effects of medical racism and segregation. Medical racism is a critical issue since it prevents individuals from accessing healthcare. This chapter advocates for widespread changes to current systems after examining their detrimental impact on Black pregnant individuals. The prevalence of birth trauma is extensive, and it can have lasting consequences for one's psychological well-being and familial connections. Empirical evidence and anecdotal accounts substantiate this claim. This chapter presents several policy reforms aimed at improving maternal health, via establishment of robust social support systems, implementation of reproductive justice initiatives, and provision of culturally appropriate healthcare services.

I. INTRODUCTION

I know, first-hand, the complicated Black birthing process because I navigated it as a legal epidemiologist, first-time mom, and maternal near-miss survivor. After the birth of my daughter, I experienced avoidable setbacks that could have ended my life. As someone whose professional work lies at the intersection of public health, healthcare systems, and legal frameworks, I have had the opportunity to work with

DOI: 10.4018/979-8-3693-4272-5.ch011

data about maternal and child deaths and illnesses that aligned with the events of my daughter's birth. This experience inspired my advocacy and commitment to informing policy decisions relating to Black birthing experiences, serving as a call to action to address these systems that threaten the health and well-being of Black birthing people and their families.

This discussion focuses on how policy decisions impact Black people before, during, and after they give birth and what birth trauma means for them. I consider family, historical, and societal frameworks to improve Black maternal and child health and present potential strategies to inform steps toward Black women's health equity. These considerations include analysis of historical injustices and barriers such as medical racism, segregation, and slavery. More recent policy decisions and healthcare system issues have altered how Black people are born and created contemporary disparities in access and quality of health care. These outcomes have affected Black families and their coping strategies to address birth trauma, policy frameworks, and global examples to see what unites and distinguishes the Black birthing experience across the world. I conclude with my journey to motherhood, offering transparency and insights into the impact of trauma on family dynamics, mental health, resilience, and policy solutions.

II. HISTORICAL ROOTS OF BLACK BIRTH TRAUMA

Segregation exacerbated health inequalities that disproportionately affected Black populations. In the past, Black individuals who gave birth found themselves in racially segregated hospital facilities with fewer resources and inferior services compared to hospitals for their white counterparts. Black women have significantly elevated rates of maternal sickness and mortality, partially due to a lack of trust and neglect resulting from segregated healthcare systems (Coley & Hall, 2012). Case Study: During the period of segregation, Black people were subjected to exploitation and mistreatment within hospital systems, as shown by the narrative of Henrietta Lacks (Skloot, 2010). Henrietta's cervical cancer cells were harvested without her consent during the 1950s (Skloot, 2010).

Historically, individuals of African descent have also endured racism, mistreatment, and medical experimentation inside the healthcare system. Medical racism has had a considerable influence on the health of Black mothers and birthing individuals, including the exploitation of Black women's bodies for gynecological research without consent and the perpetuation of harmful stereotypes and biases by medical professionals. Black people's persisting lack of faith in the medical system leads to inequalities in the use of prenatal care and maternal health outcomes (Coley & Hall, 2012). Case Study: The Tuskegee Syphilis Study, carried out by the U.S. Public

Health Service between 1932 and 1972, intentionally denied medical treatment to a cohort of African American males diagnosed with syphilis in order to examine the natural development of the illness without any intervention (Jones, 1993). The lack of informed consent led to significant health consequences and a decrease in faith in medical research within the Black community (Jones, 1993).

An Analysis of the Circumstances and Legal Measures That Have Shaped the Delivery Experiences of Black Persons Throughout History

The maternal health outcomes of Black birthing experiences have been impacted by structural and political policy issues, leading to fluctuations across time. Black Americans faced substantial obstacles in accessing high-quality healthcare due to the implementation of racial segregation legislation. African Americans were compelled to give birth in underfunded and racially segregated institutions that lacked sufficient medical equipment, proficient personnel, and essential supplies. According to Coley and Hall (2012), black individuals who give birth get medical treatment of inferior quality compared to white individuals. The detrimental consequences of segregated healthcare are seen by the demise of Mamie Odessa Hale in 1955 (Dawley, 2003). Due to the prevailing racial segregation regulations, Ms. Hale, an African American woman, was denied access to a Caucasian hospital in Georgia when she urgently required a cesarean section (Dawley, 2003).

Policies impacting access to prenatal care have had an impact on the birth experiences of Black individuals.. African Americans face difficulties in obtaining prompt and sufficient prenatal care due to factors such as insufficient insurance coverage, transportation barriers, and inequities in healthcare systems across various areas and communities. The laws regarding Medicaid expansion have also had an influence on African American persons who experience childbirth. Medicaid is crucial for guaranteeing sustainable healthcare access to persons with low incomes, particularly pregnant women and those giving birth. Nevertheless, the disparate growth of Medicaid among states, especially those that have chosen not to broaden Medicaid eligibility, has resulted in inequitable availability of prenatal care and maternal health services (Coley & Hall, 2012). Analysis of a Specific Situation: Examining the impact of Medicaid expansion on Black outcomes in different states reveals significant disparities in access to prenatal care and maternal health services. In contrast to Texas, where Medicaid was not expanded, California increased Medicaid coverage due to the implementation of the Affordable Care Act (ACA).

The experiences of Black individuals giving birth have been impacted in varying ways in response to efforts taken to promote maternal health. The absence of proportional participation of Black women in committees focused on maternal health, such as the Maternal Mortality Review Committees (MMRCs), and the failure to use their recommendations raises questions about the intention to change the system (Coley & Hall, 2012). According to Coley and Hall (2012), these factors hindered the effectiveness of MMRCs in addressing racial disparities in maternal mortality. A case study focuses on establishing the Black Mamas Matter Alliance (BMMA), a grassroots organization led by Black women (Black Mamas Matter Alliance, 2018). This group addresses racial disparities in maternal health outcomes through the implementation of community organizing and legislative campaigning (Black Mamas Matter Alliance, 2018).

Bias among medical practitioners has recently garnered attention. Implicit bias training programs for medical professionals target their biases that may lead to the unjust treatment of Black patients and potentially mitigate disparities in maternal healthcare. The effect of these training programs on the differences in maternal health outcomes is not well understood (Coley & Hall, 2012). The case study analyzes the implementation of implicit bias training programs in hospitals and healthcare organizations, with a specific focus on the program created by the American College of Obstetricians and Gynecologists (Howell & Zeitlin, 2017). These programs aim to improve healthcare providers' attitudes and behaviors toward Black patients and ensure fair and equal maternal healthcare delivery.

To summarize, several factors have contributed to the persistent disparities in the delivery experiences of individuals belonging to the Black community. It is crucial to enact laws that specifically address the significant differences in health-care accessibility, quality, and delivery in order to eliminate these inequalities. To mitigate racial differences in birth outcomes, it is crucial to implement efforts that focus on achieving equality in maternal health and giving priority to the needs of Black women, birthing individuals, and their families.

III. CONTEMPORARY REALITIES OF BLACK BIRTH TRAUMA

Black maternity and child health disparities expose significant inequalities, such as elevated rates of maternal death and morbidity, in comparison to their White counterparts. Black women have a much higher incidence of maternal mortality compared to white women. Specifically, Black women are three to four times more likely to die from problems connected to pregnancy than white women (Centers for Disease Control and Prevention [CDC], 2020; Creanga et al., 2017). Case Study: Amber Isaac, a Black mother who tragically died during childbirth on April 21, 2020, in New York City, highlights systemic inequities and racial biases that cause higher rates of Black maternal mortality (Reed, 2020). This is furthermore exemplified by her well-documented apprehensions regarding healthcare personnel who disregarded her symptoms (Reed, 2020).

Furthermore, Black women exhibit elevated rates of maternal morbidity, which give rise to significant complications during pregnancy, childbirth, and the postpartum phase (Howell et al., 2018). Tennis icon Serena Williams experienced a significant hemorrhage during childbirth due to healthcare staff disregarding her worries and neglecting to immediately identify her symptoms (Salam, 2018). This illustrates the need for improved clinical procedures that embed respect for the health concerns of all mothers and birthing people (Fair et al., 2021). Disparities in health outcomes for Black birthing people and infants are further worsened by socioeconomic position, level of education, geographic location, and immigrant status (Howell et al., 2018). Case Study: Aisha, a Black mother residing in a remote rural region with restricted healthcare availability, encountered difficulties in obtaining prenatal care and encountered childbirth complications as a result of delays in receiving medical assistance (Kozhimannil et al., 2019). This case highlights how social determinants of health can significantly influence maternal outcomes (Kozhimannil et al., 2019).

Black maternal health disparities also affect child health. Black babies are more likely to be born prematurely, have low birth weight, or experience difficulties in the neonatal period compared to white babies (Howell et al., 2018). Case Study: Malik, a Black infant delivered prematurely to a woman with untreated hypertension, experienced several health difficulties in the neonatal intensive care unit. This instance highlights the impact of intergenerational maternal health disparities on health outcomes (Huang et al., 2022). The disparities in health outcomes for Black individuals who give birth and their infants can be traced to systemic inequities strongly rooted in racism, socioeconomic adversity, and structural barriers within the healthcare system (Huang et al., 2022). This highlights the need for a comprehensive strategy that addresses social determinants of health, advocates for culturally competent healthcare, dismantles institutional racism in the healthcare system, and includes lived experiences of Black mothers, birthing people, and families in policy decision-making.

An examination of differences in healthcare access and quality, cultural influences, and structural inequities driven by current policies demonstrates the complex nature of obstacles encountered by Black persons in obtaining high-quality healthcare. Black people have substantial gaps in healthcare access, including obstacles in accessing timely and inexpensive treatment (Kaiser Family Foundation [KFF], n.d.). Case Study: Jamila, an African American woman living in a mostly African American community with few healthcare resources, encountered obstacles in locating healthcare providers who would take her insurance and endured lengthy waiting periods for her visits (KFF, n.d.). This highlights one of the challenges frequently encountered by marginalized groups when accessing high-quality healthcare (Ravi et al., 2021). Furthermore, Black people experience a reduced standard of healthcare in comparison to their white counterparts, even when accounting for factors such as wealth and insurance status (Artiga et al., 2018). Case Study: Tyrone, a Black man with a familial predisposition to heart disease, got inadequate medical attention for his high blood pressure from a healthcare practitioner who neglected to prescribe evidence-based therapies and failed to monitor his condition effectively (Ford & Airhihenbuwa, 2010). Tyrone later suffered a cardiovascular event that may have been prevented under better circumstances (Ford & Airhihenbuwa, 2010). Black people's perception of healthcare and their interactions with physicians are influenced by distrust of the healthcare system, language barriers, and cultural beliefs around illness and treatment (Sabin, 2022). Case Study: Fatima, a Black immigrant with little competence in the English language, faces difficulties in effectively expressing her symptoms and concerns to her healthcare provider (Ngo-Metzger et al., 2003). She reported that she was given an inaccurate diagnosis, resulting in a postponement of treatment for a serious medical problem (Ngo-Metzger et al., 2003). Furthermore, healthcare policies related to the funding, payment, and provision of healthcare might perpetuate systemic inequities and exacerbate healthcare disparities among individuals of Black ethnicity (Artiga et al., 2018). Case Study: Michael, a Black individual residing in a state that chose not to expand Medicaid under the ACA, experienced financial constraints that prevented him from obtaining health insurance (Commonwealth Fund, 2022; American Heart Association [AHA], 2022; American Medical Association [AMA], 2018). Consequently, he encountered obstacles in obtaining preventive care and managing chronic illnesses. This case underscores the influence of policy choices on healthcare accessibility and outcomes (Commonwealth Fund, 2022; AHA, 2022; AMA, 2018). Overall, the ability to find and receive high-quality healthcare is hindered for Black people due to gaps in healthcare access and quality, cultural influences, and structural inequities driven by current laws. A comprehensive approach is critical to effectively address these inequalities, which includes increasing availability of high-quality healthcare, tackling prejudice within the healthcare system, fostering cultural proficiency among healthcare providers, and advocating for legislation that promotes better outcomes for Black individuals giving birth and their families.

IV. FAMILIAL RESONANCE OF BLACK BIRTH TRAUMA

Traumatic events during childbirth have a considerable influence on relationships, support networks, and mental well-being within Black families. This encompasses tense relationships among partners, family members, and healthcare providers, resulting in distrust, animosity, and discord. Case Study: Jamal and Aisha, a Black couple who experienced traumatic childbirth, found it challenging to express their emotions and share their experiences with others (Rhoden, 2022). Their relationship became troubled as they struggled with ongoing shame, rage, and sadness, showing the impact that birth trauma may have on close relationships (Rhoden, 2022). In addition, Black birth trauma has the potential to undermine pre-existing support systems, as individuals may feel isolated or lack understanding from friends, family, and community members who have not had comparable issues associated with childbirth. Latoya, an African American mother, faces challenges in forming relationships with other mothers in her community after a traumatic birthing experience (Jones et al., 2015). She felt detachment and absence of assistance, leading to feelings of isolation and separation from others throughout the postpartum time (Jones et al., 2015). Case Study: Marcus, an African American parent, had symptoms consistent with PTSD after witnessing his partner's traumatic childbirth (Ertan et al., 2021). This person had difficulties associated with intrusive thoughts, anxiety, and avoidance behaviors, highlighting the impact of birth trauma on the psychological health of both partners and family members (Ertan et al., 2021). Ultimately, Black birth trauma places a heavy load on family structures, significantly affecting relationships, support systems, and mental health in deep and intricate ways (Ertan et al., 2021). It is crucial to acknowledge and address the many repercussions of birth trauma on the welfare and success of Black individuals and families, while also developing resilience, flexibility, and community support in the face of challenges.

Black families that have undergone traumatic delivery experiences face challenges in obtaining the appropriate support they may need. Black families may face obstacles when trying to access mental health care that aligns with their cultural preferences. These hurdles might include societal disapproval, financial constraints, and a lack of available local professionals. Case Study: The Johnson family faced difficulties in locating cheap mental health professionals who had expertise in their background and encounters with birth trauma (Shimodera et al., 2012). Their suffering was made worse by the lack of treatment options and long waiting times, highlighting the need of having culturally sensitive care available (Steiner et al., 2014). Social services offer vital aid to those who have faced birth trauma, such as emotional assistance, physical support, and community resources. Case Study: The Smith family took part in a local support group for parents with a distressing childbirth experience, in order to seek comfort and emotional support. (Center for Health Journalism, 2022). Spending time with Black parents who experienced similar birth trauma helped them feel better understood, affirmed, and supported during their healing process (Center for Health Journalism, 2022).

Robust reproductive justice initiatives address structural inequities, access to quality care, and resulting maternal health disparities. Case Study: Reproductive justice advocates hosted community workshops and advocacy campaigns to raise birth trauma awareness and highlight its impact on Black families (Center for Children and Families, 2022). This resulted in legislative changes that increased funding for maternal mental healthcare and access to doulas for disadvantaged groups (Center for Children and Families, 2022). In order to adequately meet the needs of individuals and families who have undergone a distressing childbirth experience, it is crucial for policy to prioritize the provision of mental health services, social support initiatives, and reproductive justice measures specifically designed for Black families impacted by birth trauma. By pursuing focused policy efforts, policymakers may promote fair results and enhance the welfare of Black communities.

Intergenerational trauma is the transfer of trauma and its consequences from one generation to another. This has significant consequences for the dynamics and overall well-being of Black communities impacted by intergenerational, which can create tension in familial ties, leading to feelings of isolation, bitterness, and unresolved discord. Case Study: Lisa, a Black mother, struggled to bond with her mother, who had gone through a traumatic childbirth experience (Grote et al., 2010; Grote et al., 2015). Lisa's ability to seek assistance and advice during her pregnancy and birthing experiences was adversely impacted by their strained relationship, highlighting the outcomes of the transfer of trauma across generations (Grote et al., 2010; Grote et al., 2015). Moreover, the presence of intergenerational trauma can have significant effects on the mental health and overall well-being of Black families, leading to melancholy, anxiety, and PTSD symptoms. Case Study: The Jackson family endured intergenerational trauma stemming from previous incidents of racial violence and prejudice (Brondolo et al., 2005). The family members had symptoms of PTSD and depression, which led to ongoing cycles of emotional distress and dysfunction over several generations (Brondolo et al., 2005). To summarize, intergenerational trauma has profound consequences for family dynamics and overall well-being in Black communities impacted by birth trauma. Policymakers and practitioners must acknowledge and tackle this issue to promote healing.

V. COPING STRATEGIES AND RESILIENCE

Black families have employed several strategies, both individually and collectively, to successfully navigate and overcome difficult circumstances. These solutions, which include components from psychological and societal viewpoints, are crucial for efficiently handling trauma and fostering resilience. People often turn to their acquaintances, family, or support networks to seek social support, seeking validation for their experiences and receiving aid (Jones, 2019). Case Study: Jessica sought peace in a support group created for Black women, where she found understanding and encouragement after a traumatic childbirth (Coy et al., 2021). Some individuals choose professional mental health therapies to address and manage trauma and create efficient coping skills (Coy et al., 2021). Case Study: David sought treatment specifically to address symptoms of despair that arose after his spouse experienced a difficult pregnancy (UT Southwestern Medical Center, 2024). He discovered a safe and supportive place where he could openly express himself and explore effective coping mechanisms (UT Southwestern Medical Center, 2024).

Some people also engage in self-care activities like mindfulness and meditation to control their emotions and enhance their overall well-being (Watts-Jones, 2010). Case Study: Maria, who experienced a traumatic childbirth, incorporated regular meditation into her schedule as a means of seeking peace during turmoil (Watts-Jones, 2010). Usually, black communities combine personal coping tactics with group resilience techniques. Close ties and cultural traditions are frequently what family groups rely on to provide support and togetherness in return. Case Study: Following a distressing delivery, the Thompson family sought solace and support from their church community (de Mendonca Lima & Kousmin Pryce, 2021). They received assistance for both their mental well-being and childcare responsibilities (de Mendonca Lima & Kousmin Pryce, 2021). Cultural practices and rituals have a vital role in enhancing resilience and facilitating the process of healing. Case Study: The Johnson family utilized storytelling and song as a method of healing, tapping into cultural customs that had been passed down through generations (Leary, 2005).

Certain families actively campaign for and promote policy enhancements by using their own experiences to raise awareness. Case Study: The Smith family advocated for improved maternal healthcare services following a distressing childbirth experience (Black Mamas Matter Alliance, 2018). They engaged in local community discussions and mobilized inhabitants to advocate for enhanced availability of medical care (Black Mamas Matter Alliance, 2018). Black families have the ability to come together and take action to bring about significant changes in the system and promote healing within their communities through grassroots movements and activities organized by the community. Case Study: The Davis family, for instance, joined a grassroots organization that focuses on advocating for maternal health (Dula, 2021). They participated in organizing demonstrations and increasing awareness of birth trauma within their community (Dula, 2021). In addition, cultural traditions and ancestral wisdom offer direction and assistance, promoting resilience throughout several generations. Case Study: The Williams family utilized their ancestral traditions of resilience to find strength and foster connection through cultural activities such as drumming circles (Child Trends, 2020; Turner, 2021; Dope Black, n.d.). Black families utilize a range of coping mechanisms and resilience methods to address birth trauma, highlighting both personal and communal resources (Child Trends, 2020; Turner, 2021; Dope Black, n.d.). Acknowledging and affirming these flexible approaches can promote resilience, empowerment, and recovery in impacted communities (Child Trends, 2020; Turner, 2021; Dope Black, n.d.). In the face of adversity, Black families have resorted to a wide spectrum of tactics, prioritizing cultural practices, social support, activism, and overall health and wellness. Black communities may be empowered by lawmakers, doctors, and community leaders who work to improve mother and child health outcomes, aid in healing, and empower Black communities.

In order to provide culturally competent treatment, healthcare providers must prioritize needs of underrepresented groups, work to achieve reproductive justice, and actively challenge and repair institutional inequities. As a result, we can ensure that all families will be able to meet their basic needs and thrive.

VI. POLICY LANDSCAPE AND GAPS

An analysis of the current policy frameworks that impact the health of Black birthing people highlights a complicated and interrelated environment influenced by healthcare policies, legislation on reproductive rights, and social welfare programs (Alker & Roygardner, 2022). The implementation of policies such as the ACA and Targeted Regulation of Abortion Providers (TRAP legislation) has had critical effects on the ability of Black women to obtain healthcare services and exercise their reproductive rights (Alker & Roygardner, 2022). The ACA increased the Medicaid eligibility criteria, improving the availability of prenatal care for low-income Black moms (Kozhimannil et al., 2016). Nevertheless, differences remain across states that chose not to expand Medicaid, highlighting the significance of policy choices made at the state level. Policies have a substantial influence on the quality of care, as demonstrated by initiatives like the Alliance for Innovation on Maternal Health (AIM). AIM's introduction of evidence-based maternal safety bundles has successfully reduced maternal mortality and morbidity rates among Black persons (Howell et al., 2018).

Notwithstanding these efforts, the existing policy frameworks exhibit substantial shortcomings that result in persistent disparities in the health of Black women, individuals giving birth, and children. Black women residing in states that have not adopted Medicaid expansion under the ACA have a significant deficiency in comprehensive maternity healthcare services, creating a severe gap (Alker & Roygardner, 2022). This disparity results in a lack of access to crucial prenatal, maternity, and postpartum care for many Black people, which worsens the existing inequalities in maternal health outcomes. For instance, in states that have not implemented Medicaid expansion, economically disadvantaged Black people may face challenges in obtaining prompt prenatal care, resulting in heightened risks throughout pregnancy and delivery.

There is a growing urgency to enhance the accountability and enforcement mechanisms of existing maternal health initiatives. The Maternal Mortality Review Committees Act and the Preventing Maternal Mortality Act of 2018 were made to make it easier to collect and look over data on maternal mortality. However, there are differences in how these rules are put into place and applied. (Congress.gov., 2018; KFF, 2020; Mount Sinai, 2024). Without adequate enforcement mechanisms and accountability measures, disparities in maternal health outcomes may persist, undermining the effectiveness of these policies in addressing systemic inequities (Congress.gov., 2018; KFF, 2020; Mount Sinai, 2024). Although MMRCs are present, disparities in maternal mortality rates persist among Black women in comparison to their counterparts from other racial/ethnic backgrounds. These disparities highlight the need for more effective implementation and enforcement of policies aimed at reducing maternal mortality (Congress.gov., 2018; KFF, 2020; Mount Sinai, 2024).

Furthermore, there is a lack of adequate allocation of resources for social welfare initiatives that especially target the socioeconomic factors that affect the health outcomes of mothers and babies. Although programs such as the Special Supplemental Nutrition Program for Women, Infants, and Children (WIC) have effectively impacted birth outcomes and addressed some inequalities, the budget allocation for these efforts is insufficient to support low-income Black families adequately (Bitler & Currie, 2005; GAO, 2017). Lack of adequate financial investment exacerbates inequalities in the health outcomes of mothers and newborns by restricting marginalized communities' access to crucial resources and support services. Insufficient financing for the WIC program might lead to restricted availability of nourishing food and healthcare oversight for economically disadvantaged Black pregnant women and children (Bitler & Currie, 2005; GAO, 2017). This has the potential to worsen the current gaps in birth outcomes and mother well-being.

In order to promote health equality and enhance the health outcomes of Black families, particularly in terms of maternal and infant health, it is crucial to address the current deficiencies in policy. Moreover, authorities must commit supplementary funds and resources to social welfare initiatives targeting socioeconomic determinants of health. Policymakers may capitalize on the chance to reduce disparities and provide equitable access to support and resources for optimum childbirth outcomes, irrespective of race or socioeconomic position.

VII. PROPOSING SOLUTIONS AND RECOMMENDATIONS

Changes in policy should be based on evidence if we want to reduce the maternal mortality rate among Black people. A successful technique is to allocate funds to community-based care initiatives including as home visiting programs, doula and nursing services, and culturally appropriate prenatal and postpartum care (Crear-Perry et al., 2021). Community-based care improves the health outcomes of mothers and infants by offering personalized support and culturally suitable resources (Crear-Perry et al., 2021). The Healthy Start program funds community-based groups that offer assorted services to pregnant persons and families, such as home visiting, breastfeeding assistance, and mental health counseling (US Department of Health and Human Services, 2023).

Similarly, support for extending Medicaid benefits is crucial; these benefits should include comprehensive healthcare services during the prenatal, pregnancy, and postpartum stages. Medicaid expansion has been linked to increased availability of prenatal care and decreased rates of maternal mortality, especially among disadvantaged and minority populations (KFF, 2022; Kozhimannil et al., 2016). States such as California have shown substantial decreases in maternal mortality rates with the expansion of Medicaid under the ACA (KFF, 2022; Kozhimannil et al., 2016).

Furthermore, unconscious bias training for healthcare personnel should be introduced with the specific goal of tackling systemic prejudices in maternity care (American Hospital Association, 2013). Culturally competent care models incorporate cultural beliefs, values, and practices into clinical practice to ensure that care is respectful, responsive, and applicable to the needs of varied patient groups (American Hospital Association, 2013). This also requires healthcare professionals to identify and address medical racism with antiracist policies (Hardeman et al., 2016). Case Study: The California Birth Equity Collaborative is a program that offers unconscious bias training to healthcare personnel. The major goals of this study are to Improve maternal health outcomes and reduce treatment disparities (California Maternal Quality Care Collaborative, n.d.; Howell et al., 2018). Case Study: The CenteringPregnancy framework offers group prenatal care that focuses on peer support and culturally suitable instruction (Centering Healthcare Institute, n.d.). This model has demonstrated effective implementation in several healthcare settings that specifically serve Black communities, resulting in improved birth outcomes and heightened satisfaction among Black participants (Centering Healthcare Institute, n.d.).

Advocating for comprehensive reproductive health education in diverse environments, such as schools and healthcare institutions, is crucial. Comprehensive reproductive health education provides individuals with the necessary knowledge and abilities to make well-informed choices regarding their reproductive health (Gavin et al., 2014; Kirby et al., 2007; Chandra-Mouli et al., 2015). The Teen Pregnancy Prevention Program (TPP) supports evidence-based, comprehensive sex education programs that share information on contraception, promote healthy relationships, and prevent pregnancy to improve reproductive health outcomes (Gavin et al., 2014).

Implementing strategies to overcome geographic barriers and shortages of maternity care professionals is also critical. The Maternal Health Access Project in Mississippi uses telemedicine to connect pregnant women in rural places with obstetricians for prenatal visits (Maternal Health Access Project, 2022). New tools like telemedicine can help lawmakers make it easier for women from underserved groups to get prenatal care. This can even out differences in maternal health (Maternal Health Access Project, 2022; Olds et al., 2014).

Promising strategies also encompass the provision of increased availability of doulas and midwives, postpartum support services, legislation promoting reproductive equity, and initiatives that encourage community involvement and collaborations. Using doula and midwifery services leads to enhanced delivery outcomes, heightened satisfaction with healthcare, and decreased healthcare expenses (Kozhimannil et al., 2016). Enacting these policies, for example, implementing Medicaid coverage for doula care, might effectively mitigate maternal and child health inequalities (Kozhimannil et al., 2016).

Additionally, it is critical to implement legislation that ensures equitable and unbiased access to midwifery services (Attanasio et al., 2019). A viable strategy to accomplish this objective is to integrate midwives into healthcare systems and invest financial resources to increase midwifery training programs. An effective legislative approach would include expanding the scope of Medicaid to encompass midwifery services (Attanasio et al., 2019; Thornton & Chavkin, 2016). This would enable a larger proportion of Black women to get midwifery care throughout the stages of pregnancy, delivery, and the postpartum period (Attanasio et al., 2019; Thornton & Chavkin, 2016).

Furthermore, it is crucial to advocate for initiatives that bolster the representation of individuals of African descent in the field of midwifery. In order to promote the involvement of Black women in the field of midwifery, it is advisable to establish scholarship programs, mentorship initiatives, and targeted outreach efforts that cater to their specific requirements and motivations (American College of Nurse-Midwives, 2024). By expanding diversity in the midwifery field, Black pregnant people are more likely to have access to culturally competent care (American College of Nurse-Midwives, 2024). This will increase their likelihood of receiving treatment tailored to their specific requirements and preferences.

Postpartum support services, such as mental health counseling and breastfeeding assistance, could be enhanced to foster mothers' and infants' health and well-being. The New Jersey Family Health Survey revealed that Black mothers who received assistance with breastfeeding from lactation consultants based in the community were more inclined to begin and sustain breastfeeding (New Jersey Department of Health, 2022). This underscores the significance of comprehensive postpartum support services in enhancing breastfeeding outcomes and maternal well-being (New Jersey Department of Health, 2022).

Advocating for reproductive justice policies that support the rights of individuals to make well-informed choices regarding their reproductive health, including the availability of contraception and abortion services, is crucial for promoting health equality and ensuring reproductive autonomy. For example, the Reproductive Health Equity Act in Oregon guarantees unrestricted access to a comprehensive array of reproductive healthcare services, including abortion treatment, for all persons, regardless of their wealth, race, or insurance status (Oregon Health Authority, n.d.).

The active involvement and collaboration of the community are vital for the progress, execution, and evaluation of programs aimed at improving the welfare of mothers and children (McLemore et al., 2018). Including people, groups, and organizations in the decision-making process may help make sure that policies and actions are in line with what the community needs (McLemore et al., 2018). As stated by the Black Mamas Matter Alliance (2018), BMMA is a group that supports and speaks for Black moms and women who are giving birth. The BMMA is a group that promotes policies prioritizing Black moms' and individuals' needs and experiences throughout childbirth. They strive to tackle maternity and infant health inequalities via community-led initiatives and advocacy endeavors (BMMA, n.d.).

Policymakers can undertake evidence-based policy interventions in the areas outlined in this chapter that promote health equality for Black mothers and infant health.

VIII. A GLOBAL PERSPECTIVE

The topic of Black birth trauma has become a significant concern that has a profound impact on the health consequences of both mothers and infants on a global scale. Although differences in mother and infant mortality have been extensively studied in some countries, such as the United States, adopting a global viewpoint provides a more comprehensive knowledge of the many elements that contribute to Black birth trauma.

Global Healthcare Disparities: Black persons who give birth experience higher rates of maternal and newborn mortality compared to white persons worldwide. Black women in countries like the United States, the United Kingdom, Brazil, and South Africa have higher rates of maternal mortality. This is frequently due to limited access to high-quality prenatal and obstetric care, encountering racial prejudice within healthcare institutions, and facing socioeconomic inequities (Knight et al., 2014; d'Oliveira et al., 2002; Heaman et al., 2014; Moodley, 2019). These inequalities continue regardless of differences in healthcare funding, delivery systems, and cultural circumstances.

Countries have taken action via legislation and policy to address Black birth trauma and promote maternal and infant health fairness. The ACA has broadened the availability of maternal healthcare coverage, encompassing services such as prenatal care and childbirth, to persons with low income (Artiga et al., 2016; Howell et al., 2016; Bryant & Haas, 2018; Howell & Zeitlin, 2017). Similarly, the National Health Service in the United Kingdom offers healthcare coverage to all persons (Majeed et al., 2018). However, there are differences in maternal mortality rates based on race. As a result, there is an increasing demand for specific actions to address racism in the healthcare system. The main objective of the Sistema Único de Saúde in Brazil is to deliver comprehensive healthcare services to everyone, including maternity and newborn care. However, there are still racial inequalities in the availability and outcomes of healthcare, mainly affecting Afro-Brazilian women living in underprivileged regions (Diniz et al., 2012). In South Africa, maternal mortality initiatives have focused on improving access to prenatal care, skilled birth attendants, and emergency obstetric services (Moodley, 2019). Nevertheless, there remain challenges in efficiently reaching rural and vulnerable groups.

A comparative review of policy and legal initiatives in many nations highlights both commonalities and variations in policies aimed at addressing Black birth trauma. Although universal healthcare coverage has been implemented in several countries, disparities in healthcare access and health outcomes persist. These discrepancies might be ascribed to fundamental structural issues such as racism, poverty, and inequitable allocation of resources (Ruger & Yach, 2009). Countries with strong and comprehensive social welfare and support systems in place, like the Nordic nations, often observe lower maternal mortality rates. Nonetheless, racial inequalities persist throughout these structures (Vohra-Gupta, 2023).

An international analysis of Black birth trauma illustrates the importance of addressing social determinants of health, allocating resources to culturally competent healthcare, and implementing policy initiatives that advance maternal and child health equity. Key takeaways from successful interventions include the necessity of community involvement, facilitating multidisciplinary cooperation, and continuously monitoring and evaluating healthcare systems to ensure responsibility and efficiency (Gross et al., 2006).

Conclusion: To summarize, analyzing global Black birth trauma reveals the pervasive presence of inequities in the health outcomes of both mothers and infants. This underscores the need for thorough and far-reaching measures to address these disparities. Analyzing these parallels and distinctions in experiences, healthcare systems, and government interventions across different nations and regions can provide crucial perspectives for creating evidence-based therapies and ensuring equitable healthcare access worldwide.

IX. PERSONAL REFLECTIONS AND LESSONS LEARNED: NAVIGATING BLACK BIRTH TRAUMA

Personal Experience: My journey with Black birth trauma began on a day that was supposed to be one of joy and celebration—the birth of my three-year old daughter. However, what should have been a moment of profound happiness quickly turned into a nightmare as life-threatening complications arose a few days after childbirth—complications that were ignored and downplayed by my medical providers. The experience was harrowing, filled with fear, pain, and uncertainty. In the aftermath of the trauma, I struggled to come to terms with what had happened, grappling with feelings of guilt, anger, and profound sadness. As a legal epidemiologist steeped in knowledge about the maternal mortality crisis, I thought I was prepared for any challenges that may arise during childbirth. However, even with this expertise, I found myself unprepared for the traumatic birth experience I encountered. My hospital stay extended to nearly a month, during which my husband slept on the couch of my hospital room, taking turns caring for me and our premature daughter down the hall in the neonatal intensive care unit.

As I began the process of healing, I leaned on my support networks—my husband, family, and friends—who provided unwavering love and encouragement during this challenging time. I learned to navigate my emotions and develop coping mechanisms to manage the lingering effects of trauma. I also found solace in connecting with other mothers who had experienced similar challenges, sharing stories of resilience and hope. Additionally, I utilized my experience to inform legislation with recommendations spoken on panel discussions, podcasts, and conferences to inform next steps and inspire improved Black maternal health outcomes.

Lessons Learned: Reflecting on my experience with Black birth trauma, I have gleaned several valuable lessons that have shaped my perspective and approach to maternal and infant health advocacy. Firstly, I have come to understand the profound impact that trauma can have on family dynamics, relationships, and mental health. The ripple effects of trauma extend far beyond the individual, impacting the entire family unit and necessitating holistic approaches to healing and support.

Secondly, I have learned the importance of accessing culturally competent care and support services. Too often, Black birthing individuals are underserved and overlooked within healthcare systems that fail to acknowledge their unique needs and experiences. Culturally competent care that is sensitive to the cultural, social, and historical context of Black birth trauma is essential for promoting healing and well-being.

Finally, my childbirth experience has underscored the critical role of policy interventions in addressing and preventing Black birth trauma. Policies that prioritize access to quality healthcare, mental health services, and support programs can make a meaningful difference in the lives of Black birthing individuals and their families. By advocating for policy solutions that center the needs of marginalized communities, we can work towards a future where every Black mother and child receives the care and support they deserve.

Impact on Advocacy and Policy Work: My personal experience with Black birth trauma has profoundly influenced my advocacy and policy work in the field of maternal and infant health. It has given me a sense of purpose and urgency in fighting for policies that address the root causes of disparities and promote equity in healthcare. I am committed to amplifying the voices of marginalized communities, advocating for policies prioritizing the well-being of Black mothers and children, and driving systemic change that leads to better outcomes for all.

Closure: In sharing my story, I hope to inspire empathy, understanding, and action. Black birth trauma is a deeply personal and often overlooked issue that requires greater attention and advocacy. By centering the voices and experiences of those affected, we can drive positive change, promote healing, and create a future where Black birthing individuals are supported, valued, and empowered.

X. CONCLUSION

This chapter offers an extensive analysis of Black birth trauma, family dynamics, and policy remedies within the framework of disparities in mother and infant health. It provides key ideas and facts about the impact of historical events, including slavery, segregation, and medical racism, on the enduring effects of Black birth trauma and its influence on current health outcomes (American Heart Association, 2020; Black et al., 2020). It examines modern inequalities in health outcomes for Black mothers and babies, especially regarding higher rates of maternal death and morbidity. This analysis shows the role of systemic factors and policy choices in contributing to these disparities. Furthermore, it explores the long-lasting effects of Black birth trauma on family dynamics, including its impact on personal relationships, support systems, and mental well-being. Furthermore, it examines the strategies utilized by Black families and grassroots organizations to manage these challenges and uncover sources of strength and flexibility.

This investigation considers contemporary policy frameworks that influence the health of Black mothers, delivering individuals, and their families. These include laws about reproductive rights, health care policies, and social aid programs. It points out major policy holes and flaws that don't do enough to fix birth trauma and unfair treatment of Black people. It also gives policymakers suggestions based on facts that can help solve the problems listed. These recommendations emphasize the importance of community-driven and participatory approaches in policy creation and implementation. The chapter ends by urging politicians, healthcare professionals, and advocacy organizations to prioritize Black families' needs in policy efforts and decision-making processes. This provides considerations to inform next steps towards better maternal and newborn health outcomes.

It is very important to recognize and treat the effects of Black birth trauma, which means looking at past, present, and family issues in a broad way. This model is very important for getting long-lasting benefits for Black people. To get a full picture, it's important to look at the historical roots of Black birth trauma, the differences that still exist, and the effects on families. Advocates, policymakers, and health care providers can create comprehensive and effective strategies to address injustices and promote equity if they put experiences and needs of Black birthing people and their families first.

For the sake of Black mothers' and children's health, policymakers should adopt a constructive approach. However, there is positive news; there are grounds for optimism on the potential of policy enhancements to ameliorate the situation. The list includes more resources and knowledge, a dedication to enhancing healthcare fairness, engaged communities, forward-thinking approaches, and the potential for lasting transformation. Implementation of these recommendations by governments might potentially result in enhanced health outcomes and the elimination of disparities affecting Black communities, particularly in the context of reproductive health for birthing individuals and their families.

REFERENCES

Alker, J., & Roygardner, L. (2022, May 12). Policymakers have more work to do to address the Black maternal health crisis. *Georgetown University Health Policy Institute Center for Children and Families*. https://ccf.georgetown.edu/2022/05/12/policymakers-have-more-work-to-do-to-address-the-black-maternal-health-crisis/

American College of Nurse-Midwives. (2024). Access to midwifery care: National chartbook. https://www.midwife.org/acnm/files/cclibraryfiles/filename/000000009191/Access%20to%20Midwifery%20Care%20National_Chartbook_20240606.pdf

American Heart Association. (2020, Nov 9). Addressing structural racism central to reducing cardiovascular disease disparities across the U.S. https://newsroom.heart.org/news/addressing-structural-racism-central-to-reducing-cardiovascular-disease-disparities-across-the-u-s

American Heart Association. (2022). Wider access to health insurance via Medicaid expansion improved cardiac care. https://newsroom.heart.org/news/addressing-structural-racism-central-to-reducing-cardiovascular-disease-disparities-across-the-u-s

American Hospital Association. (2013, Jun 18). Becoming a culturally competent health care organization. https://www.aha.org/ahahret-guides/2013-06-18-becoming-culturally-competent-health-care-organization

American Medical Association. (2018). How Medicaid expansion has improved care access, outcomes. https://www.ama-assn.org/delivering-care/public-health/how-medicaid-expansion-has-improved-care-access-outcomes

Artiga, S., Foutz, J., Cornachione, E., & Garfield, R. (2016). *Key Facts on Health and Health Care by Race and Ethnicity*. Henry J. Kaiser Family Foundation., https://files.kff.org/attachment/Chartpack-Key-Facts-on-Health-and-Health-Care-by-Race-and-Ethnicity.

Artiga, S., Orgera, K., Damico, A., & Pham, O. (2018). Disparities in Health and Health Care: Five Key Questions and Answers. *Kaiser Family Foundation*. Link: https://files.kff.org/attachment/Issue-Brief-Disparities-in-Health-and-Health-Care-Five-Key-Questions-and-Answers.

Attanasio, L. B., Hardeman, R. R., Kozhimannil, K. B., & Kjerulff, K. H. (2019). Midwifery care, social and medical risk factors, and cesarean delivery: A retrospective cohort study. *Women's Health Issues*, *29*(3), 220–226.

Bitler, M. P., & Currie, J. (2005). Does WIC work? The effects of WIC on pregnancy and birth outcomes. *Journal of Policy Analysis and Management*, *24*(1), 73–91. DOI: 10.1002/pam.20070 PMID: 15584177

Black, D. (n.d.). The impact of historical trauma on Black family dynamics. https://www.dopeblack.org/blog/the-impact-of-historical-trauma-on-black-family-dynamics

Black Mamas Matter Alliance. (2018). Black mamas matter toolkit. https://blackmamasmatter.org/wp-content/uploads/2018/05/USPA_BMMA_Toolkit_Booklet-Final-Update_Web-Pages-1.pdf

Brondolo, E., Kelly, K. P., Coakley, V., Gordon, T., Thompson, S., Levy, E., Cassells, A., Tobin, J. N., Sweeney, M., & Contrada, R. J. (2005). The Perceived Ethnic Discrimination Questionnaire: Development and Preliminary Validation of a Community Version. *Journal of Applied Social Psychology*, *35*(2), 335–365. DOI: 10.1111/j.1559-1816.2005.tb02124.x

Bryant, A. S., & Haas, J. S. (2018). Medicaid expansion and the use of prenatal care among low-income women. *Maternal and Child Health Journal*, *22*(3), 454–462.

California Maternal Quality Care Collaborative. (n.d.). Birth Equity Toolkit. https://www.cmqcc.org/resources-tool-kits/toolkits/birth-equity-toolkit

Center for Children and Families. (2022). Black Mamas Matter Alliance highlights policy change needed in honor of Black Maternal Health Week. *Georgetown University Health Policy Institute*. https://ccf.georgetown.edu/2022/04/12/black-mamas-matter-alliance-highlights-policy-change-needed-in-honor-of-black-maternal-health-week/

Center for Health Journalism. (2022). Haunted by trauma: The Black parents who nearly died in childbirth. https://centerforhealthjournalism.org/fellowships/projects/haunted-trauma-black-parents-who-nearly-died-childbirth

Centering Healthcare Institute. (n.d.). *CenteringPregnancy: Group Prenatal Care Model.*

Centers for Disease Control and Prevention (CDC). (2020). Pregnancy Mortality Surveillance System. https://www.cdc.gov/maternal-mortality/php/pregnancy-mortality-surveillance/index.html

Chandra-Mouli, V., Lane, C., & Wong, S. (2015). What does not work in adolescent sexual and reproductive health: A review of evidence on interventions commonly accepted as best practices. *Global Health, Science and Practice*, *3*(3), 333–340. DOI: 10.9745/GHSP-D-15-00126 PMID: 26374795

Commonwealth Fund. (2022). Inequities in health coverage and access: Black and Hispanic adults. https://www.commonwealthfund.org/publications/issue-briefs/2022/inequities-health-coverage-access-black-hispanic-adults

Congress.gov. (2018). H.R.1318 - Preventing Maternal Deaths Act of 2018. https://www.congress.gov/bill/115th-congress/house-bill/1318

Coy, D., Malekpour, S., Saeri, A. K., & Dargaville, R. (2021). Rethinking community empowerment in the energy transformation: A critical review of the definitions, drivers and outcomes. *Energy Research & Social Science*, *72*, 101871. DOI: 10.1016/j.erss.2020.101871

Creanga, A. A., Syverson, C., Seed, K., & Callaghan, W. M. (2017). Pregnancy-Related Mortality in the United States, 2011–2013. [Link]. *Obstetrics and Gynecology*, *130*(2), 366–373. DOI: 10.1097/AOG.0000000000002114 PMID: 28697109

Crear-Perry, J., Correa-de-Araujo, R., Lewis Johnson, T., McLemore, M. R., Neilson, E., & Wallace, M. (2021). Social and Structural Determinants of Health Inequities in Maternal Health. *Journal of Women's Health (2002)*, *30*(2), 230–235. DOI: 10.1089/jwh.2020.8882

d'Oliveira, A. F., Diniz, S. G., & Schraiber, L. B. (2002). Violence against women in health-care institutions: An emerging problem. *Lancet*, *359*(9318), 1681–1685. DOI: 10.1016/S0140-6736(02)08592-6 PMID: 12020546

Dawley, K. (2003, Mar 4). Origins of Nurse-Midwifery in the United States and its Expansion in the 1940s. *Journal of Midwifery & Women's Health*, *48*(2), 86–95. DOI: 10.1016/S1526-9523(03)00002-3 PMID: 12686940

Diniz, S. G., d'Oliveira, A. F., & Lansky, S. (2012). Equity and women's health services for contraception, abortion and childbirth in Brazil. *Reproductive Health Matters*, *20*(40), 94–101. DOI: 10.1016/S0968-8080(12)40657-7 PMID: 23245414

Dula, S. (2021, Oct 28). 6 Maternal Health Organizations Working to Support Mothers. *Pregnancy & Newborn Magazine*. https://www.pnmag.com/mom-baby/6-maternal-health-organizations-working-to-support-mothers/

Ertan, D., Hingray, C., Burlacu, E., Sterlé, A., & El-Hage, W. (2021). Post-traumatic stress disorder following childbirth. *BMC Psychiatry*, *21*(1), 155. DOI: 10.1186/s12888-021-03158-6 PMID: 33726703

Fair, F., Soltani, H., Raben, L., van Streun, Y., Sioti, E., Papadakaki, M., Burke, C., Watson, H., Jokinen, M., Shaw, E., Triantafyllou, E., van den Muijsenbergh, M., & Vivilaki, V. (2021). Midwives' experiences of cultural competency training and providing perinatal care for migrant women: A mixed methods study: Operational Refugee and Migrant Maternal Approach (ORAMMA) project. *BMC Pregnancy and Childbirth*, *21*(1), 340. DOI: 10.1186/s12884-021-03799-1 PMID: 33926420

Ford, C. L., & Airhihenbuwa, C. O. (2010). Critical Race Theory, race equity, and public health: toward antiracism praxis. *American Journal of Public Health, 100 Suppl 1*(Suppl 1), S30–S35. DOI: 10.2105/AJPH.2009.171058

Gavin, L., Moskosky, S., Carter, M., Curtis, K., Glass, E., Godfrey, E., ... & Zapata, L. (2014). Providing quality family planning services: Recommendations of CDC and the US Office of Population Affairs. *MMWR. Recommendations and Reports: Morbidity and Mortality Weekly Report. Recommendations and Reports / Centers for Disease Control, 63*(Rr-04), 1-54.

Gross, J., Power, T., & St John, W. (2006). A social marketing model for disseminating research-based interventions. *American Journal of Community Psychology*, *38*(1-2), 79–89. PMID: 16909316

Grote, N. K., Bridge, J. A., Gavin, A. R., Melville, J. L., Iyengar, S., & Katon, W. J. (2010). A meta-analysis of depression during pregnancy and the risk of preterm birth, low birth weight, and intrauterine growth restriction. *Archives of General Psychiatry*, *67*(10), 1012–1024. DOI: 10.1001/archgenpsychiatry.2010.111 PMID: 20921117

Grote, N. K., Katon, W. J., Russo, J. E., Lohr, M. J., Curran, M., Galvin, E., & Carson, K. (2015). COLLABORATIVE CARE FOR PERINATAL DEPRESSION IN SOCIOECONOMICALLY DISADVANTAGED WOMEN: A RANDOMIZED TRIAL. *Depression and Anxiety*, *32*(11), 821–834. DOI: 10.1002/da.22405 PMID: 26345179

Hardeman, R. R., Medina, E. M., & Kozhimannil, K. B. (2016). Structural Racism and Supporting Black Lives - The Role of Health Professionals. *The New England Journal of Medicine*, *375*(22), 2113–2115. DOI: 10.1056/NEJMp1609535 PMID: 27732126

Heaman, M. I., Moffatt, M., Elliott, L., Sword, W., Helewa, M. E., Morris, H., Gregory, P., Tjaden, L., & Cook, C. (2014). Barriers, motivators and facilitators related to prenatal care utilization among inner-city women in Winnipeg, Canada: A case–control study. *BMC Pregnancy and Childbirth*, *14*(1), 227. DOI: 10.1186/1471-2393-14-227 PMID: 25023478

Howell, E. A. (2018). Reducing Disparities in Severe Maternal Morbidity and Mortality. *Clinical Obstetrics and Gynecology*, *61*(2), 387–399. DOI: 10.1097/GRF.0000000000000349 PMID: 29346121

Howell, E. A., Brown, H., Brumley, J., Bryant, A. S., Caughey, A. B., Cornell, A. M., Grant, J. H., Gregory, K. D., Gullo, S. M., Kozhimannil, K. B., Mhyre, J. M., Toledo, P., D'Oria, R., Ngoh, M., & Grobman, W. A. (2018). Reduction of Peripartum Racial and Ethnic Disparities: A Conceptual Framework and Maternal Safety Consensus Bundle. *Obstetrics and Gynecology*, *131*(5), 770–782. DOI: 10.1097/AOG.0000000000002475 PMID: 29683895

Howell, E. A., Egorova, N., Balbierz, A., Zeitlin, J., & Hebert, P. L. (2016). Black-white differences in severe maternal morbidity and site of care. *American Journal of Obstetrics and Gynecology*, *214*(1), 122.e1–122.e1227. DOI: 10.1016/j.ajog.2015.08.019 PMID: 26283457

Howell, E. A., & Zeitlin, J. (2017). Improving hospital quality to reduce disparities in severe maternal morbidity and mortality. *Seminars in Perinatology*, *41*(5), 266–272. DOI: 10.1053/j.semperi.2017.04.002 PMID: 28735811

Howell, E. A., & Zeitlin, J. (2017). Quality of Care and Disparities in Obstetrics. *Obstetrics and Gynecology Clinics of North America*, *44*(1), 13–25. DOI: 10.1016/j.ogc.2016.10.002 PMID: 28160890

Huang, C., Wei, K., Lee, P. M. Y., Qin, G., Yu, Y., & Li, J. (2022). Maternal hypertensive disorder of pregnancy and mortality in offspring from birth to young adulthood: National population based cohort study. *BMJ (Clinical Research Ed.)*, *379*, e072157. DOI: 10.1136/bmj-2022-072157 PMID: 36261141

Jones, A. (2019). Help Seeking in the Perinatal Period: A Review of Barriers and Facilitators. *Social Work in Public Health*, *34*(7), 596–605. DOI: 10.1080/19371918.2019.1635947 PMID: 31242074

Jones, J. H. (1993). *Bad Blood: The Tuskegee Syphilis Experiment*. Free Press.

Jones, K. M., Power, M. L., Queenan, J. T., & Schulkin, J. (2015). Racial and ethnic disparities in breastfeeding. *Breastfeeding Medicine*, *10*(4), 186–196. DOI: 10.1089/bfm.2014.0152 PMID: 25831234

Kaiser Family Foundation. (n.d.). Mental health and substance use disorder coverage in marketplace plans. https://www.kff.org/mental-health/issue-brief/mental-health-and-substance-use-disorder-coverage-in-medicare-advantage-plans/

KFF. (2020). Analysis of Federal Bills to Strengthen Maternal Health Care. *Kaiser Family Foundation*. https://www.kff.org/womens-health-policy/fact-sheet/analysis-of-federal-bills-to-strengthen-maternal-health-care/

KFF. (2022). Medicaid Coverage of Pregnancy-Related Services: Findings from a 2021 State Survey. *Kaiser Family Foundation*. https://www.kff.org/report-section/medicaid-coverage-of-pregnancy-related-services-findings-from-a-2021-state-survey-report/

Kirby, D., Laris, B. A., & Rolleri, L. A. (2007). Sex and HIV education programs: Their impact on sexual behaviors of young people throughout the world. *The Journal of Adolescent Health*, *40*(3), 206–217. DOI: 10.1016/j.jadohealth.2006.11.143 PMID: 17321420

Knight, M., Kenyon, S., Brocklehurst, P., Neilson, J., Shakespeare, J., & Kurinczuk, J.. (2014). *Saving Lives, Improving Mothers' Care – Lessons Learned to Inform Future Maternity Care from the UK and Ireland Confidential Enquiries into Maternal Deaths and Morbidity 2009–12*. National Perinatal Epidemiology Unit, University of Oxford.

Kozhimannil, K. B., Hardeman, R. R., Alarid-Escudero, F., Vogelsang, C. A., Blauer-Peterson, C., & Howell, E. A. (2016). Modeling the Cost-Effectiveness of Doula Care Associated with Reductions in Preterm Birth and Cesarean Delivery. *Birth (Berkeley, Calif.)*, *43*(1), 20–27. DOI: 10.1111/birt.12218 PMID: 26762249

Kozhimannil, K. B., Interrante, J. D., Henning-Smith, C., & Admon, L. K. (2019). Rural-Urban Differences In Severe Maternal Morbidity And Mortality In The US, 2007-15. *Health Affairs (Project Hope)*, *38*(12), 2077–2085. DOI: 10.1377/hlthaff.2019.00805 PMID: 31794322

Leary, Joy DeGruy. (2005). *Post traumatic slave syndrome: America's legacy of enduring injury and healing*. Milwaukie, Oregon: Uptone Press.

Majeed, A., Allwood, D., Foley, K., & Bindman, A. (2018). Healthcare outcomes and quality in the NHS: How do we compare and how might the NHS improve? *BMJ (Clinical Research Ed.)*, *362*, k3036. DOI: 10.1136/bmj.k3036 PMID: 30006368

McLemore, M. R., Altman, M. R., Cooper, N., Williams, S., Rand, L., & Franck, L. (2018). Health care experiences of pregnant, birthing and postnatal women of color at risk for preterm birth. *Social Science & Medicine*, *201*, 127–135. DOI: 10.1016/j.socscimed.2018.02.013 PMID: 29494846

Moodley, J., Fawcus, S., & Pattinson, R. (2019). Improvements in maternal mortality in South Africa. *South African Medical Journal*, *108*(3a), s4–s8.

New Jersey Department of Health. (2022). *New Jersey breastfeeding strategic plan 2022* [PDF]. https://www.nj.gov/health/fhs/wic/documents/FINAL%20New%20Jersey%20Breastfeeding%20Strategic%20Plan%202022.pdf

Ngo-Metzger, Q., Massagli, M. P., Clarridge, B. R., Manocchia, M., Davis, R. B., Iezzoni, L. I., & Phillips, R. S. (2003). Linguistic and cultural barriers to care. *Journal of General Internal Medicine*, *18*(1), 44–52. DOI: 10.1046/j.1525-1497.2003.20205.x PMID: 12534763

Olds, D. L., Kitzman, H., Knudtson, M. D., Anson, E., Smith, J. A., & Cole, R. (2014). Effect of Home Visiting by Nurses on Maternal and Child Mortality: Results of a 2-Decade Follow-Up of a Randomized Clinical Trial. *JAMA Pediatrics*, *168*(9), 800–806. DOI: 10.1001/jamapediatrics.2014.472 PMID: 25003802

Oregon Health Authority. (n.d.). Reproductive Health Equity Act. https://www.oregon.gov/oha/ph/healthypeoplefamilies/reproductivesexualhealth/pages/reproductive-health-equity-act.aspx

Ravi, D., Iacob, A., & Profit, J. (2021). Unequal care: Racial/ethnic disparities in neonatal intensive care delivery. *Seminars in Perinatology*, *45*(4), 151411. DOI: 10.1016/j.semperi.2021.151411 PMID: 33902931

Reed, B. (2020, May 2). “New York mother dies after raising alarm on hospital neglect.” *The Guardian*. https://www.theguardian.com/us-news/2020/may/02/amber-rose-isaac-new-york-childbirth-death

Rhoden, R. J. (2022). Look at us as people too: The phenomenological experiences of traumatic childbirth in primi- and multiparous Black women (Doctoral dissertation, Rutgers University). Retrieved from https://doi.org/doi:10.7282/t3-8aze-b741

Salam, M. (2018, Jan 11). “Serena Williams Reveals Health Scare After Giving Birth to Her Daughter.” *The New York Times*.

Shimodera, S., Furukawa, T. A., Mino, Y., Shimazu, K., Nishida, A., & Inoue, S. (2012). Cost-effectiveness of family psychoeducation to prevent relapse in major depression: Results from a randomized controlled trial. *BMC Psychiatry*, *12*(1), 40. DOI: 10.1186/1471-244X-12-40 PMID: 22583708

Sinai, M. (2024). The Preventing Maternal Deaths Act of 2018 and Why it is Important. https://health.mountsinai.org/blog/the-preventing-maternal-deaths-act-of-2018-and-why-it-is-important/

Steiner, C. A., Barrett, M. L., Weiss, A. J., ... (2006, Feb). Trends and Projections in Hospital Stays for Adults With Multiple Chronic Conditions, 2003–2014. 2014 Nov. In: Healthcare Cost and Utilization Project (HCUP) Statistical Briefs [Internet]. Rockville (MD): Agency for Healthcare Research and Quality (US); Statistical Brief #183.https://www.ncbi.nlm.nih.gov/books/NBK264314/

Thornton, A. C., & Chavkin, W. (2016). The role of midwives in reducing maternal and neonatal mortality in Haiti. *Journal of Midwifery & Women's Health, 61*(1), 71–77.

Trends, C. (2020). Reimagining Black families' cultural assets can inform policies and practices that enhance their well-being. https://www.childtrends.org/publications/reimagining-black-families-cultural-assets-can-inform-policies-and-practices-that-enhance-their-well-being

Turner, E. A. (2021). Building resilience in Black youth. *Psychology Today*. https://www.psychologytoday.com/us/blog/building-resilience-black-youth/202101/building-resilience-in-black-youth

US Department of Health and Human Services. (2023). Healthy Start Initiative: Eliminating disparities in perinatal health. Retrieved from https://www.hrsa.gov/grants/find-funding/HRSA-24-033

US Government Accountability Office (GAO). (2017). Women, Infants, and Children (WIC) Program: Action needed to address challenges in administering nutrition services and monitoring. *GAO-17-435*. https://www.gao.gov/products/gao-02-142

Vohra-Gupta, S., Petruzzi, L., Jones, C., & Cubbin, C. (2023). An Intersectional Approach to Understanding Barriers to Healthcare for Women. *Journal of Community Health, 48*(1), 89–98. DOI: 10.1007/s10900-022-01147-8 PMID: 36273069

KEYWORD DEFINITIONS

- **Culturally competent care:** Healthcare that identifies and embraces differences amongst all patient populations, and implements treatment tailored to the needs of these groups
- **Healthcare disparities:** Disproportionate healthcare outcomes incurred by minority populations due to unfair access and treatment
- **Implicit bias:** An unconscious feeling of negativity towards patients belonging to minority populations that adversely impacts treatment

- **Intergenerational trauma:** Stress, caused by historical and modern systems of racism, that is passed down from one generation to the next and adversely impacts patient outcomes
- **Medical racism:** Healthcare inequities implemented via systemic and institutionalized racism
- **Policy reform:** Policy and legislative amendments needed to improve Black maternal health outcomes and help affected Black families
- **Reproductive justice:** A maternal health framework that emphasizes the relationship between medical racism and disproportionate rates of morbidity and mortality, highlighting the right for all birthing people to have access to competent healthcare that meets their individual needs
- **Social support systems:** Communities that help parents navigate Black birth trauma and help facilitate the journey to healing

Compilation of References

Abdullah, T., Graham-LoPresti, J. R., Tahirkheli, N. N., Hughley, S. M., & Watson, L. T. J. (2021). Microaggressions and posttraumatic stress disorder symptom scores among Black Americans: Exploring the link. *Traumatology*, *27*(3), 244–253. DOI: 10.1037/trm0000259

Abrams, J. A., Hill, A., & Maxwell, M. (2019). Underneath the mask of the strong Black woman schema: Disentangling influences of strength and self-silencing on depressive symptoms among US Black women. *Sex Roles*, *80*(9-10), 517–526. DOI: 10.1007/s11199-018-0956-y PMID: 31086431

Adeyemo, E. O., Oluwole, E. O., Kanma-Okafor, O. J., Izuka, O. M., & Odeyemi, K. A. (2020). Prevalence and predictors of postpartum depression among postnatal women in Lagos, Nigeria. *African Health Sciences*, *20*(4), 1943–1954. DOI: 10.4314/ahs.v20i4.53 PMID: 34394261

Ajayi, K. V., & Garney, W. R. (2023). What Black Mothers with Preterm Infants Want for Their Mental Health Care: A Qualitative Study. *Women's Health Reports (New Rochelle, N.Y.)*, *4*(1), 39–47. DOI: 10.1089/whr.2022.0088 PMID: 36893324

Alang, S. M. (2019). Mental health care among blacks in America: Confronting racism and constructing solutions. *Health Services Research*, *54*(2), 346–355. DOI: 10.1111/1475-6773.13115 PMID: 30687928

Alhusen, J. L., Bower, K. M., Epstein, E., & Sharps, P. (2016). Racial Discrimination and Adverse Birth Outcomes: An Integrative review. *Journal of Midwifery & Women's Health*, *61*(6), 707–720. DOI: 10.1111/jmwh.12490 PMID: 27737504

Alio, A. P., Dillion, T., Hartman, S., Johnson, T., Turner, S., Bullock, S., & Dozier, A. (2022). A community collaborative for the exploration of local factors affecting Black mothers' experiences with perinatal care. *Maternal and Child Health Journal*, *26*(4), 751–760. DOI: 10.1007/s10995-022-03422-5 PMID: 35316456

Ali, S. H., Mohsin, F. M., Banks, A., Lynn, P., & Lim, S. (2022). Peer-led, remote intervention to improve mental health outcomes using a holistic, spirituality-based approach: Results from a pilot study. *Community Mental Health Journal, 58*(5), 862–874. DOI: 10.1007/s10597-021-00893-8 PMID: 34561834

Alker, J., & Roygardner, L. (2022, May 12). Policymakers have more work to do to address the Black maternal health crisis. *Georgetown University Health Policy Institute Center for Children and Families*. https://ccf.georgetown.edu/2022/05/12/policymakers-have-more-work-to-do-to-address-the-black-maternal-health-crisis/

Almeida, J., Belanoff, C., & Erbetta, K. F. (2021). The Time has Come for All States to Measure Racial Discrimination: A Call to Action for the Pregnancy Risk Assessment Monitoring System (PRAMS). *Maternal and Child Health Journal, 26*(1), 7–11. DOI: 10.1007/s10995-021-03160-0 PMID: 33945082

Altman, M. R., McLemore, M. R., Oseguera, T., Lyndon, A., & Franck, L. S. (2020). Listening to Women: Recommendations from Women of Color to Improve Experiences in Pregnancy and Birth Care. *Journal of Midwifery & Women's Health, 65*(4), 466–473. DOI: 10.1111/jmwh.13102 PMID: 32558179

American College of Nurse-Midwives. (2024). Access to midwifery care: National chartbook. https://www.midwife.org/acnm/files/cclibraryfiles/filename/000000009191/Access%20to%20Midwifery%20Care%20National_Chartbook_20240606.pdf

American Heart Association. (2020, Nov 9). Addressing structural racism central to reducing cardiovascular disease disparities across the U.S. https://newsroom.heart.org/news/addressing-structural-racism-central-to-reducing-cardiovascular-disease-disparities-across-the-u-s

American Heart Association. (2022). Wider access to health insurance via Medicaid expansion improved cardiac care. https://newsroom.heart.org/news/addressing-structural-racism-central-to-reducing-cardiovascular-disease-disparities-across-the-u-s

American Hospital Association. (2013, Jun 18). Becoming a culturally competent health care organization. https://www.aha.org/ahahret-guides/2013-06-18-becoming-culturally-competent-health-care-organization

American Medical Association. (2018). How Medicaid expansion has improved care access, outcomes. https://www.ama-assn.org/delivering-care/public-health/how-medicaid-expansion-has-improved-care-access-outcomes

Ammerman, R. T., Putnam, F. W., Altaye, M., Chen, L., Holleb, L. J., Stevens, J., & Van Ginkel, J. B. (2010). Changes in depressive symptoms in first-time mothers in home visitation. *Child Abuse & Neglect, 34*(9), 639–649. PMID: 20638720

Anderson, K., Thompson, L., & Raikes, H. (2017). Home-based care and early childhood development. *Journal of Child Health Care, 21*(3), 270–280.

Anderson, R. E., Jones, S., Anyiwo, N., McKenny, M., & Gaylord-Harden, N. (2019). What's race got to do with it? Racial socialization's contribution to Black adolescent coping. *Journal of Research on Adolescence, 29*(4), 822–831. DOI: 10.1111/jora.12440 PMID: 30099797

Anstey, E. H., Shoemaker, M. L., Barrera, C. M., O'Neil, M. E., Verma, A. B., & Holman, D. M. (2017). Breastfeeding and breast cancer risk reduction: Implications for black mothers. *American Journal of Preventive Medicine, 53*(3), S40–S46. DOI: 10.1016/j.amepre.2017.04.024 PMID: 28818244

Antilla, J. M., & Johnson, T. S. (2024). Life stressors and mental well-being: Experiences of African American women navigating perinatal loss and pregnancy subsequent to loss. *The Journal of Black Psychology, 0*(0), 326–364. DOI: 10.1177/00957984241230670

Aoki, A., Togoobaatar, G., Tseveenjav, A., Nyam, N., Zuunnast, K., & Takehara, K. (2022). Quality of life of mothers of children and adolescents with mental health problems in Mongolia: Associations with the severity of children's mental health problems and family structure. *Global Mental Health (Cambridge, England), 9*, 298–305. DOI: 10.1017/gmh.2022.34 PMID: 36618750

Araji, S., Griffin, A., Dixon, L., Spencer, S. K., Peavie, C., & Wallace, K. (2020). An overview of maternal anxiety during pregnancy and the post-partum period. *Journal of Mental Health & Clinical Psychology, 4*(4). https://www.mentalhealthjournal.org/articles/an-overview-of-maternal-anxiety-during-pregnancy-and-the-post-partum-period.pdf

Arteaga, S., Hubbard, E., Arcara, J., Cuentos, A., Armstead, M., Jackson, A., Gomez, A. M., & Marshall, C. (2023). "They're gonna be there to advocate for me so I'm not by myself": A qualitative analysis of Black women's motivations for seeking and experiences with community doula care. *Women and Birth; Journal of the Australian College of Midwives, 36*(3), 257–263. DOI: 10.1016/j.wombi.2022.08.007 PMID: 36089498

Artiga, S., Orgera, K., Damico, A., & Pham, O. (2018). Disparities in Health and Health Care: Five Key Questions and Answers. *Kaiser Family Foundation*. Link: https://files.kff.org/attachment/Issue-Brief-Disparities-in-Health-and-Health-Care-Five-Key-Questions-and-Answers.

Artiga, S., Foutz, J., Cornachione, E., & Garfield, R. (2016). *Key Facts on Health and Health Care by Race and Ethnicity*. Henry J. Kaiser Family Foundation., https://files.kff.org/attachment/Chartpack-Key-Facts-on-Health-and-Health-Care-by-Race-and-Ethnicity.

Asiodu, I. V., Bugg, K., & Palmquist, A. E. (2021). Achieving breastfeeding equity and justice in Black communities: Past, present, and future. *Breastfeeding Medicine*, *16*(6), 447–451. DOI: 10.1089/bfm.2020.0314 PMID: 33979550

Asiodu, I. V., Waters, C. M., Dailey, D. E., Lee, K. A., & Lyndon, A. (2015). Breastfeeding and use of social media among first-time African American mothers. *Journal of Obstetric, Gynecologic, and Neonatal Nursing : JOGNN*, *44*(2), 268–278. DOI: 10.1111/1552-6909.12552 PMID: 25712127

Attanasio, L. B., Hardeman, R. R., Kozhimannil, K. B., & Kjerulff, K. H. (2019). Midwifery care, social and medical risk factors, and cesarean delivery: A retrospective cohort study. *Women's Health Issues*, *29*(3), 220–226.

Atzl, V. M., Narayan, A. J., Rivera, L. M., & Lieberman, A. F. (2019). Adverse childhood experiences and prenatal mental health: Type of ACEs and age of maltreatment onset. *Journal of Family Psychology*, *33*(3), 304–314. DOI: 10.1037/fam0000510 PMID: 30802085

Baffour, T. D., & Chonody, J. M. (2009). African-American women's conceptualizations of health disparities: A community-based participatory research approach. *American Journal of Community Psychology*, *44*(3-4), 374–381. DOI: 10.1007/s10464-009-9260-x PMID: 19838795

Baiden, D., & Evans, M. (2021). Black African newcomer women's perception of postpartum mental health services in Canada. *Canadian Journal of Nursing Research*, *53*(3), 202–210. DOI: 10.1177/0844562120934273 PMID: 32551939

Baiden, D., & Evans, M. (2022). Recruitment Strategies to Engage Newcomer Mothers of African Descent in Maternal Mental Health Research in Canada. *Journal of Transcultural Nursing*, *33*(4), 467–474. DOI: 10.1177/10436596221090268 PMID: 35466798

Bailey, Z. D., Krieger, N., Agénor, M., Graves, J., Linos, N., & Bassett, M. T. (2017). Structural racism and health inequities in the USA: Evidence and interventions. *The Lancet, 389*(10077), 1453-1463. https://ajph.aphapublications.org/doi/pdf/10.2105/AJPH.2014.302200

Bains, K., Bicknell, S., Jovanović, N., Conneely, M., McCabe, R., Copello, A., Fletcher-Rogers, J., Priebe, S., & Janković, J. (2023). Healthcare professionals' views on the accessibility and acceptability of perinatal mental health services for South Asian and Black women: A qualitative study. *BMC Medicine, 21*(1), 370. DOI: 10.1186/s12916-023-02978-5 PMID: 37784145

Baker, C. E., & Iruka, I. U. (2013). Supporting families in home-based care. *Early Childhood Research Quarterly, 28*(4), 784–794.

Baker, C. E., & Iruka, I. U. (2013). Supporting parents of African American children through parent education: Promising approaches and opportunities for research. *Journal of Child and Family Studies, 22*(1), 87–100.

Balaji, A. B., Claussen, A. H., Smith, D. C., Visser, S. N., Morales, M. J., & Perou, R. (2007). Social support networks and maternal mental health and well-being. *Journal of Women's Health, 16*(10), 1386–1396. DOI: 10.1089/jwh.2007.CDC10 PMID: 18062754

Banks, A. Black adolescent experiences with COVID-19 and mental health services utilization. J Racial Ethn Heal Disparities. 2021; 1–9. In.

Bargai, N., Ben-Shakhar, G., & Shalev, A. Y. (2007). Posttraumatic stress disorder and depression in battered women: The mediating role of learned helplessness. *Journal of Family Violence, 22*(5), 267–275. DOI: 10.1007/s10896-007-9078-y

Barnet, B., Liu, J., & DeVoe, M. (2008). Double jeopardy: Depressive symptoms and rapid subsequent pregnancy in adolescent mothers. *Archives of Pediatrics & Adolescent Medicine, 162*(3), 246–252. DOI: 10.1001/archpediatrics.2007.60 PMID: 18316662

Bashir, S. A. (2002). Home is where the harm is: Inadequate housing as a public health crisis. *American Journal of Public Health, 92*(5), 733–738. DOI: 10.2105/AJPH.92.5.733 PMID: 11988437

Bauer, A., Knapp, M., & Parsonage, M. (2014). Lifetime costs of perinatal anxiety and depression. *Journal of Affective Disorders, 163*, 134–141.

Baylor, Scott, & White Health. (2023). *Is mom brain real? Understanding and coping with postpartum brain fog*. https://www.bswhealth.com/blog/is-mom-brain-real

Beauchamp, T. L., & Childress, J. F. (2001). *Principles of Biomedical Ethics*. Oxford University Press.

Beauregard, J. L. (2019). Racial disparities in breastfeeding initiation and duration among US infants born in 2015. *MMWR. Morbidity and Mortality Weekly Report*, 68. PMID: 31465319

Beck, C. T., McSweeney, M., Reed, P., & Moots, B. (2006). Psychometric properties of the Postpartum Depression Screening Scale in African American mothers. *Journal of Obstetric, Gynecologic, and Neonatal Nursing : JOGNN*, *35*(1), 117–123.

BeLue, R., Halgunseth, L. C., Abiero, B., & Bediako, P.BeLue. (2015). Maternal health status and parenting stress in low-income, ethnic-minority mothers of children with conduct disorder problems: The role of daily parenting hassles. *Journal of Racial and Ethnic Health Disparities*, *2*(4), 501–509. DOI: 10.1007/s40615-015-0098-7 PMID: 26863556

Bhui, K., Warfa, N., Edonya, P., McKenzie, K., & Bhugra, D. (2007). Cultural competence in mental health care: A review of model evaluations. *BMC Health Services Research*, *7*(1), 1–10. DOI: 10.1186/1472-6963-7-15 PMID: 17266765

Biello, K. B., Sipsma, H. L., & Kershaw, T. (2010). Effect of teenage parenthood on mental health trajectories: Does sex matter? *American Journal of Epidemiology*, *172*(3), 279–287. DOI: 10.1093/aje/kwq128 PMID: 20576756

Bitler, M. P., & Currie, J. (2005). Does WIC work? The effects of WIC on pregnancy and birth outcomes. *Journal of Policy Analysis and Management*, *24*(1), 73–91. DOI: 10.1002/pam.20070 PMID: 15584177

Black Mamas Matter Alliance. (2018). Black mamas matter toolkit. https://blackmamasmatter.org/wp-content/uploads/2018/05/USPA_BMMA_Toolkit_Booklet-Final-Update_Web-Pages-1.pdf

Black Mamas Matter Alliance. (n.d.). *Our work*. https://blackmamasmatter.org/our-work/

Black, D. (n.d.). The impact of historical trauma on Black family dynamics. https://www.dopeblack.org/blog/the-impact-of-historical-trauma-on-black-family-dynamics

Black, A. R., Murry, V. M., Cutrona, C. E., & Chen, Y. (2009). Multiple roles, multiple lives: The protective effects of role responsibilities on the health functioning of African American mothers. *Women & Health*, *49*(2-3), 144–163. DOI: 10.1080/03630240902915051 PMID: 19533507

Black, M. M., Papas, M. A., Hussey, J. M., Dubowitz, H., Kotch, J. B., & Starr, R. H. (2002). Behavior problems among preschool children born to adolescent mothers: Effects of maternal depression and perceptions of partner relationships. *Journal of Clinical Child and Adolescent Psychology, 31*(1), 16–26. DOI: 10.1207/S15374424JCCP3101_04 PMID: 11845646

Bohren, M. A., Tunçalp, Ö., & Miller, S. (2020). Transforming intrapartum care: Respectful maternity care. *Best Practice & Research. Clinical Obstetrics & Gynaecology, 67*, 113–126. DOI: 10.1016/j.bpobgyn.2020.02.005 PMID: 32245630

Borrelli, S., Ramasamy, R., Wong, R., & Spiby, H. (2023). Care and support during maternity for mothers affected by modern slavery: A scoping review. *International Journal of Nursing Studies Advances, 5*, 100139. DOI: 10.1016/j.ijnsa.2023.100139 PMID: 38746591

Bourassa, C., Billan, J., Starblanket, D., Anderson, S., Legare, M., Hagel, M. C., Oakes, N., Jardine, M., Boehme, G., Dubois, E., Spencer, O., Hotomani, M., & McKenna, B. (2020). Ethical research engagement with Indigenous communities. *Journal of Rehabilitation and Assistive Technologies Engineering, 7*, 2055668320922706. DOI: 10.1177/2055668320922706 PMID: 32612848

Bower, K. M., Geller, R. J., Jeffers, N., McDonald, M., & Alhusen, J. (2023). Experiences of racism and perinatal depression: Findings from the pregnancy risk assessment monitoring system, 2018. *Journal of Advanced Nursing, 79*(5), 1982–1993. DOI: 10.1111/jan.15519 PMID: 36630188

Bowers, B., Jacobson, N., & Krupp, A. (2017). Can lay community advisors improve the clarity of research participant recruitment materials and increase the likelihood of participation? *Research in Nursing & Health, 40*(1), 63–69. DOI: 10.1002/nur.21752 PMID: 27686332

Bowlby, J. (1982). Attachment and loss: Retrospect and prospect. *The American Journal of Orthopsychiatry, 52*(4), 664–678. DOI: 10.1111/j.1939-0025.1982.tb01456.x PMID: 7148988

Brantley, M. (2023). Black feminist theory in maternal health research: A review of concepts and future directions. *Sociology Compass, 17*(5), e13083. DOI: 10.1111/soc4.13083 PMID: 37859646

Braveman, P., Heck, K., Egerter, S., Dominguez, T. P., Rinki, C., Marchi, K. S., & Curtis, M. (2017). Worry about racial discrimination: A missing piece of the puzzle of Black-White disparities in preterm birth? *PLoS One, 12*(10), e0186151. DOI: 10.1371/journal.pone.0186151 PMID: 29020025

Brondolo, E., Kelly, K. P., Coakley, V., Gordon, T., Thompson, S., Levy, E., Cassells, A., Tobin, J. N., Sweeney, M., & Contrada, R. J. (2005). The perceived ethnic discrimination questionnaire: Development and preliminary validation of a community version 1. *Journal of Applied Social Psychology, 35*(2), 335–365. DOI: 10.1111/j.1559-1816.2005.tb02124.x

Bronfenbrenner, U. (1979). *The ecology of human development: Experiments by nature and design.* Harvard University Press. DOI: 10.4159/9780674028845

Brown, D. R., & Gary, L. E. (1987). Stressful life events, social support networks, and the physical and mental health of urban black adults. *Journal of Human Stress, 13*(4), 165–174. DOI: 10.1080/0097840X.1987.9936810 PMID: 3448130

Brown, H. L., Small, M. J., Clare, C. A., & Hill, W. C. (2021). Black women health inequity: The origin of perinatal health disparity. *Journal of the National Medical Association, 113*(1), 105–113. DOI: 10.1016/j.jnma.2020.11.008 PMID: 33339616

Brown, J. D., Harris, S. K., Woods, E. R., Buman, M. P., & Cox, J. E. (2012). Longitudinal study of depressive symptoms and social support in adolescent mothers. *Maternal and Child Health Journal, 16*(4), 894–901. DOI: 10.1007/s10995-011-0814-9 PMID: 21556696

Bryant, A. S., & Haas, J. S. (2018). Medicaid expansion and the use of prenatal care among low-income women. *Maternal and Child Health Journal, 22*(3), 454–462.

Bryant-Davis, T., & Adams, T. (2016). A psychocultural exploration of womanism, activism, and social justice. In Bryant-Davis, T., & Comas-Díaz, L. (Eds.), *Womanist and mujerista psychologies: Voices of fire, acts of courage* (pp. 219–236). American Psychological Association., DOI: 10.1037/14937-010

Burke, T., Arnkoff, D., Staser, A., & Cook, J. M. (2020). Perinatal trauma: A trauma-informed approach to obstetrics. *Journal of Clinical Psychology in Medical Settings, 27*(1), 69–78. DOI: 10.1007/s10880-019-09664-4

Business and Professional Women Foundation. (2008). *Successful workplaces digest.* https://bpwfoundation.org/wp-content/uploads/2015/02/BPW_Foundation_Successful_Workplaces_Digest.pdf

Butterworth, P., Olesen, S. C., & Leach, L. S. (2012). The role of hardship in the association between socioeconomic position and depression. *The Australian and New Zealand Journal of Psychiatry, 46*(4), 364–373. DOI: 10.1177/0004867411433215 PMID: 22508596

Byrd, W. M., Fletcher, J. M., Menachemi, N., & Kiefe, C. I. (2020). Health disparities, COVID-19, and a way forward: The case for investment in health equity. *The Milbank Quarterly*, *98*(3), 472–499.

Byrnes, L. (2018). Perinatal mood and anxiety disorders. *The Journal for Nurse Practitioners*, *14*(7), 507–513. DOI: 10.1016/j.nurpra.2018.03.010

California Maternal Quality Care Collaborative. (n.d.). Birth Equity Toolkit. https://www.cmqcc.org/resources-tool-kits/toolkits/birth-equity-toolkit

Callaghan, M., Ford, N., & Schneider, H. (2010). A systematic review of task-shifting for HIV treatment and care in Africa. *Human Resources for Health*, *8*(1), 1–9. DOI: 10.1186/1478-4491-8-8 PMID: 20356363

Campbell, C. (2021). Medical violence, obstetric racism, and the limits of informed consent for Black women. *Michigan Journal of Race & Law*, *26*(0), 47. DOI: 10.36643/mjrl.26.sp.medical

Çankaya, S., & Can, R. (2021). The effect of continuous supportive care on birth pain, birth fear, midwifery care perception, oxytocin use, and delivery time during the intrapartum period: An experimental study. *Nigerian Journal of Clinical Practice*, *24*(11), 1624–1632. DOI: 10.4103/njcp.njcp_147_20 PMID: 34782500

Capers, M. (2019). The experiences of Black women during perinatal loss: A literature review. *MCN. The American Journal of Maternal Child Nursing*, *44*(6), 334–341.

Carrington, C. H. (2006). Clinical depression in African American women: Diagnoses, treatment, and research. *Journal of Clinical Psychology*, *62*(7), 779–791. DOI: 10.1002/jclp.20289 PMID: 16703605

Carvalho, K., Kheyfets, A., Maleki, P., Miller, B., Abouhala, S., Anwar, E., & Amutah-Onukagha, N. (2021). A systematic policy review of Black maternal health-related policies proposed federally and in Massachusetts: 2010–2020. *Frontiers in Public Health*, *9*, 664659. DOI: 10.3389/fpubh.2021.664659 PMID: 34746071

Carver, C. S. (1997). You want to measure coping but your protocol is too long: Consider the brief COPE. *International Journal of Behavioral Medicine*, *4*(1), 92–100. DOI: 10.1207/s15327558ijbm0401_6 PMID: 16250744

Castelin, S., & White, G. (2022). "I'm a Strong Independent Black Woman": The Strong Black Woman Schema and Mental Health in College-Aged Black Women. *Psychology of Women Quarterly*, *46*(2), 196–208. DOI: 10.1177/03616843211067501

Center for Children and Families. (2022). Black Mamas Matter Alliance highlights policy change needed in honor of Black Maternal Health Week. *Georgetown University Health Policy Institute*. https://ccf.georgetown.edu/2022/04/12/black-mamas-matter-alliance-highlights-policy-change-needed-in-honor-of-black-maternal-health-week/

Center for Health Journalism. (2022). Haunted by trauma: The Black parents who nearly died in childbirth. https://centerforhealthjournalism.org/fellowships/projects/haunted-trauma-black-parents-who-nearly-died-childbirth

Centering Healthcare Institute. (n.d.). *CenteringPregnancy: Group Prenatal Care Model*.

Centers for Disease Control and Prevention (CDC). (2020). Pregnancy Mortality Surveillance System. https://www.cdc.gov/maternal-mortality/php/pregnancy-mortality-surveillance/index.html

Centers for Disease Control and Prevention. (2021). *About teen pregnancy*. Reproductive Health: Teen Pregnancy. https://www.cdc.gov/vitalsigns/teenpregnancy/index.html

Centers for Disease Control and Prevention. (2024). *Impact of racism on our nation's health*. https://www.cdc.gov/minority-health/racism-health/index-1.html

Centers for Disease Control and Prevention. (2024, May 8). Infant mortality. https://www.cdc.gov/reproductivehealth/maternalinfanthealth/infantmortality.htm

Chambers, B. D., Erausquin, J. T., Tanner, A. E., Nichols, T. R., & Brown-Jeffy, S. (2018). Testing the association between traditional and novel indicators of county-level structural racism and birth outcomes among Black and White women. *Journal of Racial and Ethnic Health Disparities*, *5*(5), 966–977. DOI: 10.1007/s40615-017-0444-z PMID: 29218496

Chandra-Mouli, V., Lane, C., & Wong, S. (2015). What does not work in adolescent sexual and reproductive health: A review of evidence on interventions commonly accepted as best practices. *Global Health, Science and Practice*, *3*(3), 333–340. DOI: 10.9745/GHSP-D-15-00126 PMID: 26374795

Chang, M.-Y., Chen, C.-H., & Huang, K.-F. (2008). Effects of music therapy on psychological health of women during pregnancy. *Journal of Clinical Nursing*, *17*(19), 2580–2587. DOI: 10.1111/j.1365-2702.2007.02064.x PMID: 18298503

Charette, M. F., & Heller, D. (2018). Implementing trauma-informed care in a women's hospital: A pilot study. *Journal of Obstetric, Gynecologic, and Neonatal Nursing : JOGNN*, *47*(1), S18–S19.

Chaudron, L. H., Szilagyi, P. G., Tang, W., Anson, E., Talbot, N. L., Wadkins, H. I. M., Tu, X., & Wisner, K. L. (2010). Accuracy of Depression Screening Tools for Identifying Postpartum Depression Among Urban Mothers. *Pediatrics*, *125*(3), e609–e617. DOI: 10.1542/peds.2008-3261 PMID: 20156899

Chen, G. M. (1989). Relationships of the dimensions of intercultural communication competence. *Communication Quarterly*, *37*(2), 118–133. DOI: 10.1080/01463378909385533

Childs, G. D., Knight, C., & White, R. (2015). Never-pregnant African American adolescent girls' perceptions of adolescent pregnancy. *Journal of Pediatric Nursing*, *30*(2), 310–320. DOI: 10.1016/j.pedn.2014.08.012 PMID: 25236337

Chinn, J. J., Martin, I. K., & Redmond, N. (2020). Health equity among Black women in the United States. *Journal of Women's Health*, *30*(2), 212–219. DOI: 10.1089/jwh.2020.8868 PMID: 33237831

Choi, K. R., Records, K., Low, L. K., Alhusen, J. L., Kenner, C., Bloch, J. R., Premji, S. S., Hannan, J., Anderson, C. M., Yeo, S., & Cynthia Logsdon, M. (2020). Promotion of Maternal–Infant Mental Health and Trauma-Informed Care During the COVID-19 Pandemic. *Journal of Obstetric, Gynecologic, and Neonatal Nursing : JOGNN*, *49*(5), 409–415. DOI: 10.1016/j.jogn.2020.07.004 PMID: 32795425

Clark, A. E., Macey, E., Irby, A., Stone, C., Pell Abernathy, M., & Turman, J. E.Jr. (2023). Diverse Perspectives to Support a Human Rights Approach to Reduce Indiana's Maternal Mortality Rate. *Humanity & Society*, *47*(1), 69–94. DOI: 10.1177/01605976221109785

Cleveland Clinic. (2024). *Advanced maternal age*. https://my.clevelandclinic.org/health/diseases/22438-advanced-maternal-age

Cohen, S., & Hoberman, H. M. (1983). Positive events and social supports as buffers of life change stress. *Journal of Applied Social Psychology*, *13*(2), 99–125. DOI: 10.1111/j.1559-1816.1983.tb02325.x

Cohen, S., Janicki-Deverts, D., & Miller, G. E. (2007). Psychological stress and disease. *Journal of the American Medical Association*, *298*(14), 1685–1687. DOI: 10.1001/jama.298.14.1685 PMID: 17925521

Cohen, S., & McKay, G. (1984). Social support, stress and the buffering hypothesis: A theoretical analysis. In Baum, A., Taylor, S. E., & Singer, J. E. (Eds.), Vol. 4, pp. 253–267). Handbook of Psychology and Health. Erlbaum., DOI: 10.4324/9781003044307

Collins, C., Gonzalez, M., & Angell, B. (2010). A community support approach to HIV/AIDS in Black communities. *Social Work in Public Health, 25*(1), 20–39.

Collins, E., McGuinness, S., & O'Sullivan, A. (2021). Understanding the experiences of Black women following perinatal loss: A qualitative study. *Journal of Psychosocial Nursing and Mental Health Services, 59*(8), 26–32. DOI: 10.3928/02793695-20210615-03

Collins, P. H. (2000). *Black feminist thought: Knowledge, consciousness, and the politics of empowerment.* Routledge.

Collins, P. Y., Patel, V., Joestl, S. S., March, D., Insel, T. R., Daar, A. S., Bordin, I. A., Costello, E. J., Durkin, M., Fairburn, C., Glass, R. I., Hall, W., Huang, Y., Hyman, S. E., Jamison, K., Kaaya, S., Kapur, S., Kleinman, A., Ogunniyi, A., & Walport, M. (2010). Grand challenges in global mental health. *Nature, 475*(7354), 27–30. DOI: 10.1038/475027a PMID: 21734685

Commonwealth Fund. (2022). Inequities in health coverage and access: Black and Hispanic adults. https://www.commonwealthfund.org/publications/issue-briefs/2022/inequities-health-coverage-access-black-hispanic-adults

Congress.gov. (2018). H.R.1318 - Preventing Maternal Deaths Act of 2018. https://www.congress.gov/bill/115th-congress/house-bill/1318

Cortezzo, D. E., Ellis, K., & Schlegel, A. (2020). Perinatal palliative care birth planning as advance care planning. *Frontiers in Pediatrics, 8*, 556. DOI: 10.3389/fped.2020.00556 PMID: 33014940

Côté-Arsenault, D., Denney-Koelsch, E. M., McCoy, T. P., & Kavanaugh, K. (2019). African American and Latino bereaved parent health outcomes after receiving perinatal palliative care: A comparative mixed methods case study. *Applied Nursing Research, 50*, 151200. DOI: 10.1016/j.apnr.2019.151200 PMID: 31735485

Cox, J. E., Buman, M., Valenzuela, J., Joseph, N. P., Mitchell, A., & Woods, E. R. (2008). Depression, parenting attributes, and social support among adolescent mothers attending a teen tot program. *Journal of Pediatric and Adolescent Gynecology, 21*(5), 275–281. DOI: 10.1016/j.jpag.2008.02.002 PMID: 18794023

Cox, J. L., Holden, J. M., & Sagovsky, R. (1987). Detection of Postnatal Depression: Development of the 10-item Edinburgh Postnatal Depression Scale. *The British Journal of Psychiatry, 150*(6), 782–786. DOI: 10.1192/bjp.150.6.782 PMID: 3651732

Coy, D., Malekpour, S., Saeri, A. K., & Dargaville, R. (2021). Rethinking community empowerment in the energy transformation: A critical review of the definitions, drivers and outcomes. *Energy Research & Social Science*, *72*, 101871. DOI: 10.1016/j.erss.2020.101871

Creanga, A. A., Syverson, C., Seed, K., & Callaghan, W. M. (2017). Pregnancy-Related Mortality in the United States, 2011–2013. [Link]. *Obstetrics and Gynecology*, *130*(2), 366–373. DOI: 10.1097/AOG.0000000000002114 PMID: 28697109

Crear-Perry, J., Correa-de-Araujo, R., Lewis Johnson, T., McLemore, M. R., Neilson, E., & Wallace, M. (2021). Social and structural determinants of health inequities in maternal health. *Journal of Women's Health*, *30*(2), 230–235. DOI: 10.1089/jwh.2020.8882 PMID: 33181043

Crenshaw, K. (1989). Demarginalizing the intersection of race and sex: A Black feminist critique of antidiscrimination doctrine, feminist theory and antiracist politics. *University of Chicago Legal Forum*, *1989*(1), 139–167.

Cross, C. J., Taylor, R. J., & Chatters, L. M. (2018). Family social support networks of African American and Black Caribbean adolescents. *Journal of Child and Family Studies*, *27*(9), 2757–2771. DOI: 10.1007/s10826-018-1116-2 PMID: 30344428

d'Oliveira, A. F., Diniz, S. G., & Schraiber, L. B. (2002). Violence against women in health-care institutions: An emerging problem. *Lancet*, *359*(9318), 1681–1685. DOI: 10.1016/S0140-6736(02)08592-6 PMID: 12020546

Dabney, K. P., & Glover, M. (2019). Perinatal loss in Black women: A qualitative study of coping strategies. *Journal of Loss and Trauma*, *24*(1), 34–49. DOI: 10.1080/15325024.2018.1494196

Dagher, R. K., & Linares, D. E. (2022). A Critical Review on the Complex Interplay between Social Determinants of Health and Maternal and Infant Mortality. *Children (Basel, Switzerland)*, *9*(3), 394. DOI: 10.3390/children9030394 PMID: 35327766

Dagher, R. K., Pérez-Stable, E. J., & James, R. S. (2021). Socioeconomic and racial/ethnic disparities in postpartum consultation for mental health concerns among US mothers. *Archives of Women's Mental Health*, *24*(5), 781–791. DOI: 10.1007/s00737-021-01132-5 PMID: 33855652

Dailey, D. (2008). Conceptualizing perceived racism and its effect on the health of African- Americans: Implications for practice and research. *Journal of National Black Nurses' Association. Journal of National Black Nurses' Association*, *19*, 73–80. DOI: 10.1177/1054773808314636 PMID: 18807782

Dalal, A. K., & Schnipper, J. L. (2016). Care team identification in the electronic health record: A critical first step for patient-centered communication. *Journal of Hospital Medicine*, *11*(5), 381–385. DOI: 10.1002/jhm.2542 PMID: 26762584

Dalsania, A. K., Fastiggi, M. J., Kahlam, A., Shah, R., Patel, K., Shiau, S., Rokicki, S., & DallaPiazza, M. (2021). The relationship between social determinants of health and racial disparities in COVID-19 mortality. *Journal of Racial and Ethnic Health Disparities*, *9*(1), 288–295. DOI: 10.1007/s40615-020-00952-y PMID: 33403652

Damschroder, L. J., Aron, D. C., Keith, R. E., Kirsh, S. R., Alexander, J. A., & Lowery, J. C. (2009). Fostering implementation of health services research findings into practice: A consolidated framework for advancing implementation science. *Implementation Science : IS*, *4*(1), 50. DOI: 10.1186/1748-5908-4-50 PMID: 19664226

Danasekaran, R., Mani, G., & Annadurai, K. (2015). Growing concern about maternal mental health disorders. *Clinical Obstetrics, Gynecology and Reproductive Medicine*, *1*(1), 19. DOI: 10.15761/COGRM.1000106

Davis, C., Villalobos, A. V. K., Turner, M. M., Long, S., & Lapinski, M. K. (2021). Racism and resistance: A qualitative study of bias as a barrier to breastfeeding. *Breastfeeding Medicine*, *16*(6), 471–480. DOI: 10.1089/bfm.2020.0307 PMID: 33784475

Davis, J. A., Finlay-Jones, A. L., Bear, N., Prescott, S. L., Silva, D. T., & Ohan, J. L. (2023). Time-out for well-being: A mixed methods evaluation of attitudes and likelihood to engage in different types of online emotional well-being programmes in the perinatal period. *Women's Health (London, England)*, *19*, DOI: 10.1177/17455057231184507 PMID: 37431205

Dawley, K. (2003, Mar 4). Origins of Nurse-Midwifery in the United States and its Expansion in the 1940s. *Journal of Midwifery & Women's Health*, *48*(2), 86–95. DOI: 10.1016/S1526-9523(03)00002-3 PMID: 12686940

Delles, M. (2021, Oct 29). Case Study – Angela C – Maternal Fetal Issues - Center for Practical Bioethics. Retrieved August 28, 2024, from Center for Practical Bioethics website: https://www.practicalbioethics.org/shared-decision-making-and-advance-care-planning/advance-care-planning/case-study-angela-c-maternal-fetal-issues/

Denney-Koelsch, E., Black, B. P., Côté-Arsenault, D., Wool, C., Kim, S., & Kavanaugh, K. (2016). A survey of perinatal palliative care programs in the United States: Structure, processes, and outcomes. *Journal of Palliative Medicine*, *19*(10), 1080–1086. DOI: 10.1089/jpm.2015.0536 PMID: 27559768

Dimes, M. o. (2024). *40% of Black women experience maternal mental health symptoms, nearly twice the rate of all women.* March of Dimes. https://www.marchofdimes.org/black-maternal-mental-health-week

Diniz, S. G., d'Oliveira, A. F., & Lansky, S. (2012). Equity and women's health services for contraception, abortion and childbirth in Brazil. *Reproductive Health Matters, 20*(40), 94–101. DOI: 10.1016/S0968-8080(12)40657-7 PMID: 23245414

DuBois, J. M., Bailey-Burch, B., Bustillos, D., Campbell, J., Cottler, L., Fisher, C. B., Hadley, W. B., Hoop, J. G., Roberts, L., Salter, E. K., Sieber, J. E., & Stevenson, R. D. (2011). Ethical issues in mental health research: The case for community engagement. *Current Opinion in Psychiatry, 24*(3), 208–214. DOI: 10.1097/YCO.0b013e3283459422 PMID: 21460643

Dula, S. (2021, Oct 28). 6 Maternal Health Organizations Working to Support Mothers. *Pregnancy & Newborn Magazine.* https://www.pnmag.com/mom-baby/6-maternal-health-organizations-working-to-support-mothers/

Dunkel Schetter, C., Schafer, P., Lanzi, R. G., Clark-Kauffman, E., Raju, T. N., & Hillemeier, M. M. (2013). Shedding light on the mechanisms underlying health disparities through community participatory methods: The stress pathway. *Perspectives on Psychological Science, 8*(6), 613–633. DOI: 10.1177/1745691613506016 PMID: 26173227

Dwarakanath, M., Hossain, F., Balascio, P., Moore, M. C., Hill, A. V., & De Genna, N. M. (2023). Experiences of postpartum mental health sequelae among black and biracial women during the COVID-19 pandemic. *BMC Pregnancy and Childbirth, 23*(1), 636. DOI: 10.1186/s12884-023-05929-3 PMID: 37667206

Economic Policy Institute. (2020). The cost of child care in the United States. Retrieved from https://www.epi.org/child-care-costs-in-the-united-states/

Engle, P. L. (2009). Maternal mental health: Program and policy implications. *The American Journal of Clinical Nutrition, 89*(3), 963S–966S. DOI: 10.3945/ajcn.2008.26692G PMID: 19176734

Ertan, D., Hingray, C., Burlacu, E., Sterlé, A., & El-Hage, W. (2021). Post-traumatic stress disorder following childbirth. *BMC Psychiatry, 21*(1), 155. DOI: 10.1186/s12888-021-03158-6 PMID: 33726703

Estriplet, T., Morgan, I., Davis, K., Perry, J. C., & Matthews, K. (2022). Black Perinatal Mental Health: Prioritizing maternal mental health to optimize infant health and wellness. *Frontiers in Psychiatry, 13*, 807235. DOI: 10.3389/fpsyt.2022.807235 PMID: 35573337

Etowa, J. B., Beagan, B. L., Eghan, F., & Bernard, W. T. (2017). "You feel you have to be made of steel": The strong Black woman, health, and well-being in Nova Scotia. *Health Care for Women International, 38*(4), 379–393. DOI: 10.1080/07399332.2017.1290099 PMID: 28151098

Etowa, J., Nare, H., Dubula-Majola, V., Edet, O., John, M., Nkwocha, C. R., Stephens, C., Mbewu, N., Hannan, J., & Etowa, E. (2022). Male Partners' Roles in Infant Feeding Practices: Perspectives of Black Mothers Living with HIV in Three Countries. Healthcare, Falako, S., Okoli, N., Boateng, M.-O., Sandoval, J., Gumudavelly, D., Larsuel, S., & Opara, I. (2023). Utilizing community-centered approaches to address Black maternal mortality. *Health Education & Behavior, 50*(4), 500–504.

Evans, N. M., Hsu, Y.-L., Kabasele, C. M., Kirkland, C., Pantuso, D., & Hicks, S. (2023). A qualitative exploration of stressors: Voices of African American women who have experienced each type of fetal/infant loss: Miscarriage, stillbirth, and infant mortality. *The Journal of Black Psychology, 49*(2), 236–263. DOI: 10.1177/00957984221127833

Fair, F., Soltani, H., Raben, L., van Streun, Y., Sioti, E., Papadakaki, M., Burke, C., Watson, H., Jokinen, M., Shaw, E., Triantafyllou, E., van den Muijsenbergh, M., & Vivilaki, V. (2021). Midwives' experiences of cultural competency training and providing perinatal care for migrant women: A mixed methods study: Operational Refugee and Migrant Maternal Approach (ORAMMA) project. *BMC Pregnancy and Childbirth, 21*(1), 340. DOI: 10.1186/s12884-021-03799-1 PMID: 33926420

Fancourt, D., & Perkins, R. (2018). The effects of mother–infant singing on emotional closeness, affect, anxiety, and stress hormones. *Music & Science, 1*, 2059204317745746. DOI: 10.1177/2059204317745746

Fante-Coleman, T., & Jackson-Best, F. (2020). Barriers and facilitators to accessing mental healthcare in Canada for Black youth: A scoping review. *Adolescent Research Review, 5*(2), 115–136. DOI: 10.1007/s40894-020-00133-2

Farley, C. L., DeSisto, M. C., Hawkins, J. W., & West, M. (2018). Implementing a trauma-informed care model for perinatal loss. *MCN. The American Journal of Maternal Child Nursing, 43*(4), 218–224. DOI: 10.1097/NMC.0000000000000434 PMID: 29553946

Fawcett, E., & Taylor, S. (2018). Trauma-informed care in maternity services: A critical review. *Midwifery, 56*, 121–127. DOI: 10.1016/j.midw.2017.10.015

Feldman, N., & Pattani, A. (2019, Dec 6). *Black Mothers Get Less Treatment For Postpartum Depression Than Other Moms. KFF Health News.* https://kffhealthnews.org/news/black-mothers-get-less-treatment-for-postpartum-depression-than-other-moms/_

Firima, E., Gonzalez, L., Huber, J., Belus, J. M., Raeber, F., Gupta, R., Mokhohlane, J., Mphunyane, M., Amstutz, A., & Labhardt, N. D. (2021). Community-based models of care for management of type 2 diabetes mellitus among non-pregnant adults in sub-Saharan Africa: A scoping review protocol. *F1000 Research*, 10. PMID: 35387273

Firouzbakht, M., Rahmani, N., Sharif Nia, H., & Omidvar, S. (2022). Coping strategies and depression during the COVID-19 pandemic in pregnant women: A cross sectional study. *BMC Psychiatry*, *22*(1), 153. DOI: 10.1186/s12888-022-03792-8 PMID: 35232424

Flanagan, K., & Daniels, K. (2017). Perinatal bereavement: Implementing a hospital-wide program. *Nursing for Women's Health*, *21*(4), 296–304. DOI: 10.1016/j.nwh.2017.06.007

Floyd James, K., Chen, K., Hindra, S. S., Gray, S., Robinson, M. N., Tobin, C. S. T., Choi, K., & Saint Arnault, D. (2024). Racism-related stress and mental health among black women living in Los Angeles County, California: A comparison of postpartum mood and anxiety disorder screening scales. *Archives of Women's Mental Health*, *27*(5), 1–10. DOI: 10.1007/s00737-024-01458-w PMID: 38561564

Floyd James, K., Smith, B. E., Robinson, M. N., Thomas Tobin, C. S., Bulles, K. F., & Barkin, J. L. (2023). Factors Associated with Postpartum Maternal Functioning in Black Women: A Secondary Analysis. *Journal of Clinical Medicine*, *12*(2), 647. DOI: 10.3390/jcm12020647 PMID: 36675575

Ford, C. L., & Airhihenbuwa, C. O. (2010). Critical Race Theory, race equity, and public health: toward antiracism praxis. *American Journal of Public Health, 100 Suppl 1*(Suppl 1), S30–S35. DOI: 10.2105/AJPH.2009.171058

Fothergill, K. E., Ensminger, M. E., Robertson, J., Green, K. M., Thorpe, R. J., & Juon, H.-S. (2011). Effects of social integration on health: A prospective study of community engagement among African American women. *Social Science & Medicine*, *72*(2), 291–298. DOI: 10.1016/j.socscimed.2010.10.024 PMID: 21131117

Franks, W., Henwood, K., & Bowden, G. (2007). Promoting maternal mental health: Women's strategies for presenting a positive identity and the implications for mental health promotion. *Journal of Public Mental Health*, *6*(2), 40–51. DOI: 10.1108/17465729200700013

Fulton, J. I., Singh, H., Pakkal, O., Uleryk, E. M., & Nelson, M. L. (2022). Community-based culturally tailored education programmes for black adults with cardiovascular disease, diabetes, hypertension and stroke: A systematic review protocol of primary empirical studies. *BMJ Open*, *12*(6), e059883. DOI: 10.1136/bmjopen-2021-059883 PMID: 35688600

Furtado-Eraso, S., Escalada-Hernández, P., & Marín-Fernández, B. (2021). Integrative review of emotional care following perinatal loss. *Western Journal of Nursing Research*, *43*(5), 489–504. DOI: 10.1177/0193945920954448 PMID: 32886030

Gadson, A., Akpovi, E., & Mehta, P. K. (2017). Exploring the social determinants of racial/ethnic disparities in prenatal care utilization and maternal outcome. *Seminars in Perinatology*, *41*(5), 308–317. DOI: 10.1053/j.semperi.2017.04.008 PMID: 28625554

Gaston, M. H., Porter, G. K., & Thomas, V. G. (2007). Prime Time Sister Circles: Evaluating a gender-specific, culturally relevant health intervention to decrease major risk factors in mid-life African-American women. *Journal of the National Medical Association*, *99*(4), 428–438. PMID: 17444433

Gausman, J., & Langer, A. (2020). Sex and Gender Disparities in the COVID-19 Pandemic. *Journal of Women's Health*, *29*(4), 465–466. DOI: 10.1089/jwh.2020.8472 PMID: 32320331

Gavin, L., Moskosky, S., Carter, M., Curtis, K., Glass, E., Godfrey, E., ... & Zapata, L. (2014). Providing quality family planning services: Recommendations of CDC and the US Office of Population Affairs. *MMWR. Recommendations and Reports: Morbidity and Mortality Weekly Report. Recommendations and Reports / Centers for Disease Control, 63*(Rr-04), 1-54.

Gavin, N. I., Gaynes, B. N., Lohr, K. N., Meltzer-Brody, S., Gartlehner, G., & Swinson, T. (2005). Perinatal depression: A systematic review of prevalence and incidence. *Obstetrics and Gynecology*, *106*(5), 1071–1083. DOI: 10.1097/01.AOG.0000183597.31630.db PMID: 16260528

Gaylord-Harden, N. K., & Cunningham, J. A. (2009). The impact of racial discrimination and coping strategies on internalizing symptoms in African American youth. *Journal of Youth and Adolescence*, *38*(4), 532–543. DOI: 10.1007/s10964-008-9377-5 PMID: 19636726

Gee, G. C., & Ford, C. L. (2011). Structural racism and health inequities. *Du Bois Review*, *8*(1), 115–132. DOI: 10.1017/S1742058X11000130 PMID: 25632292

Gerber, M. R. (2019). Trauma-informed maternity care. In Gerber, M. R. (Ed.), *Trauma-informed healthcare approaches: A guide for primary care* (pp. 145–155). Springer. DOI: 10.1007/978-3-030-04342-1_8

Geronimus, A. T. (1992). The weathering hypothesis and the health of African-American women and infants: Evidence and speculations. *Ethnicity & Disease*, *2*(3), 207–221. PMID: 1467758

Geronimus, A. T. (1996). Black/white differences in the relationship of maternal age to birthweight: A population-based test of the weathering hypothesis. *Social Science & Medicine*, *42*(4), 589–597. DOI: 10.1016/0277-9536(95)00159-X PMID: 8643983

Geronimus, A. T., Hicken, M., Keene, D., & Bound, J. (2006). "Weathering" and age patterns of allostatic load scores among blacks and whites in the United States. *American Journal of Public Health*, *96*(5), 826–833. DOI: 10.2105/AJPH.2004.060749 PMID: 16380565

Getahun, D., Oyelese, Y., Peltier, M., Yeh, M., Chiu, V. Y., Takhar, H., Khadka, N., Mensah, N., Avila, C., & Fassett, M. J. (2023). Trends in Postpartum Depression by Race/Ethnicity and Pre-pregnancy Body Mass Index. *American Journal of Obstetrics and Gynecology*, *228*(1), S122–S123. DOI: 10.1016/j.ajog.2022.11.248

Gholizadeh Shamasbi, S., Barkin, J. L., Ghanbari-Homayi, S., Eyvazzadeh, O., & Mirghafourvand, M. (2020). The relationship between maternal functioning and mental health after childbirth in Iranian women. *International Journal of Environmental Research and Public Health*, *17*(5), 1558. DOI: 10.3390/ijerph17051558 PMID: 32121286

Gilmore, A. D., Osho, G. S., & Heads, A. B. (2013). Stress, anxiety, depression and psychological responses among African Americans: Empirical investigation and coping strategies. *American Journal of Health Sciences*, *4*(3), 121–130. DOI: 10.19030/ajhs.v4i3.8008

Giurgescu, C., Misra, D. P., Sealy-Jefferson, S., Caldwell, C. H., Templin, T. N., Slaughter-Acey, J. C., & Osypuk, T. L. (2015). The impact of neighborhood quality, perceived stress, and social support on depressive symptoms during pregnancy in African American women. *Social Science & Medicine*, *130*, 172–180. DOI: 10.1016/j.socscimed.2015.02.006 PMID: 25703670

Gjerdingen, D., & Center, B. (2003). First-time parents' postpartum changes in employment, child care, and housework responsibilities. *Social Science Research*, *32*(1), 20–43.

Glanz, K., Rimer, B. K., & Viswanath, K. (2008). *Health behavior and health education: Theory, research, and practice* (4th ed.). Jossey-Bass.

Glickman, C. P., Le, H.-N., Robertson, H., Arbit, R., Danielson, A., Patchen, L., Fries, M., Scott, R., & Biel, M. (2020). Black women's preferences for embedding mental health services in an obstetrics setting.

Goddard-Durant, S. K., Doucet, A., Tizaa, H., & Sieunarine, J. A. (2023). "I don't have the energy": Racial stress, young Black motherhood, and Canadian social policies. *Canadian Review of Sociology/Revue canadienne de sociologie, 60*(4), 542-566.

Gold, K. J., & Johnson, T. R. B. (2020). Integrating perinatal and pediatric bereavement care: A summary of key recommendations from a national meeting of bereavement experts. *Journal of Perinatology, 40*, 8–12. DOI: 10.1038/s41372-019-0548-5

Gómez, J. E., Johnson, B. A., Selva, M., & Sallis, J. F. (2004). Violent crime and outdoor physical activity among inner-city youth. *Preventive Medicine, 39*(5), 876–881. DOI: 10.1016/j.ypmed.2004.03.019 PMID: 15475019

Gonzalez, C., Ramirez, M., Diaz, A., Duran, M., & Areán, P. (2021). Expanding virtual postpartum mental health care for latina women: A participatory research and policy agenda. *Women's Health Issues, 31*(2), 96–99. DOI: 10.1016/j.whi.2020.10.005 PMID: 33250342

Goodman, L., Choi, J. H., & Zhu, J. (2021). *More women have become homeowners and heads of households. Could the pandemic undo that progress?* Urban Institute. https://www.urban.org/urban-wire/more-women-have-become-homeowners-and-heads-household-could-pandemic-undo-progress

Gopalan, P., Spada, M. L., Shenai, N., Brockman, I., Keil, M., Livingston, S., Moses-Kolko, E., Nichols, N., O'Toole, K., Quinn, B., & Glance, J. B. (2022). Postpartum depression—Identifying risk and access to intervention. *Current Psychiatry Reports, 24*(12), 889–896. DOI: 10.1007/s11920-022-01392-7 PMID: 36422834

Greene, M. C., Huang, T. T., Giusto, A., Lovero, K. L., Stockton, M. A., Shelton, R. C., Dos Santos, P., Saúte, F., & Wainberg, M. L. (2021). Leveraging systems science to promote the implementation and sustainability of mental health and psychosocial interventions in low-and middle-income countries. *Harvard Review of Psychiatry, 29*(4), 262–277. DOI: 10.1097/HRP.0000000000000306 PMID: 34241978

Gross, J., Power, T., & St John, W. (2006). A social marketing model for disseminating research-based interventions. *American Journal of Community Psychology, 38*(1-2), 79–89. PMID: 16909316

Grote, N. K., Bridge, J. A., Gavin, A. R., Melville, J. L., Iyengar, S., & Katon, W. J. (2010). A meta-analysis of depression during pregnancy and the risk of preterm birth, low birth weight, and intrauterine growth restriction. *Archives of General Psychiatry*, *67*(10), 1012–1024. DOI: 10.1001/archgenpsychiatry.2010.111 PMID: 20921117

Grote, N. K., Katon, W. J., Russo, J. E., Lohr, M. J., Curran, M., Galvin, E., & Carson, K. (2015). COLLABORATIVE CARE FOR PERINATAL DEPRESSION IN SOCIOECONOMICALLY DISADVANTAGED WOMEN: A RANDOMIZED TRIAL. *Depression and Anxiety*, *32*(11), 821–834. DOI: 10.1002/da.22405 PMID: 26345179

Guille, C., Henrich, N., Brinson, A. K., & Jahnke, H. R. (2024). Improving the Management of Maternal Mental Health with Digital Health Care. *Psychiatric Research and Clinical Practice*, *6*(1), 23–32. DOI: 10.1176/appi.prcp.20230035 PMID: 38510485

Gur, R. E., White, L. K., Waller, R., Barzilay, R., Moore, T. M., Kornfield, S., Njoroge, W. F. M., Duncan, A. F., Chaiyachati, B. H., Parish-Morris, J., Maayan, L., Himes, M. M., Laney, N., Simonette, K., Riis, V., & Elovitz, M. A. (2020). The Disproportionate Burden of the COVID-19 Pandemic Among Pregnant Black Women. *Psychiatry Research*, *293*, 113475. DOI: 10.1016/j.psychres.2020.113475 PMID: 33007683

Guruge, S., Thomson, M. S., George, U., & Chaze, F. (2015). Social support, social conflict, and immigrant women's mental health in a C anadian context: A scoping review. *Journal of Psychiatric and Mental Health Nursing*, *22*(9), 655–667. DOI: 10.1111/jpm.12216 PMID: 26031541

Guttmacher Institute. (2017). *Sex and HIV education.* State Laws and Policies. https://www.guttmacher.org/state-policy/explore/sex-and-hiv-education

H.R.2902 – Maternal CARE Act. 116th Congress (2019-2020) (2019, May 22). https://www.congress.gov/bill/116th-congress/house-bill/2902

Hankerson, S. H., Suite, D., & Bailey, R. K. (2018). Treatment disparities among African American men with depression: Implications for clinical practice. *Journal of Health Care for the Poor and Underserved*, *26*(1), 21–34. DOI: 10.1353/hpu.2015.0012 PMID: 25702724

Hardeman, R. R., Medina, E. M., & Kozhimannil, K. B. (2016). Structural Racism and Supporting Black Lives - The Role of Health Professionals. *The New England Journal of Medicine*, *375*(22), 2113–2115. DOI: 10.1056/NEJMp1609535 PMID: 27732126

Harrell, T., Howell, E. A., Balbierz, A., Guel, L., Pena, J., Janevic, T., & Gorbenko, K. (2022). Improving postpartum care: Identifying opportunities to reduce postpartum emergency room visits among publicly-insured women of color. *Maternal and Child Health Journal, 26*(4), 913–922. DOI: 10.1007/s10995-021-03282-5 PMID: 34982328

Harris, J. R. A. (2021). Community-based participatory research with Black churches. *Counseling and Values, 66*(1), 2–20. DOI: 10.1002/cvj.12141

Harvey, S. T., Bennett, J. A., Burmeister, E., & Wyder, M. (2018). Evaluating a nurse-led community model of service for perinatal mental health. *Collegian (Royal College of Nursing, Australia), 25*(5), 525–531. DOI: 10.1016/j.colegn.2017.12.005

Haslam, D. M., Pakenham, K. I., & Smith, A. (2006). Social support and postpartum depressive symptomatology: The mediating role of maternal self-efficacy. *Infant Mental Health Journal, 27*(3), 276–291. DOI: 10.1002/imhj.20092 PMID: 28640472

Hassoun Ayoub, L., Partridge, T., & Gómez, J. M. (2023). Two sides of the same coin: A mixed methods study of black mothers' experiences with violence, stressors, parenting, and coping during the COVID-19 pandemic. *The Journal of Social Issues, 79*(2), 667–693. DOI: 10.1111/josi.12526 PMID: 36249547

Hatton-Bowers, H., Clark, C., Parra, G., Calvi, J., Bird, M. Y., Avari, P., Foged, J., & Smith, J. (2023). Promising findings that the cultivating healthy intentional mindful educators' program (CHIME) strengthens early childhood teachers' emotional resources: An iterative study. *Early Childhood Education Journal, 51*(7), 1291–1304. DOI: 10.1007/s10643-022-01386-3 PMID: 35967911

Heaman, M. I., Moffatt, M., Elliott, L., Sword, W., Helewa, M. E., Morris, H., Gregory, P., Tjaden, L., & Cook, C. (2014). Barriers, motivators and facilitators related to prenatal care utilization among inner-city women in Winnipeg, Canada: A case–control study. *BMC Pregnancy and Childbirth, 14*(1), 227. DOI: 10.1186/1471-2393-14-227 PMID: 25023478

Hernandez, N. D., Dorsey, J., Glass, D. M., Pope, E., Worthy, N., Blasingame, E., Gooding, J., Braxton, P., Whitfield, M., & Dotson, Y. (2019). Community-engaged approaches to address the ethical concerns of maternal mental health disparities research. *Journal of Health Care for the Poor and Underserved, 30*(4, Suppl), 12–20. DOI: 10.1353/hpu.2019.0110 PMID: 31735713

Hernandez, N. D., Francis, S., Allen, M., Bellamy, E., Sims, O. T., Oh, H., Guillaume, D., Parker, A., & Chandler, R. (2022). Prevalence and predictors of symptoms of perinatal mood and anxiety disorders among a sample of urban black women in the south. *Maternal and Child Health Journal*, *26*(4), 770–777. DOI: 10.1007/s10995-022-03425-2 PMID: 35344149

Herrick, C. L., & Burkhard, J. (2024). Black Maternal Mental Health. *Journal of Prenatal & Perinatal Psychology & Health*, *38*(1).

Hodgkinson, S. C., Colantuoni, E., Roberts, D., Berg-Cross, L., & Belcher, H. M. (2010). Depressive symptoms and birth outcomes among pregnant teenagers. *Journal of Pediatric and Adolescent Gynecology*, *23*(1), 16–22. DOI: 10.1016/j.jpag.2009.04.006 PMID: 19679498

Hodgkinson, S., Beers, L., Southammakosane, C., & Lewin, A. (2014). Addressing the mental health needs of pregnant and parenting adolescents. *Pediatrics*, *133*(1), 114–122. DOI: 10.1542/peds.2013-0927 PMID: 24298010

Hoffman, K. M., Trawalter, S., Axt, J. R., & Oliver, M. N. (2016). Racial bias in pain assessment and treatment recommendations, and false beliefs about biological differences between blacks and whites. *Proceedings of the National Academy of Sciences of the United States of America*, *113*(16), 4296–4301. DOI: 10.1073/pnas.1516047113 PMID: 27044069

Holiday, J. M. (2010). The word, the body, and the kinfolk: The intersection of transpersonal thought with womanist approaches to psychology. *International Journal of Transpersonal Studies*, *29*(2), 10. DOI: 10.24972/ijts.2010.29.2.103

Holland, M. L., Yoo, B. K., Kitzman, H., Chaudron, L., Szilagyi, P. G., & Temkin-Greener, H. (2011). Self-efficacy as a mediator between maternal depression and child hospitalizations in low-income urban families. *Maternal and Child Health Journal*, *15*(7), 1011–1019. DOI: 10.1007/s10995-010-0662-z PMID: 20706866

Horan, H., Ryu, J., Stone, J., & Thurston, L. (2023). Healing trauma with interprofessional collaboration and trauma-informed perinatal care: A qualitative case study. *Birth (Berkeley, Calif.)*, *50*(3), 525–534. DOI: 10.1111/birt.12672 PMID: 36039484

House, T. S., Alnajjar, E., Mulekar, M., & Spiryda, L. B. (2020). Mommy meltdown: Understanding racial differences between black and white women in attitudes about postpartum depression and treatment modalities. *Journal of Clinical Gynecology and Obstetrics*, *9*(3), 37–42. DOI: 10.14740/jcgo664 PMID: 33732401

Howell, E. A. (2018). Reducing disparities in severe maternal morbidity and mortality. *Clinical Obstetrics and Gynecology, 61*(2), 387–399. DOI: 10.1097/GRF.0000000000000349 PMID: 29346121

Howell, E. A., Brown, H., Brumley, J., Bryant, A. S., Caughey, A. B., Cornell, A. M., Grant, J. H., Gregory, K. D., Gullo, S. M., Kozhimannil, K. B., Mhyre, J. M., Toledo, P., D'Oria, R., Ngoh, M., & Grobman, W. A. (2018). Reduction of Peripartum Racial and Ethnic Disparities: A Conceptual Framework and Maternal Safety Consensus Bundle. *Obstetrics and Gynecology, 131*(5), 770–782. DOI: 10.1097/AOG.0000000000002475 PMID: 29683895

Howell, E. A., Egorova, N. N., Balbierz, A., Zeitlin, J., & Hebert, P. L. (2018). Site of delivery contribution to black-white severe maternal morbidity disparity. *American Journal of Obstetrics and Gynecology*. Advance online publication. DOI: 10.1016/j.ajog.2016.05.007 PMID: 27179441

Howell, E. A., Egorova, N., Balbierz, A., Zeitlin, J., & Hebert, P. L. (2016). Black-white differences in severe maternal morbidity and site of care. *American Journal of Obstetrics and Gynecology, 214*(1), 122.e1–122.e1227. DOI: 10.1016/j.ajog.2015.08.019 PMID: 26283457

Howell, E. A., & Zeitlin, J. (2017). Improving hospital quality to reduce disparities in severe maternal morbidity and mortality. *Seminars in Perinatology, 41*(5), 266–272. DOI: 10.1053/j.semperi.2017.04.002 PMID: 28735811

Howell, E. A., & Zeitlin, J. (2017). Quality of Care and Disparities in Obstetrics. *Obstetrics and Gynecology Clinics of North America, 44*(1), 13–25. DOI: 10.1016/j.ogc.2016.10.002 PMID: 28160890

Hoyert, D. L. (2022). *Maternal mortality rates in the United States, 2022*. Centers for Disease Control and Prevention. https://www.cdc.gov/nchs/data/hestat/maternal-mortality/2022/maternal-mortality-rates-2022.htm

Huang, C. Y., Costeines, J., Kaufman, J. S., & Ayala, C. (2014). Parenting stress, social support, and depression for ethnic minority adolescent mothers: Impact on child development. *Journal of Child and Family Studies, 23*(2), 255–262. DOI: 10.1007/s10826-013-9807-1 PMID: 24653641

Huang, C., Wei, K., Lee, P. M. Y., Qin, G., Yu, Y., & Li, J. (2022). Maternal hypertensive disorder of pregnancy and mortality in offspring from birth to young adulthood: National population based cohort study. *BMJ (Clinical Research Ed.), 379*, e072157. DOI: 10.1136/bmj-2022-072157 PMID: 36261141

Huang, H. Y., Li, H., & Hsu, Y. C. (2022). Coping, COVID knowledge, communication, and HBCU student's emotional well-being: Mediating role of perceived control and social connectedness. *Journal of Community Psychology, 50*(6), 2703–2725. DOI: 10.1002/jcop.22824 PMID: 35187691

Hutchison, E. D. (2014). *Dimensions of human behavior: Person and environment* (5th ed.). SAGE Publications.

Insan, N., Weke, A., Rankin, J., & Forrest, S. (2022). Perceptions and attitudes around perinatal mental health in Bangladesh, India and Pakistan: A systematic review of qualitative data. *BMC Pregnancy and Childbirth, 22*(1), 293. DOI: 10.1186/s12884-022-04642-x PMID: 35387619

Iradukunda, F., & Canty, L. (2023). Decolonizing nursing education and research to address racial disparities in maternal health. *Journal of Advanced Nursing, 79*(7), 2465–2469. DOI: 10.1111/jan.15624 PMID: 36882975

Jackson, A. P. (2000). Maternal self-efficacy and children's influence on stress and parenting among single black mothers in poverty. *Journal of Family Issues, 21*(1), 3–16. DOI: 10.1177/019251300021001001

Jalloh, M. F., & Gebreamlak, W. (2021). Black women's experiences with perinatal loss: A systematic review. *Journal of Obstetric, Gynecologic, and Neonatal Nursing : JOGNN, 50*(3), 255–264. DOI: 10.1016/j.jogn.2021.02.007

James, K. F., Klomhaus, A. M., Elliott, T., Mensah, M., Jeffers, K. S., & Choi, K. R. (2023). Structural factors in health care associated with the mental health needs of Black women in California during the perinatal period. *Journal of Obstetric, Gynecologic, and Neonatal Nursing : JOGNN, 52*(6), 481–490. DOI: 10.1016/j.jogn.2023.08.002 PMID: 37634545

Jankovic, J., Parsons, J., Jovanović, N., Berrisford, G., Copello, A., Fazil, Q., & Priebe, S. (2020). Differences in access and utilisation of mental health services in the perinatal period for women from ethnic minorities—A population-based study. *BMC Medicine, 18*(1), 1–12. DOI: 10.1186/s12916-020-01711-w PMID: 32912196

Jidong, D. E., Husain, N., Roche, A., Lourie, G., Ike, T. J., Murshed, M., Park, M. S., Karick, H., Dagona, Z. K., Pwajok, J. Y., Gumber, A., Francis, C., Nyam, P. P., & Mwankon, S. B. (2021). Psychological interventions for maternal depression among women of African and Caribbean origin: A systematic review. *BMC Women's Health, 21*(1), 1–14. DOI: 10.1186/s12905-021-01202-x PMID: 33637070

Jimah, T., Borg, H., Kehoe, P., Pimentel, P., Turner, A., Labbaf, S., Asgari Mehrabadi, M., Rahmani, A. M., Dutt, N., & Guo, Y. (2021). A technology-based pregnancy health and wellness intervention (two happy hearts): Case study. *JMIR Formative Research, 5*(11), e30991. DOI: 10.2196/30991 PMID: 34787576

Johnson, A. D. R. (2020). Implicit Provider Bias and its Implications for Black/African American Mental Health. In *The International Handbook of Black Community Mental Health* (pp. 113–134). Emerald Publishing Limited. DOI: 10.1108/978-1-83909-964-920201008

Johnson, A., Hoffman, C., Julian, M., Bengal, C., Issa, M., Kenneally, M., Harris, S. D., Rosenblum, K. L., & Muzik, M. (2023). Holding the whole person: Perinatal women's perspectives on the integrated infant mental health care model in obstetrical care during COVID-19 pandemic. *Journal of Psychiatry and Psychiatric Disorders, 7*, 248–259.

Johnson, A., Kirk, R., Rosenblum, K. L., & Muzik, M. (2015). Enhancing breastfeeding rates among African American women: A systematic review of current psychosocial interventions. *Breastfeeding Medicine, 10*(1), 45–62. DOI: 10.1089/bfm.2014.0023 PMID: 25423601

Johnson, D. M., Worrell, J., & Chandler, R. K. (2005). Assessing psychological health and empowerment in women: The personal progress scale revised. *Women & Health, 5*(1), 109–129. DOI: 10.1300/J013v41n01_07 PMID: 16048871

Johnson, M., & Molineux, M. (2020). The impact of home care on child development. *Developmental Psychology, 56*(8), 1423–1434.

Jones, A. (2019). Help Seeking in the Perinatal Period: A Review of Barriers and Facilitators. *Social Work in Public Health, 34*(7), 596–605. DOI: 10.1080/19371918.2019.1635947 PMID: 31242074

Jones, D. J., Forehand, R., Brody, G., & Armistead, L. (2019). Positive parenting and child psychosocial outcomes: A longitudinal study in a rural African American sample. *Journal of Child and Family Studies, 28*(2), 308–318.

Jones, J. (2010). *Suffering in silence? Intrapersonal communication regarding female empowerment and healthcare access for breast cancer screening in Cape Town*. Publication No.

Jones, J. H. (1993). *Bad Blood: The Tuskegee Syphilis Experiment*. Free Press.

Jones, K. M., Power, M. L., Queenan, J. T., & Schulkin, J. (2015). Racial and ethnic disparities in breastfeeding. *Breastfeeding Medicine, 10*(4), 186–196. DOI: 10.1089/bfm.2014.0152 PMID: 25831234

Jones, K., McAlister, B. S., Haas, B. K., & Duke, G. (2021). Experiences of African American mothers following the death of their infants. *Nursing for Women's Health, 25*(6), 412–418. DOI: 10.1016/j.nwh.2021.09.004 PMID: 34717892

Kaiser Family Foundation. (n.d.). Mental health and substance use disorder coverage in marketplace plans. https://www.kff.org/mental-health/issue-brief/mental-health-and-substance-use-disorder-coverage-in-medicare-advantage-plans/

Kantor, L. M., Cruz, N., Adams, C., Akhimien, C., Allibay Abdulkadir, F., Battle, C., Oluwayemi, M., Salimon, O., Won, S. H., & Niraula, S. (2023). Black Women's Maternal Health: Insights From Community Based Participatory Research in Newark, New Jersey. *Behavioral Medicine (Washington, D.C.)*, 1–8. PMID: 37382100

Karatsoreos, I. N., & McEwen, B. S. (2011). Psychobiological allostasis: Resistance, resilience and vulnerability. *Trends in Cognitive Sciences, 15*(12), 576–584. DOI: 10.1016/j.tics.2011.10.005 PMID: 22078931

Kathree, T., Selohilwe, O. M., Bhana, A., & Petersen, I. (2014). Perceptions of postnatal depression and health care needs in a South African sample: The "mental" in maternal health care. *BMC Women's Health, 14*(1), 1–11. DOI: 10.1186/s12905-014-0140-7 PMID: 25389015

Kearney, M. S., & Levine, P. B. (2012). Why is the teen birth rate in the United States so high and why does it matter? *The Journal of Economic Perspectives, 26*(2), 141–166. DOI: 10.1257/jep.26.2.141 PMID: 22792555

Keith, V. M., Lincoln, K. D., Taylor, R. J., & Jackson, J. S. (2010). Discriminatory experiences and depressive symptoms among African American women: Do skin tone and mastery matter? *Sex Roles, 62*(1-2), 48–59. DOI: 10.1007/s11199-009-9706-5 PMID: 21151821

Kemet, S., Yang, Y., Nseyo, O., Bell, F., Gordon, A. Y. A., Mays, M., Fowler, M., & Jackson, A. (2022). "When I think of mental healthcare, I think of no care." Mental Health Services as a Vital Component of Prenatal Care for Black Women. *Maternal and Child Health Journal, 26*(4), 1–10. DOI: 10.1007/s10995-021-03226-z PMID: 34519952

Kenney, L. J., & Ross, E. C. (2020). Implementation and evaluation of a perinatal bereavement program: A trauma-informed approach. *Journal of Obstetric, Gynecologic, and Neonatal Nursing : JOGNN, 49*(5), 493–501. DOI: 10.1016/j.jogn.2020.04.005

Kessler, R. C., Chiu, W. T., Demler, O., & Walters, E. E. (2005). Prevalence, severity, and comorbidity of 12-month DSM-IV disorders in the National Comorbidity Survey Replication. *Archives of General Psychiatry*, *62*(6), 617–627. DOI: 10.1001/archpsyc.62.6.617 PMID: 15939839

KFF. (2020). Analysis of Federal Bills to Strengthen Maternal Health Care. *Kaiser Family Foundation*. https://www.kff.org/womens-health-policy/fact-sheet/analysis-of-federal-bills-to-strengthen-maternal-health-care/

KFF. (2022). Medicaid Coverage of Pregnancy-Related Services: Findings from a 2021 State Survey. *Kaiser Family Foundation*. https://www.kff.org/report-section/medicaid-coverage-of-pregnancy-related-services-findings-from-a-2021-state-survey-report/

Kiernan, F., Chmiel, A., Garrido, S., Hickey, M., & Davidson, J. W. (2021). The role of artistic creative activities in navigating the COVID-19 pandemic in Australia. *Frontiers in Psychology*, *12*, 696202. DOI: 10.3389/fpsyg.2021.696202 PMID: 34512453

Kim, T. H., Connolly, J. A., & Tamim, H. (2014). The effect of social support around pregnancy on postpartum depression among Canadian teen mothers and adult mothers in the maternity experiences survey. *BMC Pregnancy and Childbirth*, *14*(1), 162. DOI: 10.1186/1471-2393-14-162 PMID: 24884410

Kirby, D., Laris, B. A., & Rolleri, L. A. (2007). Sex and HIV education programs: Their impact on sexual behaviors of young people throughout the world. *The Journal of Adolescent Health*, *40*(3), 206–217. DOI: 10.1016/j.jadohealth.2006.11.143 PMID: 17321420

Knight, M., Kenyon, S., Brocklehurst, P., Neilson, J., Shakespeare, J., & Kurinczuk, J.. (2014). *Saving Lives, Improving Mothers' Care – Lessons Learned to Inform Future Maternity Care from the UK and Ireland Confidential Enquiries into Maternal Deaths and Morbidity 2009–12*. National Perinatal Epidemiology Unit, University of Oxford.

Kozhimannil, K. B., Hardeman, R. R., Alarid-Escudero, F., Vogelsang, C. A., Blauer-Peterson, C., & Howell, E. A. (2016). Modeling the Cost-Effectiveness of Doula Care Associated with Reductions in Preterm Birth and Cesarean Delivery. *Birth (Berkeley, Calif.)*, *43*(1), 20–27. DOI: 10.1111/birt.12218 PMID: 26762249

Kozhimannil, K. B., Hardeman, R. R., Attanasio, L. B., Blauer-Peterson, C., & O'Brien, M. (2013). Doula care, birth outcomes, and costs among Medicaid beneficiaries. *American Journal of Public Health*, *103*(4), e113–e121. DOI: 10.2105/AJPH.2012.301201 PMID: 23409910

Kozhimannil, K. B., Interrante, J. D., Henning-Smith, C., & Admon, L. K. (2019). Rural-Urban Differences In Severe Maternal Morbidity And Mortality In The US, 2007-15. *Health Affairs (Project Hope)*, *38*(12), 2077–2085. DOI: 10.1377/hlthaff.2019.00805 PMID: 31794322

Kozhimannil, K. B., Vogelsang, C. A., & Hardeman, R. R. (2011). Disrupting the pathways of social determinants of health: The role of Black women physicians in addressing reproductive health disparities. *Women's Health Issues*, *21*(5), 458–464.

Kumar, N. R., Arias, M. P., Leitner, K., Wang, E., Clement, E. G., & Hamm, R. F. (2023, Feb). Assessing the impact of telehealth implementation on postpartum outcomes for Black birthing people. *American Journal of Obstetrics & Gynecology MFM*, *5*(2), 100831. DOI: 10.1016/j.ajogmf.2022.100831 PMID: 36496115

Kuzma, E. K., Pardee, M., & Morgan, A. (2020). Implementing patient-centered trauma-informed care for the perinatal nurse. *The Journal of Perinatal & Neonatal Nursing*, *34*(4), E23–E31. DOI: 10.1097/JPN.0000000000000520 PMID: 33079811

Lähdepuro, A., Lahti-Pulkkinen, M., Girchenko, P., Villa, P. M., Heinonen, K., Lahti, J., Pyhälä, R., Laivuori, H., Kajantie, E., & Räikkönen, K. (2023). Positive maternal mental health during pregnancy and psychiatric problems in children from early childhood to late childhood. *Development and Psychopathology*, 1–13. PMID: 37814418

Lähdepuro, A., Lahti-Pulkkinen, M., Pyhälä, R., Tuovinen, S., Lahti, J., Heinonen, K., Laivuori, H., Villa, P. M., Reynolds, R. M., Kajantie, E., Girchenko, P., & Räikkönen, K. (2023). Positive maternal mental health during pregnancy and mental and behavioral disorders in children: A prospective pregnancy cohort study. *Journal of Child Psychology and Psychiatry, and Allied Disciplines*, *64*(5), 807–816. DOI: 10.1111/jcpp.13625 PMID: 35524467

Laister, D., Vivanti, G., Marschik, P. B., Fellinger, J., & Holzinger, D. (2021). Enhancement of social communication behaviors in young children with autism affects maternal stress. *Frontiers in Psychiatry*, *12*, 797148. DOI: 10.3389/fpsyt.2021.797148 PMID: 34950076

Landor, C. (2023). Right to Informed Consent, Right to a Doula: An Evidence-Based Solution to the Black Maternal Mortality Crisis in the United States. *Michigan Journal of Gender & Law*, *30*(30.1), 61. DOI: 10.36641/mjgl.30.1.right

Lathan, E. C., Britt, A., Ravi, M., Ash, M. J., McAfee, E., Wallace, S., Johnson, C. B.II, Woods-Jaeger, B., Powers, A., & Michopoulos, V. (2023). When Reproduction Is No Longer Autonomous: Feeling Respected by Maternity Care Providers Moderates the Association Between Autonomy in Decision Making and Birth-Related Ptsd Symptoms in a Community Sample of Postpartum Black Women. *Journal of Trauma & Dissociation*, *24*(4), 520–537. DOI: 10.1080/15299732.2023.2212406 PMID: 37233983

Lê Cook, B., Doksum, T., Chen, C., Carle, A., & Alegría, M. (2013). The role of provider supply and organization in reducing racial/ethnic disparities in mental health care in the US. *Social Science & Medicine*, *84*, 102–109. DOI: 10.1016/j.socscimed.2013.02.006 PMID: 23466259

Leahy-Warren, P., McCarthy, G., & Corcoran, P. (2012). First-time mothers: Social support, maternal parental self-efficacy and postnatal depression. *Journal of Clinical Nursing*, *21*(3-4), 388–397. DOI: 10.1111/j.1365-2702.2011.03701.x PMID: 21435059

Leary, Joy DeGruy. (2005). *Post traumatic slave syndrome: America's legacy of enduring injury and healing*. Milwaukie, Oregon: Uptone Press.

Lee King, P. A. (2012). Replicability of structural models of the Edinburgh Postnatal Depression Scale (EPDS) in a community sample of postpartum African American women with low socioeconomic status. *Archives of Women's Mental Health*, *15*(2), 77–86. DOI: 10.1007/s00737-012-0260-8 PMID: 22297555

Le, H. N., & Lambert, S. F. (2008). Culture, context, and maternal self-efficacy in Latina mothers. *Applied Developmental Science*, *12*(4), 198–201. DOI: 10.1080/10888690802388136

Leon, I. G. (1992). Perinatal loss: A critique of current hospital practices. *Clinical Pediatrics*, *31*(6), 366–374. DOI: 10.1177/000992289203100611 PMID: 1628472

Levis, B., Negeri, Z., Sun, Y., Benedetti, A., & Thombs, B. D. (2020). Accuracy of the Edinburgh Postnatal Depression Scale (EPDS) for screening to detect major depression among pregnant and postpartum women: Systematic review and meta-analysis of individual participant data. *BMJ (Clinical Research Ed.)*, *371*, m4022. DOI: 10.1136/bmj.m4022 PMID: 33177069

Libby, P. M., Fallon, M. M., & Jarris, P. E. (2008). Public health practice and health equity: Challenges and opportunities. *Journal of Public Health Management and Practice, 14*(S), S53–S55.

Liese, K., Stewart, K., Pearson, P., Lofton, S., Mbande, T., Patil, C., Liu, L., & Geller, S. (2022). Melanated group midwifery care: Centering the voices of the Black birthing community. *Journal of Midwifery & Women's Health, 67*(6), 696–700. DOI: 10.1111/jmwh.13438 PMID: 36480019

Lindsey, M. A., & Marcell, A. V. (2012). "We're Going Through a Lot of Struggles That People Don't Even Know About" The Need to Understand African American Males' Help-Seeking for Mental Health on Multiple Levels. *American Journal of Men's Health, 6*(5), 354–364. DOI: 10.1177/1557988312441520 PMID: 22457264

Link, B. G., Northridge, M. E., Phelan, J. C., & Ganz, M. L. (2008). Social epidemiology and the fundamental cause concept: On the structuring of effective cancer screens by socioeconomic status. *The Milbank Quarterly, 76*(3), 375–402. DOI: 10.1111/1468-0009.00096 PMID: 9738168

López-Morales, H., del Valle, M. V., Canet-Juric, L., Andrés, M. L., Galli, J. I., Poó, F., & Urquijo, S. (2021). Mental health of pregnant women during the COVID-19 pandemic: A longitudinal study. *Psychiatry Research, 295*, 113567. DOI: 10.1016/j.psychres.2020.113567 PMID: 33213933

Louis-Jacques, A. F., Applequist, J., Perkins, M., Williams, C., Joglekar, R., Powis, R., Daniel, A., & Wilson, R. (2024). Florida Doulas' Perspectives on Their Role in Reducing Maternal Morbidity and Health Disparities. *Women's Health Issues, 34*(4), 417–428. DOI: 10.1016/j.whi.2024.01.003 PMID: 38503681

Lowe, N. K. (2021). Black Women's Lives Matter. *Journal of Obstetric, Gynecologic, and Neonatal Nursing : JOGNN, 50*(4), 363–368. DOI: 10.1016/j.jogn.2021.06.001 PMID: 34153227

Ludwig, M. (2018). Maternal / Fetal Conflict | UW Department of Bioethics & Humanities. https://depts.washington.edu/bhdept/ethics-medicine/bioethics-topics/detail/69

Madden, K., Bostock, L., & Devaraj, T. (2018). Trauma-informed care in maternity services: A scoping review. *Women and Birth; Journal of the Australian College of Midwives, 31*(2), 159–167. DOI: 10.1016/j.wombi.2017.09.007

Majeed, A., Allwood, D., Foley, K., & Bindman, A. (2018). Healthcare outcomes and quality in the NHS: How do we compare and how might the NHS improve? *BMJ (Clinical Research Ed.), 362*, k3036. DOI: 10.1136/bmj.k3036 PMID: 30006368

Malcome, M. L., Fedock, G., Garthe, R. C., Golder, S., Higgins, G., & Logan, T. (2019). Weathering probation and parole: The protective role of social support on Black women's recent stressful events and depressive symptoms. *The Journal of Black Psychology*, *45*(8), 661–688. DOI: 10.1177/0095798419889755

Markin, R. D., & Coleman, M. N. (2023). Intersections of gendered racial trauma and childbirth trauma: Clinical interventions for Black women. *Psychotherapy (Chicago, Ill.)*, *60*(1), 27–38. DOI: 10.1037/pst0000403 PMID: 34843315

Marmot, M., & Allen, J. (2014). Social determinants of health equity. *American Journal of Public Health*, *104*(4), 517–519. DOI: 10.2105/AJPH.2014.302200 PMID: 25100411

Matthews, K., Morgan, I., Davis, K., Estriplet, T., Perez, S., & Crear-Perry, J. A. (2021). Pathways To Equitable And Antiracist Maternal Mental Health Care: Insights From Black Women Stakeholders: Study examines pathways to equitable and antiracist maternal mental health care. *Health Affairs*, *40*(10), 1597–1604.

McCarthy, D. (2024). Gendered anti-blackness, maternal health & chattel slavery: OB/Gyn knowledge as a determinant of death of black women. *Social Science & Medicine*, *353*, 117038. DOI: 10.1016/j.socscimed.2024.117038 PMID: 38936105

McDowell, I. (2006). *Measuring health: A guide to rating scales and questionnaires* (3rd ed.). Oxford University Press. DOI: 10.1093/acprof:oso/9780195165678.001.0001

McEwen, B. S. (2004). Protection and damage from acute and chronic stress: Allostasis and allostatic load overload and allostatic load. *Annals of the New York Academy of Sciences*, *1032*(1), 1–7. DOI: 10.1196/annals.1314.001 PMID: 15677391

McEwen, B. S., & Seeman, T. (1999). Protective and damaging effects of mediators of stress. *Annals of the New York Academy of Sciences*, *896*(1), 30–47. DOI: 10.1111/j.1749-6632.1999.tb08103.x PMID: 10681886

McLemore, M. R., Altman, M. R., Cooper, N., Williams, S., Rand, L., & Franck, L. (2018). Health care experiences of pregnant, birthing and postnatal women of color at risk for preterm birth. *Social Science & Medicine*, *201*, 127–135. DOI: 10.1016/j.socscimed.2018.02.013 PMID: 29494846

Mehra, R., Boyd, L. M., Magriples, U., Kershaw, T. S., Ickovics, J. R., & Keene, D. E. (2020). Black Pregnant Women "Get the Most Judgment": A Qualitative Study of the Experiences of Black Women at the Intersection of Race, Gender, and Pregnancy. *Women's Health Issues*, *30*(6), 484–492. DOI: 10.1016/j.whi.2020.08.001 PMID: 32900575

Mehra, R., Keene, D. E., Kershaw, T. S., Ickovics, J. R., & Warren, J. L. (2019). Racial and ethnic disparities in adverse birth outcomes: Differences by racial residential segregation. *SSM - Population Health, 8*, 1–10. DOI: 10.1016/j.ssmph.2019.100417 PMID: 31193960

Melillo, G. (2020, Dec 3). US Ranks Worst in Maternal Care, Mortality Compared With 10 Other Developed Nations. https://www.ajmc.com/view/us-ranks-worst-in-maternal-care-mortality-compared-with-10-other-developed-nations

Melnyk, B. M., Gennaro, S., Szalacha, L. A., Hoying, J., O'Connor, C., Cooper, A., & Gibeau, A. (2020). Randomized controlled trial of the COPE-P intervention to improve mental health, healthy lifestyle behaviors, birth and post-natal outcomes of minority pregnant women: Study protocol with implications. *Contemporary Clinical Trials, 98*, 106090. DOI: 10.1016/j.cct.2020.106090 PMID: 32745703

Mendenhall, R., Henderson, L., Scott, B., Butler, L., Turi, K. N., Greenlee, A., Robinson, G. E., Roberts, B. W., Rodriguez-Zas, S. L., & Brooks, J. E. (2020). Involving Urban Single Low-Income African American Mothers in Genomic Research: Giving Voice to How Place Matters in Health Disparities and Prevention Strategies. *Family Medicine and Primary Care — Open Access, 4*(2). PMID: 35373191

Mendez, D. D., Hogan, V. K., & Culhane, J. F. (2013). Stress during Pregnancy: The Role of Institutional Racism. *Stress and Health, 29*(4), 266–274. DOI: 10.1002/smi.2462 PMID: 23055409

Mendez, D. D., Thorpe, R. J., Amutah, N., Davis, E. M., Walker, R. E., Chapple-McGruder, T., & Bodnar, L. (2016). Neighborhood racial composition and poverty in association with pre-pregnancy weight and gestational weight gain. *SSM - Population Health, 2*, 692–699. Advance online publication. DOI: 10.1016/j.ssmph.2016.09.008 PMID: 29349180

Mersky, J. P., Choi, C., Plummer Lee, C., & Janczewski, C. E. (2021). Disparities in adverse childhood experiences by race/ethnicity, gender, and economic status: Intersectional analysis of a nationally representative sample. *Child Abuse & Neglect, 117*, 105066. DOI: 10.1016/j.chiabu.2021.105066 PMID: 33845239

Miller, G. E., Chen, E., & Zhou, E. S. (2007). If it goes up, must it come down? Chronic stress and the hypothalamic-pituitary-adrenocortical axis in humans. *Psychological Bulletin, 133*(1), 25–45. DOI: 10.1037/0033-2909.133.1.25 PMID: 17201569

Mirowsky, J., & Ross, C. E. (2002). Depression, parenthood, and age at first birth. *Social Science & Medicine, 54*(8), 1281–1298. DOI: 10.1016/S0277-9536(01)00096-X PMID: 11989963

Mi, T., Hung, P., Li, X., McGregor, A., He, J., & Zhou, J. (2022). Racial and Ethnic Disparities in Postpartum Care in the Greater Boston Area During the COVID-19 Pandemic. *JAMA Network Open*, *5*(6), e2216355. DOI: 10.1001/jamanetworkopen.2022.16355 PMID: 35737390

Mitchell, G. K., Burridge, L., Zhang, J., Donald, M., Scott, I. A., Dart, J., & Jackson, C. L. (2015). Systematic review of integrated models of health care delivered at the primary–secondary interface: How effective is it and what determines effectiveness? *Australian Journal of Primary Health*, *21*(4), 391–408. DOI: 10.1071/PY14172 PMID: 26329878

Mollard, E., Elya, A., Gaines, C., Salahshurian, E., Riordan, E., Moore, T., Maloney, S., Balas, M. C., Shah, N., & Cooper Owens, D. (2024). Reclaiming narratives of empowerment around Black maternal health: A strengths-based, community-informed focus group study. *Ethnicity & Health*, *29*(6), 1–17. DOI: 10.1080/13557858.2024.2359384 PMID: 38805258

Mollborn, S., & Morningstar, E. (2009). Investigating the relationship between teenage childbearing and psychological distress using longitudinal evidence. *Journal of Health and Social Behavior*, *50*(3), 310–326. DOI: 10.1177/002214650905000305 PMID: 19711808

Monaghan, S., Akale, M. A., Demeke, B., & Darmstadt, G. L. (2021). Prevalence and stigma of postpartum common mental disorders in the Gurage region of Ethiopia: A mixed-methods observational cohort study. *Frontiers in Psychology*, *12*, 626797. DOI: 10.3389/fpsyg.2021.626797 PMID: 33897534

Montalmant, K. E., & Ettinger, A. K. (2023). The Racial Disparities in Maternal Mortality and Impact of Structural Racism and Implicit Racial Bias on Pregnant Black Women: A Review of the Literature. *Journal of Racial and Ethnic Health Disparities*, 1–20. PMID: 37957536

Moodley, J., Fawcus, S., & Pattinson, R. (2019). Improvements in maternal mortality in South Africa. *South African Medical Journal*, *108*(3a), s4–s8.

Moore, J. E., McLemore, M. R., Glenn, N., & Zivin, K. (2021). Policy Opportunities To Improve Prevention, Diagnosis, And Treatment Of Perinatal Mental Health Conditions: Study examines policy opportunities to improve prevention, diagnosis, and treatment of perinatal mental health. *Health Affairs*, *40*(10), 1534–1542. DOI: 10.1377/hlthaff.2021.00779 PMID: 34606359

Moreno, O., & Cardemil, E. (2013). Religiosity and mental health services: An exploratory study of help seeking among Latinos. *Journal of Latina/o Psychology*, *1*(1), 53–67. DOI: 10.1037/a0031376

Morrissey, T. W. (2017). Child care and parent labor force participation: A review of the research literature. *Review of Economics of the Household*, *15*(1), 1–24. DOI: 10.1007/s11150-016-9331-3

Mosley, E. A., Lindsey, A., Turner, D., Shah, P., Sayyad, A., Mack, A., & Lindberg, K. (2023). "I want… to serve those communities…[but] my price tag is… not what they can afford": The community-engaged Georgia doula study. *Perspectives on Sexual and Reproductive Health*, *55*(3), 200–209. DOI: 10.1363/psrh.12241 PMID: 37533301

Murray, K. R., Dulli, L. S., Ridgeway, K., Dal Santo, L., Darrow de Mora, D., Olsen, P., Silverstein, H., & McCarraher, D. R. (2017). Improving retention in HIV care among adolescents and adults in low-and middle-income countries: A systematic review of the literature. *PLoS One*, *12*(9), e0184879. DOI: 10.1371/journal.pone.0184879 PMID: 28961253

National Alliance on Mental Illness. (2022). *Mental health by the numbers*. About Mental Health. https://www.nami.org/mhstats

National Birth Equity Collaborative. (n.d.). *National Birth Equity Collaborative (NBEC): General Operating Support*. https://www.commonwealthfund.org/grants/national-birth-equity-collaborative-nbec-general-operating-support

National Partnership for Women & Families. (2018). Maternal mental health in the United States: A review of the literature. https://www.nationalpartnership.org/

National Partnership for Women and Families. (2023, Nov). *Black women's maternal health: A* multifaceted *approach to addressing persistent and dire health disparities*. https://nationalpartnership.org/report/black-womens-maternal-health/

Neal-Barnett, A., Stadulis, R., Murray, M., Payne, M. R., Thomas, A., & Salley, B. B. (2011). Sister Circles as a Culturally Relevant Intervention for Anxious African American Women. *Clinical Psychology : a Publication of the Division of Clinical Psychology of the American Psychological Association*, *18*(3), 266–273. DOI: 10.1111/j.1468-2850.2011.01258.x PMID: 22081747

Neblett, E. W.Jr, Bernard, D. L., & Banks, K. H. (2016). The moderating roles of gender and socioeconomic status in the association between racial discrimination and psychological adjustment. *Cognitive and Behavioral Practice*, *23*(3), 385–397. DOI: 10.1016/j.cbpra.2016.05.002

Nelson, T., Ernst, S. C., Tirado, C., Fisse, J. L., & Moreno, O. (2022). Psychological Distress and Attitudes Toward Seeking Professional Psychological Services Among Black Women: The Role of Past Mental Health Treatment. *Journal of Racial and Ethnic Health Disparities*, *9*(2), 527–537. DOI: 10.1007/s40615-021-00983-z PMID: 33559107

Nelson, T., Ernst, S. C., & Watson-Singleton, N. N. (2023). Perinatal complications, poor hospital treatment, and positive screen for postpartum depressive symptoms among black women. *Journal of Racial and Ethnic Health Disparities*, *10*(3), 1371–1378. DOI: 10.1007/s40615-022-01322-6 PMID: 35513596

Nepal, A., Dangol, S. K., & van Der Kwaak, A. (2020). Improving maternal health services through social accountability interventions in Nepal: An analytical review of existing literature. *Public Health Reviews*, *41*(1), 1–24. DOI: 10.1186/s40985-020-00147-0 PMID: 33349273

Neufeld, A., Harrison, M. J., Stewart, M., Hughes, K., & Spitzer, D. (2008). Immigrant women: Making connections to community resources for support in family caregiving. *Qualitative Health Research*, *18*(7), 913–922. PMID: 18552318

New Jersey Department of Health. (2022). *New Jersey breastfeeding strategic plan 2022* [PDF]. https://www.nj.gov/health/fhs/wic/documents/FINAL%20New%20Jersey%20Breastfeeding%20Strategic%20Plan%202022.pdf

Ngo-Metzger, Q., Massagli, M. P., Clarridge, B. R., Manocchia, M., Davis, R. B., Iezzoni, L. I., & Phillips, R. S. (2003). Linguistic and cultural barriers to care. *Journal of General Internal Medicine*, *18*(1), 44–52. DOI: 10.1046/j.1525-1497.2003.20205.x PMID: 12534763

Njoku, A., Evans, M., Nimo-Sefah, L., & Bailey, J. (2023, Feb 3). Listen to the Whispers before They Become Screams: Addressing Black Maternal Morbidity and Mortality in the United States. *Healthcare (Basel)*, *11*(3), 438. DOI: 10.3390/healthcare11030438 PMID: 36767014

Norris, C. M., & Mitchell, F. D. (2014). Exploring the stress-support-distress process among Black women. *Journal of Black Studies*, *45*(1), 3–18. DOI: 10.1177/0021934713517898

Novacek, D. M., Hampton-Anderson, J. N., Ebor, M. T., Loeb, T. B., & Wyatt, G. E. (2020). Mental health ramifications of the COVID-19 pandemic for Black Americans: Clinical and research recommendations. *Psychological Trauma: Theory, Research, Practice, and Policy*, *12*(5), 449–451. DOI: 10.1037/tra0000796 PMID: 32525370

Novoa, C., & Taylor, J. (2018). Quality, affordable child care is critical to Black families. Center for American Progress. https://www.americanprogress.org/

Nuru-Jeter, A., Dominguez, T. P., Hammond, W. P., Leu, J., Skaff, M., Egerter, S., Jones, C. P., & Braveman, P. (2009). "It's the skin you're in": African American women talk about their experiences of racism. An exploratory study to develop measures of racism for birth outcome studies. *Maternal and Child Health Journal*, *13*(1), 29–39. DOI: 10.1007/s10995-008-0357-x PMID: 18463971

O'Brien, E., & Rich, M. (2022). Obstetric violence in historical perspective. *Lancet*, *399*(10342), 2183–2185. DOI: 10.1016/S0140-6736(22)01022-4 PMID: 35691313

O'Donnell, K. J., & Meaney, M. J. (2017). Fetal origins of mental health: The developmental origins of health and disease hypothesis. *The American Journal of Psychiatry*, *174*(4), 319–328. DOI: 10.1176/appi.ajp.2016.16020138 PMID: 27838934

Oburota, C. S., Okungbowa, E. F., & Eke, F. A. (2023). Socioeconomic Inequalities in Maternal Health Care Utilization and Delivery Channels in Nigeria. [JPSS]. *Journal of Population and Social Studies*, *31*, 672–695. DOI: 10.25133/JPSSv312023.037

Office of Disease Prevention and Health Promotion. (n.d.). Social Determinants of Health—Healthy People 2030 | health.gov. Retrieved November 10, 2023, from https://health.gov/healthypeople/priority-areas/social-determinants-health

Ogunwole, S. M., Bennett, W. L., Williams, A. N., & Bower, K. M. (2020). Community-based Doulas and COVID-19: addressing structural and institutional barriers to maternal health equity.

Ogunwole, S. M., & Starks, F. D. (2024). Cultivating Critical Love to Improve Black Maternal Health Outcomes. *AMA Journal of Ethics*, *26*(1), 72–83. DOI: 10.1001/amajethics.2024.72 PMID: 38180861

Olds, D. L., Kitzman, H., Knudtson, M. D., Anson, E., Smith, J. A., & Cole, R. (2014). Effect of Home Visiting by Nurses on Maternal and Child Mortality: Results of a 2-Decade Follow-Up of a Randomized Clinical Trial. *JAMA Pediatrics*, *168*(9), 800–806. DOI: 10.1001/jamapediatrics.2014.472 PMID: 25003802

Oliver-Williams, C., & Viruell-Fuentes, E. (2021). Lessons about postpartum depression from the woman-centered health home. *Women's Health Issues*, *31*(3), 204–211. PMID: 33707142

Opara, I., Mayberry, B., Abu-Baker, K., & Ghaji, N. (2020). The impact of maternal stress on maternal-child health outcomes among Black mothers: A systematic review. *Journal of Women's Health*, *29*(1), 33–42.

Oregon Health Authority. (n.d.). Reproductive Health Equity Act. https://www.oregon.gov/oha/ph/healthypeoplefamilies/reproductivesexualhealth/pages/reproductive-health-equity-act.aspx

Organization for Economic Co-operation and Development. (2024). *Paid parental leave: Big differences for mothers and fathers*. https://oecdstatistics.blog/2023/01/12/paid-parental-leave-big-differences-for-mothers-and-fathers/

Owens, D. C. (2017). *Medical bondage: Race, gender, and the origins of American gynecology*. University of Georgia Press. DOI: 10.2307/j.ctt1pwt69x

Owens, D. C., & Fett, S. M. (2019). Black maternal and infant health: Historical legacies of slavery. *American Journal of Public Health, 109*(10), 1342–1345. DOI: 10.2105/AJPH.2019.305243 PMID: 31415204

Owens, D., & Denney-Koelsch, E. M. (2023). African American culture and perinatal loss. In Denney-Koelsch, E. M. (Ed.), *Perinatal bereavement rituals and practices among U.S. cultural groups* (pp. 248–262). Springer., DOI: 10.1007/978-3-031-47203-9_5

Panzarine, S., Slater, E., & Sharps, P. (1995). Coping, social support, and depressive symptoms in adolescent mothers. *The Journal of Adolescent Health, 17*(2), 113–119. DOI: 10.1016/1054-139X(95)00064-Y PMID: 7495822

Paremoer, L., Nandi, S., Serag, H., & Baum, F. (2021). Covid-19 pandemic and the social determinants of health. *BMJ (Clinical Research Ed.), 372*(129), n129. DOI: 10.1136/bmj.n129 PMID: 33509801

Parker, A. (2021). Reframing the narrative: Black maternal mental health and culturally meaningful support for wellness. *Infant Mental Health Journal*, *42*(4), 502–516. DOI: 10.1002/imhj.21910 PMID: 33470438

Parker, A. (2022). Just Help Me: A Research Poem by Black Mothers. *Qualitative Inquiry*, *28*(10), 1092–1093. DOI: 10.1177/10778004221087684

Penner, F., Wall, K. M., Guan, K. W., Huang, H. J., Richardson, L., Dunbar, A. S., Groh, A. M., & Rutherford, H. J. (2023). Racial disparities in EEG research and their implications for our understanding of the maternal brain. *Cognitive, Affective & Behavioral Neuroscience*, *23*(1), 1–16. DOI: 10.3758/s13415-022-01040-w PMID: 36414837

Perez, N. B., Melkus, G. D. E., Wright, F., Yu, G., Vorderstrasse, A. A., Sun, Y. V., & Taylor, J. Y. (2023). Latent class analysis of depressive symptom phenotypes among Black/African American mothers. *Nursing Research*, *72*(2), 93–102. DOI: 10.1097/NNR.0000000000000635 PMID: 36729771

Perinatal depression. (n.d.). National Institute of Mental Health (NIMH). https://www.nimh.nih.gov/health/publications/perinatal-depression#:~:text=Perinatal%20depression%20includes%20depression%20that,caring%20for%20themselves%20or%20others

Perry, B., Pollard, R., Blakley, T., Baker, W., & Vigilante, D. (2016). Childhood trauma, the neurobiology of adaptation, and "use-dependent" development of the brain: How "states" become "traits.". *Infant Mental Health Journal*, *16*(4), 271–291. DOI: 10.1002/1097-0355(199524)16:4<271::AID-IMHJ2280160404>3.0.CO;2-B

Petersen, E. E., Davis, N. L., Goodman, D., Cox, S., Syverson, C., Seed, K., Shapiro-Mendoza, S., Callaghan, W. M., & Barfield, W. (2019). Racial/ethnic disparities in pregnancy-related deaths - United States, 2007–2016. *MMWR. Morbidity and Mortality Weekly Report*, *68*(35), 762–765. DOI: 10.15585/mmwr.mm6835a3 PMID: 31487273

Petersen, R., Gillespie, S. L., & Hamoda, H. M. (2020). Addressing disparities in perinatal loss: A qualitative study of Black women's experiences and needs. *Maternal and Child Health Journal*, *24*(8), 1047–1056. DOI: 10.1007/s10995-020-02921-3 PMID: 32335805

Policy Center for Maternal Mental Health. (2023). Black Maternal Mental Health [Report]. www.policycentermmh.org/black-maternal-mental-health-issue-brief

Ponting, C., Urizar Jr, G. G., & Dunkel Schetter, C. (2022). Psychological interventions for prenatal anxiety in Latinas and Black women: A scoping review and recommendations. *Frontiers in Psychiatry*, *13*, 820343. DOI: 10.3389/fpsyt.2022.820343 PMID: 35370831

Powell, B. J., Waltz, T. J., Chinman, M. J., Damschroder, L. J., Smith, J. L., Matthieu, M. M., Proctor, E. K., & Kirchner, J. E. (2015). A refined compilation of implementation strategies: Results from the expert recommendations for implementing change (ERIC) project. *Implementation Science : IS*, *10*(1), 21. Advance online publication. DOI: 10.1186/s13012-015-0209-1 PMID: 25889199

Powers, A., Woods-Jaeger, B., Stevens, J. S., Bradley, B., Patel, M. B., Joyner, A., Smith, A. K., Jamieson, D. J., Kaslow, N., & Michopoulos, V. (2020). Trauma, psychiatric disorders, and treatment history among pregnant African American women. *Psychological Trauma: Theory, Research, Practice, and Policy*, *12*(2), 138–146. DOI: 10.1037/tra0000507 PMID: 31464464

Prady, S. L., Endacott, C., Dickerson, J., Bywater, T. J., & Blower, S. L. (2021). Inequalities in the identification and management of common mental disorders in the perinatal period: An equity focused re-analysis of a systematic review. *PLoS One*, *16*(3), e0248631. DOI: 10.1371/journal.pone.0248631 PMID: 33720994

Prather, C., Fuller, T. R., Jeffries, W. L.IV, Marshall, K. J., Howell, A. V., Belyue-Umole, A., & King, W. (2018). Racism, African American women, and their sexual and reproductive health: A review of historical and contemporary evidence and implications for health equity. *Health Equity*, *2*(1), 249–259. DOI: 10.1089/heq.2017.0045 PMID: 30283874

Price, S. K., Proctor, E. K., & Kinghorn, A. M. (2017). Trauma-informed care: Opportunities for high-quality, trauma-informed care and implications for policy. Report to the Missouri Foundation for Health.

Proctor, E., Silmere, H., Raghavan, R., Hovmand, P., Aarons, G., Bunger, A., & Hensley, M. (2011). Outcomes for implementation research: Conceptual distinctions, measurement challenges, and research agenda. *Administration and Policy in Mental Health*, *38*(2), 65–76. DOI: 10.1007/s10488-010-0319-7 PMID: 20957426

Prom, M. C., Denduluri, A., Philpotts, L. L., Rondon, M. B., Borba, C. P., Gelaye, B., & Byatt, N. (2022). A systematic review of interventions that integrate perinatal mental health care into routine maternal care in low-and middle-income countries. *Frontiers in Psychiatry*, *13*, 859341. DOI: 10.3389/fpsyt.2022.859341 PMID: 35360136

Proper, K. I., Picavet, H. S. J., Bogers, R. P., Verschuren, W. M., & Bemelmans, W. J. (2013). The association between adverse life events and body weight change: Results of a prospective cohort study. *BMC Public Health*, *13*(1), 957. DOI: 10.1186/1471-2458-13-957 PMID: 24125054

Quick, A. D., Tung, I., Keenan, K., & Hipwell, A. E. (2023). Psychological well-being across the perinatal period: Life satisfaction and flourishing in a longitudinal study of Young Black and White American women. *Journal of Happiness Studies*, *24*(3), 1283–1301. DOI: 10.1007/s10902-023-00634-6 PMID: 37273506

Quinless, F. W., & Nelson, M. A. M. (1988). Development of a measure of learned helplessness. *Nursing Research*, *37*(1), 11–15. DOI: 10.1097/00006199-198801000-00003 PMID: 3340571

Rafizadeh, E. B., Rice, E., Smith, J., Bell, J., & Harvath, T. A. (2023). Understanding How Community Health Workers Build Trust with Low-Income Women of Color At-Risk for Maternal Child Health Disparities: A Grounded Theory Study. *Journal of Community Health Nursing*, *40*(3), 219–231. DOI: 10.1080/07370016.2023.2168124 PMID: 36999664

Rainford, M. (2023). *Pregnant while Black: Advancing justice for maternal health in America*. Broadleaf Books. DOI: 10.2307/j.ctv2phpsbz

Ramey-Collier, K., Jackson, M., Malloy, A., McMillan, C., Scraders-Pyatt, A., & Wheeler, S. M. (2023). Doula care: A review of outcomes and impact on birth experience. *Obstetrical & Gynecological Survey*, *78*(2), 124–127. DOI: 10.1097/OGX.0000000000001103 PMID: 36786720

Ravi, D., Iacob, A., & Profit, J. (2021). Unequal care: Racial/ethnic disparities in neonatal intensive care delivery. *Seminars in Perinatology*, *45*(4), 151411. DOI: 10.1016/j.semperi.2021.151411 PMID: 33902931

Reddy, S., Patel, N., Saxon, M., Amin, N., & Biviji, R. (2021). Innovations in US health care delivery to reduce disparities in maternal mortality among African American and American Indian/Alaskan Native women. *Journal of Patient-Centered Research and Reviews*, *8*(2), 140–145. DOI: 10.17294/2330-0698.1793 PMID: 33898647

Reed, B. (2020, May 2). "New York mother dies after raising alarm on hospital neglect." *The Guardian*. https://www.theguardian.com/us-news/2020/may/02/amber-rose-isaac-new-york-childbirth-death

Reeves, W. C., Pratt, L. A., Thompson, W., Ahluwalia, I. B., Dhingra, S. S., McKnight-Eily, L. R., ... & Safran, M. A. (2011). Mental illness surveillance among adults in the United States. DOI: 10.15585/mmwr.su6003a1

Renbarger, K. M., Abebe, S., Place, J. M., Goldsby, E., Hall, G., & Kroot, A. (2023). Perspectives of infant mortality from African American community members. *Women's Health Reports (New Rochelle, N.Y.)*, *4*(1), 423–430. DOI: 10.1089/whr.2023.0017 PMID: 37638331

Rhoden, R. J. (2022). Look at us as people too: The phenomenological experiences of traumatic childbirth in primi- and multiparous Black women (Doctoral dissertation, Rutgers University). Retrieved from https://doi.org/doi:10.7282/t3-8aze-b741

Rhodes, A., & Segre, L. (2013). Perinatal Depression: A Review of U.S. Legislation and Law. *Archives of Women's Mental Health*, *16*(4), 259–270. DOI: 10.1007/s00737-013-0359-6 PMID: 23740222

Ribeiro Brown, B., Williams, E.-D. G., Abelson, J. M., Chandrakapure, A., & Watkins, D. C. (2022). An Exploratory Case Study of the Types of Resources Black Boys Use to Support Their Mental Health. Healthcare, Roberts, D., Jackson, L., Davie, P., Zhao, C., Harrold, J. A., Fallon, V., & Silverio, S. A. (2023). Exploring the reasons why mothers do not breastfeed, to inform and enable better support. *Frontiers in Global Women's Health*, *4*, 1148719.

Riddle, J. N., Hopkins, T., Yeaton-Massey, A., & Hellberg, S. (2023). No baby to bring home: Perinatal loss, infertility, and mental illness—Overview and recommendations for care. *Current Psychiatry Reports*, *25*(6), 747–757. DOI: 10.1007/s11920-023-01469-x PMID: 37878138

Ríos-Salas, V., & Larson, A. (2015). Perceived discrimination, socioeconomic status, and mental health among Latino adolescents in US immigrant families. *Children and Youth Services Review*, *56*, 116–125. DOI: 10.1016/j.childyouth.2015.07.011

Roberts, D. (1997). *Killing the black body: Race, reproduction, and the meaning of liberty*. Doubleday Publishing Group.

Roberts, E. M., Moskowitz, D., & Nugent, C. (2020). Racial and ethnic disparities in mental health treatment. *Health Services Research*, *55*(2), 104–113.

Robinson, A., Davis, M., Hall, J., Lauckner, C., & Anderson, A. K. (2019). It takes an e-village: Supporting African American mothers in sustaining breastfeeding through Facebook communities. *Journal of Human Lactation*, *35*(3), 569–582. DOI: 10.1177/0890334419831652 PMID: 30889373

Rocca, C. H., Doherty, I., Padian, N. S., Hubbard, A. E., & Minnis, A. M. (2010). Pregnancy intentions and teenage pregnancy among Latinas: A mediation analysis. *Perspectives on Sexual and Reproductive Health*, *42*(3), 186–196. DOI: 10.1363/4218610 PMID: 20887287

Ross, C. E., & Mirowsky, J. (2001). Neighborhood disadvantage, disorder, and health. *Journal of Health and Social Behavior*, *42*(3), 258–276. DOI: 10.2307/3090214 PMID: 11668773

Sabin, J. (2020). *How we fail Black patients in pain*. Association of American Medical Colleges. https://www.aamc.org/news/how-we-fail-black-patients-pain

Sackey, D., Jones, M., & Farley, R. (2021). Reconceptualising specialisation: Integrating refugee health in primary care. *Australian Journal of Primary Health*, *26*(6), 452–457. DOI: 10.1071/PY20138 PMID: 33243370

Salam, M. (2018, Jan 11). "Serena Williams Reveals Health Scare After Giving Birth to Her Daughter." *The New York Times*.

Salinas, J. L., Salinas, M., & Kahn, M. (2022). Doulas, racism, and whiteness: How birth support workers process advocacy towards women of color. *Societies (Basel, Switzerland), 12*(1), 19. DOI: 10.3390/soc12010019

SAMHSA's Concept of Trauma and Guidance for a Trauma-Informed Approach. (n.d.). https://ncsacw.acf.hhs.gov/userfiles/files/SAMHSA_Trauma.pdf

Sánchez-Hucles, J. V. (2016). Womanist therapy with Black women. In Bryant-Davis, T., & Comas-Díaz, L. (Eds.), *Womanist and Mujerista Psychologies: Voices of Fire, Acts of Courage* (pp. 69–92). American Psychological Association., DOI: 10.1037/14937-004

Santiago-Warner, S. (2024). Social work practice in perinatal palliative care: An overview. *Social Work in Health Care, 63*(4-5), 248–262. DOI: 10.1080/00981389.2024.2316697 PMID: 38357813

Schneiderman, N., Ironson, G., & Siegel, S. D. (2005). Stress and health: Psychological, behavioral, and biological determinants. *Annual Review of Clinical Psychology, 1*(1), 607–628. DOI: 10.1146/annurev.clinpsy.1.102803.144141 PMID: 17716101

Schuster, A. L., Perraillon, M. C., Paul, J. J., Leiferman, J. A., Battaglia, C., & Morrato, E. H. (2022). The Effect of the Affordable Care Act (ACA) on Women's Postpartum Insurance and Depression in Five States that Did Not Expand Medicaid, 2012–2015. *Medical Care, 60*(1), 22–28. DOI: 10.1097/MLR.0000000000001652 PMID: 34670222

Schuyler Center for Analysis and Advocacy. (2008). *Teenage births: Outcomes for young parents and their children.* http://www.scaany.org/documents/teen_pregnancy_dec08.pdf

Scott, K. A., Britton, L., & McLemore, M. R. (2019). The ethics of perinatal care for Black women: Dismantling the structural racism in "mother blame" narratives. *The Journal of Perinatal & Neonatal Nursing, 33*(2), 108–115. DOI: 10.1097/JPN.0000000000000394 PMID: 31021935

Scott, K. A., & Davis, D. A. (2022). Destigmatizing and democratizing postpartum care: A "Black woman-person first" approach. *Clinical Obstetrics and Gynecology, 65*(3), 663–675. DOI: 10.1097/GRF.0000000000000729 PMID: 35723647

Segerstrom, S. C., & Miller, G. E. (2004). Psychological stress and the human immune system: A meta-analytic study of 30 years of inquiry. *Psychological Bulletin, 130*(4), 601–630. DOI: 10.1037/0033-2909.130.4.601 PMID: 15250815

Sellers, R. M., Copeland-Linder, N., Martin, P. P., & Lewis, R. H. (2006). Racial identity matters: The relationship between racial discrimination and psychological functioning in African American adolescents. *Journal of Research on Adolescence, 16*(2), 187–216. DOI: 10.1111/j.1532-7795.2006.00128.x

Shakibazadeh, E., Namadian, M., Bohren, M., Vogel, J., Rashidian, A., Nogueira Pileggi, V., Madeira, S., Leathersich, S., Tunçalp, ., Oladapo, O., Souza, J., & Gülmezoglu, A. (2018). Respectful care during childbirth in health facilities globally: A qualitative evidence synthesis. *BJOG, 125*(8), 932–942. DOI: 10.1111/1471-0528.15015 PMID: 29117644

Shanok, A. F., & Miller, L. (2007). Stepping up to motherhood among inner-city teens. *Psychology of Women Quarterly, 31*(3), 252–261. DOI: 10.1111/j.1471-6402.2007.00368.x

Shields, R., & Wailoo, K. (2002). *Childhood and Adolescence in Society*. McGraw-Hill Education.

Shimodera, S., Furukawa, T. A., Mino, Y., Shimazu, K., Nishida, A., & Inoue, S. (2012). Cost-effectiveness of family psychoeducation to prevent relapse in major depression: Results from a randomized controlled trial. *BMC Psychiatry, 12*(1), 40. DOI: 10.1186/1471-244X-12-40 PMID: 22583708

Shorey, S., Ng, E. D., & Downe, S. (2021). Cultural competence and experiences of maternity health care providers on care for migrant women: A qualitative meta-synthesis. *Birth (Berkeley, Calif.), 48*(4), 458–469. DOI: 10.1111/birt.12581 PMID: 34363236

Shrestha, S. D., Pradhan, R., Tran, T. D., Gualano, R. C., & Fisher, J. R. W. (2016). Reliability and validity of the Edinburgh Postnatal Depression Scale (EPDS) for detecting perinatal common mental disorders (PCMDs) among women in low-and lower-middle-income countries: A systematic review. *BMC Pregnancy and Childbirth, 16*(1), 72. DOI: 10.1186/s12884-016-0859-2 PMID: 27044437

Siegel, R. S., & Brandon, A. R. (2014). Adolescents, pregnancy, and mental health. *Journal of Pediatric and Adolescent Gynecology, 27*(3), 138–150. DOI: 10.1016/j.jpag.2013.09.008 PMID: 24559618

Silas, M. J., & Seward, D. X. (2023). Black women's help-seeking and self-care strategies: A phenomenological exploration. *Journal of Counseling and Development, 101*(2), 157–166. DOI: 10.1002/jcad.12465

Simpson, K. R. (2021). *Racism in maternity care is a public health crisis in the United States* (Vol. 46). LWW.

Sinai, M. (2024). The Preventing Maternal Deaths Act of 2018 and Why it is Important. https://health.mountsinai.org/blog/the-preventing-maternal-deaths-act-of-2018-and-why-it-is-important/

Slaughter-Acey, J. C., Caldwell, C. H., Misra, D. P., & Giurgescu, C. (2019). The influence of personal and group racism on entry into prenatal care among African American women. *Women's Health Issues*, *29*(2), 157–164. PMID: 24041828

Smith, J., Brown, L., & Johnson, A. (2020). Culturally competent care for Black mothers: Addressing postpartum depression through tailored home care services. *Journal of Maternal Health*, *15*(2).

Smith, M. V., & Kruse-Austin, A. (2015). A gender-informed model to train community health workers in maternal mental health. *Evaluation and Program Planning*, *51*, 59–62. DOI: 10.1016/j.evalprogplan.2014.12.008 PMID: 25534578

Smith, S. A., & Blumenthal, D. S. (2012). Community Health Workers Support Community-based Participatory Research Ethics: Lessons Learned along the Research-to-Practice-to-Community Continuum. *Journal of Health Care for the Poor and Underserved*, *23*(4, Suppl), 77–87. DOI: 10.1353/hpu.2012.0156 PMID: 23124502

Social Determinants of Health - Healthy People 2030 (n.d.). https://health.gov/healthypeople/priority-areas/social-determinants-health

Social determinants of health. (n.d.). https://www.who.int/health-topics/social-determinants-of-health

Society for Human Resource Management. (2022). *Leveling the parental-leave playing field*. https://www.shrm.org/topics-tools/news/benefits-compensation/leveling-parental-leave-playing-field

Sroka, A. W., Mbayiwa, K., Ilyumzhinova, R., Meyer, W., Fowle, J., Gipson, C. J., Norcott, C., Hipwell, A. E., & Keenan, K. (2023). Depression screening may not capture significant sources of prenatal stress for Black women. *Archives of Women's Mental Health*, *26*(2), 211–217. DOI: 10.1007/s00737-023-01297-1 PMID: 36797547

Steiner, C. A., Barrett, M. L., Weiss, A. J., ... (2006, Feb). Trends and Projections in Hospital Stays for Adults With Multiple Chronic Conditions, 2003–2014. 2014 Nov. In: Healthcare Cost and Utilization Project (HCUP) Statistical Briefs [Internet]. Rockville (MD): Agency for Healthcare Research and Quality (US); Statistical Brief #183.https://www.ncbi.nlm.nih.gov/books/NBK264314/

Structural Racism and Discrimination. (n.d.). NIMHD. https://www.nimhd.nih.gov/resources/understanding-health-disparities/srd.html

Suarez, E. A. (2020). Midwifery and Black maternal health: Claiming our power, resilience, and liberation. *Journal of Midwifery & Women's Health, 65*(5), 655–657. DOI: 10.1111/jmwh.13164

Surjaningrum, E. R., Minas, H., Jorm, A. F., & Kakuma, R. (2018). The feasibility of a role for community health workers in integrated mental health care for perinatal depression: A qualitative study from Surabaya, Indonesia. *International Journal of Mental Health Systems, 12*(1), 1–16. DOI: 10.1186/s13033-018-0208-0 PMID: 29881450

Tandon, S. D., Cluxton-Keller, F., Colon, L., Vega, P., & Alonso, A. (2013). Improved adequacy of prenatal care and healthcare utilization among low-income Latinas receiving group prenatal care. *Journal of Women's Health, 22*(12), 1056–1061. DOI: 10.1089/jwh.2013.4352 PMID: 24117000

Taylor, J., Novoa, C., Hamm, K., & Phadke, S. (2022, May 5). *Eliminating racial disparities in maternal and infant mortality*. Center for American Progress. https://www.americanprogress.org/article/eliminating-racial-disparities-maternal-infant-mortality/

Taylor, J. K. (2020). Structural racism and maternal health among Black women. *The Journal of Law, Medicine & Ethics, 48*(3), 506–517. DOI: 10.1177/1073110520958875 PMID: 33021163

Taylor, R. J., Chatters, L. M., & Joe, S. (2019). Social support networks and the mental health of Black mothers: A review of the literature. *Clinical Psychology Review, 69*, 116–127.

Teti, D. M., & Gelfand, D. M. (1991). Behavioral competence among mothers of infants in the first year: The mediational role of maternal self-efficacy. *Child Development, 62*(5), 918–929. DOI: 10.2307/1131143 PMID: 1756667

The National Campaign to Prevent Teen and Unplanned Pregnancy. (2021). *Texas data.* Power to Decide. https://thenationalcampaign.org/data/state/texas

The Texas Campaign to Prevent Teen Pregnancy. (2021a). *Teen birth in Texas.* https://txcampaign.org/research-data/teen-birth-in-texas/

The Texas Campaign to Prevent Teen Pregnancy. (2021b). *Disparities.* https://txcampaign.org/research-data/disparities/

Thomas, J. L., Carter, S. E., Schetter, C. D., & Sumner, J. A. (2021). Racial and ethnic disparities in posttraumatic psychopathology among postpartum women. *Journal of Psychiatric Research, 137*, 36–40. DOI: 10.1016/j.jpsychires.2021.02.030 PMID: 33647727

Thomas, M. P., Ammann, G., Brazier, E., Noyes, P., & Maybank, A. (2020). Doula services within a healthy start program: Increasing access for an underserved population. *Maternal and Child Health Journal, 24*(1), 76–83. PMID: 29198051

Thomas, T. L., Eberly, D., Smith, M. A., & Solis, J. M. (2019). Advancing health equity in public health systems. *Journal of Public Health Management and Practice, 25*(6), 563–569.

Thornicroft, G., Deb, T., & Henderson, C. (2016). Community mental health care worldwide: Current status and further developments. *World Psychiatry; Official Journal of the World Psychiatric Association (WPA), 15*(3), 276–286. DOI: 10.1002/wps.20349 PMID: 27717265

Thornton, A. C., & Chavkin, W. (2016). The role of midwives in reducing maternal and neonatal mortality in Haiti. *Journal of Midwifery & Women's Health, 61*(1), 71–77.

Thornton, R. L., Glover, C. M., Cené, C. W., Glik, D. C., Henderson, J. A., & Williams, D. R. (2017). Evaluating strategies for reducing health disparities by addressing the social determinants of health. *Health Affairs, 36*(6), 997–1004. PMID: 27503966

Tikkanen, R., Gunja, M., Fitzgerald, M., & Zephyrin, L. (2020, Nov 18). Maternal Mortality and Maternity Care in the United States Compared to 10 Other Developed Countries. https://www.commonwealthfund.org/publications/issue-briefs/2020/nov/maternal-mortality-maternity-care-us-compared-10-countries

Timmins, F., & Caldeira, S. (2017). Assessing the spiritual needs of patients. *Nursing Standard, 31*(29), 47–53. DOI: 10.7748/ns.2017.e10312 PMID: 28294021

Tindana, P. O., Singh, J. A., Tracy, C. S., Upshur, R. E. G., Daar, A. S., Singer, P. A., Frohlich, J., & Lavery, J. V. (2007). Grand challenges in global health: Community engagement in research in developing countries. *PLoS Medicine, 4*(9), e273. DOI: 10.1371/journal.pmed.0040273 PMID: 17850178

Toomey, R. B., Umaña-Taylor, A. J., Updegraff, K. A., & Jahromi, L. B. (2013). Ethnic identity development and ethnic discrimination: Examining longitudinal associations with adjustment for Mexican-origin adolescent mothers. *Journal of Adolescence, 36*(5), 825–833. DOI: 10.1016/j.adolescence.2013.06.004 PMID: 24011098

Trailhead Institute. (2023). *Restore: The Colorado blueprint for innovative public health workforce development*. https://trailhead.institute/wp-content/uploads/2023/05/Trailhead-CO-Blueprint-Report-Final-Web.pdf

Traylor, C. S., Johnson, J. D., Kimmel, M. C., & Manuck, T. A. (2020). Effects of psychological stress on adverse pregnancy outcomes and nonpharmacologic approaches for reduction: An expert review. *American Journal of Obstetrics & Gynecology MFM*, *2*(4), 100229. DOI: 10.1016/j.ajogmf.2020.100229 PMID: 32995736

Trends, C. (2020). Reimagining Black families' cultural assets can inform policies and practices that enhance their well-being. https://www.childtrends.org/publications/reimagining-black-families-cultural-assets-can-inform-policies-and-practices-that-enhance-their-well-being

Tsega, D., Admas, M., Talie, A., Tsega, T. B., Birhanu, M. Y., Alemu, S., & Mengist, B. (2022). Maternity continuum care completion and its associated factors in Northwest Ethiopia. *Journal of Pregnancy*, *2022*, 2022. DOI: 10.1155/2022/1309881 PMID: 35223099

Tuck, S. G., Summers, A. C., Bowie, J., Fife-Stallworth, D., Alston, C., Hayes, S., & Alexander, S. (2017). B'More Fit for Healthy Babies: Using Trauma-Informed Care Policies to Improve Maternal Health in Baltimore City. *Women's Health Issues*, *27*, S38–S45. DOI: 10.1016/j.whi.2017.09.002 PMID: 29050657

Tuohey, J. F. (1991, Dec). Terminal care and the pregnant woman: ethical reflections on In Re: A.C. *Pediatrics*, *88*(6), 1268–1273. DOI: 10.1542/peds.88.6.1268 PMID: 1956747

Turner, E. A. (2021). Building resilience in Black youth. *Psychology Today*. https://www.psychologytoday.com/us/blog/building-resilience-black-youth/202101/building-resilience-in-black-youth

Tyler, E. T. (2022). Black mothers matter: The social, political and legal determinants of Black maternal health across the lifespan. *Journal of Health Care Law & Policy*, *25*, 49.

University, S. C. (2021, May 4). Biases and System Failures Affecting U.S. Maternal Mortality. https://www.scu.edu/ethics/healthcare-ethics-blog/biases-and-system-failures-affecting-us-maternal-mortality/

US Department of Health and Human Services. (2023). Healthy Start Initiative: Eliminating disparities in perinatal health. Retrieved from https://www.hrsa.gov/grants/find-funding/HRSA-24-033

US Government Accountability Office (GAO). (2017). Women, Infants, and Children (WIC) Program: Action needed to address challenges in administering nutrition services and monitoring. *GAO-17-435*. https://www.gao.gov/products/gao-02-142

Versey, H. S., & Russell, C. N. (2023). The impact of COVID-19 and housing insecurity on lower-income Black women. *The Journal of Social Issues*, *79*(2), 773–793. DOI: 10.1111/josi.12555 PMID: 36711011

Vines, A. I., Baird, D. D., McNeilly, M., Hertz-Picciotto, I., Light, K. C., & Stevens, J. (2006). Social correlates of the chronic stress of perceived racism among Black women. *Ethnicity & Disease*, *16*, 101. DOI: 10.1016/j.eatdis.2006.01.009 PMID: 16599356

Vissing, H. (2024). *Somatic maternal healing: Psychodynamic and somatic trauma treatment for perinatal mental health.* Routledge.

Vohra-Gupta, S., Petruzzi, L., Jones, C., & Cubbin, C. (2023). An Intersectional Approach to Understanding Barriers to Healthcare for Women. *Journal of Community Health*, *48*(1), 89–98. DOI: 10.1007/s10900-022-01147-8 PMID: 36273069

Wainaina, C. W., Sidze, E. M., Maina, B. W., Badillo-Amberg, I., Anyango, H. O., Kathoka, F., Khasowa, D., & Okoror, C. E. (2021). Psychosocial challenges and individual strategies for coping with mental stress among pregnant and postpartum adolescents in Nairobi informal settlements: A qualitative investigation. *BMC Pregnancy and Childbirth*, *21*(1), 1–11. DOI: 10.1186/s12884-021-04128-2 PMID: 34583684

Walker, L. O., & Murry, N. (2022). Maternal stressors and coping strategies during the extended Postpartum Period: A retrospective analysis with contemporary implications. *Women's Health Reports (New Rochelle, N.Y.)*, *3*(1), 104–114. DOI: 10.1089/whr.2021.0134 PMID: 35136882

Walker, R. E., Keane, C. R., & Burke, J. G. (2010). Disparities and access to healthy food in the United States: A review of food deserts literature. *Health & Place*, *16*(5), 876–884. DOI: 10.1016/j.healthplace.2010.04.013 PMID: 20462784

Walker, R. E., Williams, J. H., & Egede, L. E. (2021). The impact of social determinants of health on Black maternal mental health. *Health Equity*, *5*(1), 56–62.

Wallace, M. E., Green, C., Richardson, L., Theall, K., & Crear-Perry, J. (2017). "Look at the whole me": A mixed-methods examination of Black infant mortality in the US through women's lived experiences and community context. *International Journal of Environmental Research and Public Health*, *14*(7), 727. DOI: 10.3390/ijerph14070727 PMID: 28678200

Walsh, T. B., Thomas, A., Quince, H., Buck, J., Tamkin, V., & Blackwell, D. (2023). Black fathers' contributions to maternal mental health. *Archives of Women's Mental Health*, *26*(1), 117–126. DOI: 10.1007/s00737-022-01284-y PMID: 36525158

Walter, A. W., Julce, C., Sidduri, N., Yinusa-Nyahkoon, L., Howard, J., Reichert, M., Bickmore, T., & Jack, B. W. (2020). Study protocol for the implementation of the Gabby Preconception Care System-an evidence-based, health information technology intervention for Black and African American women. *BMC Health Services Research, 20*(1), 1–14. DOI: 10.1186/s12913-020-05726-0 PMID: 32958031

Ward, E. C., Clark, L. O., & Heidrich, S. (2009). African American women's beliefs, coping behaviors, and barriers to seeking mental health services. *Qualitative Health Research, 19*(11), 1589–1601. DOI: 10.1177/1049732309350686 PMID: 19843967

Washington, H. A. (2006). *Medical apartheid: The dark history of medical experimentation on black Americans from colonial times to the present.* Doubleday Publishing Group.

Watson, H., Harrop, D., Walton, E., Young, A., & Soltani, H. (2019). A systematic review of ethnic minority women's experiences of perinatal mental health conditions and services in Europe. *PLoS One, 14*(1), 1–19. DOI: 10.1371/journal.pone.0210587 PMID: 30695019

Watson, N. N., & Hunter, C. D. (2015). Anxiety and depression among African American women: The costs of strength and negative attitudes toward psychological help-seeking. *Cultural Diversity & Ethnic Minority Psychology, 21*(4), 604–612. DOI: 10.1037/cdp0000015 PMID: 25602466

Weinstock, M. (2005). The potential influence of maternal stress hormones on development and mental health of the offspring. *Brain, Behavior, and Immunity, 19*(4), 296–308. DOI: 10.1016/j.bbi.2004.09.006 PMID: 15944068

Werchan, D. M., Hendrix, C. L., Ablow, J. C., Amstadter, A. B., Austin, A. C., Babineau, V., Anne Bogat, G., Cioffredi, L.-A., Conradt, E., Crowell, S. E., Dumitriu, D., Fifer, W., Firestein, M. R., Gao, W., Gotlib, I. H., Graham, A. M., Gregory, K. D., Gustafsson, H. C., Havens, K. L., & Brito, N. H. (2022). Behavioral coping phenotypes and associated psychosocial outcomes of pregnant and postpartum women during the COVID-19 pandemic. *Scientific Reports, 12*(1), 1209. DOI: 10.1038/s41598-022-05299-4 PMID: 35075202

Williams, D. R., & Mohammed, S. A. (2013). Racism and health I: Pathways and scientific evidence. *The American Behavioral Scientist, 57*(8), 1152–1173. DOI: 10.1177/0002764213487340 PMID: 24347666

Wiltz, T. (2015, Mar 3). *Racial, ethnic disparities persist in teen pregnancy rates.* The PEW Charitable Trusts. https://www.pewtrusts.org/en/research-and-analysis/blogs/stateline/2015/3/03/racial-and-ethnic-disparities-persist-in-teen-pregnancy-rates

Winters, L. I., & Winters, P. C. (2012). Black teenage pregnancy. *A Dynamic. SAGE Open*, *2*(1), 2158244012436563. Advance online publication. DOI: 10.1177/2158244012436563

Wisner, K. L., Sit, D. K. Y., McShea, M. C., Rizzo, D. M., Zoretich, R. A., Hughes, C. L., Eng, H. F., Luther, J. F., Wisniewski, S. R., Costantino, M. L., Confer, A. L., Moses-Kolko, E. L., Famy, C. S., & Hanusa, B. H. (2013). Onset Timing, Thoughts of Self-harm, and Diagnoses in Postpartum Women With Screen-Positive Depression Findings. *JAMA Psychiatry*, *70*(5), 490–498. DOI: 10.1001/jamapsychiatry.2013.87 PMID: 23487258

Witcraft, S. M., Johnson, E., Eitel, A. E., Moreland, A. D., King, C., Terplan, M., & Guille, C. (2024). Listening to Black Pregnant and Postpartum People: Using Technology to Enhance Equity in Screening and Treatment of Perinatal Mental Health and Substance Use Disorders. *Journal of Racial and Ethnic Health Disparities*. DOI: 10.1007/s40615-024-01989-z PMID: 38605223

Women of Color Network. (2006). *Domestic violence.* Women of Color Network Facts and Stats Collection: Communities of Color. https://www.doj.state.or.us/wp-content/uploads/2017/08/women_of_color_network_facts_domestic_violence_2006.pdf

Womersley, K., Ripullone, K., & Hirst, J. E. (2021). Tackling inequality in maternal health: Beyond the postpartum. *Future Healthcare Journal*, *8*(1), 31–35. DOI: 10.7861/fhj.2020-0275 PMID: 33791457

Woodhead, S., Marley, C., Calia, C., Guerra, C., Reid, C., Burke, J. P., & Amos, A. (2023). Maternal Mental Health in Sub-Saharan Africa: A Systematic Review of Interventions for Common Perinatal Mental Health Disorders.

Woods-Giscombé, C. L., Lobel, M., Zimmer, C., Wiley Cené, C., & Corbie-Smith, G. (2015). Whose stress is making me sick? Network-stress and emotional distress in African-American women. *Issues in Mental Health Nursing*, *36*(9), 710–717. DOI: 10.3109/01612840.2015.1011759 PMID: 26440874

Woods-Giscombe, C. L., Williams, K. P., Conklin, J., Dodd, A., Bravo, L., Anderson, A. M., & Hood, D. B. (2023). A scoping review of the concept of resilience among African American women. *Archives of psychiatric nursing*, 46, 107-120. DOI: 10.1016/j.apnu.2023.04.008

Woolhouse, H., Gartland, D., Mensah, F., & Brown, S. (2015). Maternal depression from early pregnancy to 4 years postpartum in a prospective pregnancy cohort study: Implications for primary health care. *BJOG*, *122*(3), 312–321. DOI: 10.1111/1471-0528.12837 PMID: 24844913

World Health Organization. (2013). Investing in mental health: Evidence for action. https://www.who.int/mental_health/en/

Wright, P. M. (2020). Perinatal loss and spirituality: A metasynthesis of qualitative research. *Illness, Crises, and Loss*, *28*(2), 99–118. DOI: 10.1177/1054137317698660

Yakovi Gan-Or, N. (2020, Oct 6). Going solo: The law and ethics of childbirth during the COVID-19 pandemic. *Journal of Law and the Biosciences*, *7*(1), lsaa079. DOI: 10.1093/jlb/lsaa079 PMID: 33235802

Yang, M., Li, L., Zhu, H., Alexander, I. M., Liu, S., Zhou, W., & Ren, X. (2009). Music Therapy To Relieve Anxiety In Pregnant Women On Bedrest: A Randomized, Controlled Trial. *MCN. The American Journal of Maternal Child Nursing*, *34*(5), 316–323. DOI: 10.1097/01.NMC.0000360425.52228.95 PMID: 19713801

Yehudah, S., & Tadros, E. (2022). Counseling advocacy: Seeking justice for black birth equity. *Journal of Counselor Leadership and Advocacy*, *9*(1), 3–20. DOI: 10.1080/2326716X.2021.2018067

Zelon, H. L., Forray, A., Knudson-Martin, C., & Johnson, S. M. (2021). Transforming perinatal bereavement care: A qualitative study of a trauma-informed group intervention. *Journal of Social Work in End-of-Life & Palliative Care*, *17*(3), 261–278. DOI: 10.1080/15524256.2021.1969292

Zigmond, A. S., & Snaith, R. P. (1983). The hospital anxiety and depression scale. *Acta Psychiatrica Scandinavica*, *67*(6), 361–370. DOI: 10.1111/j.1600-0447.1983.tb09716.x PMID: 6880820

About the Contributors

Rahmatu Kassimu, also known as Dr. K., is a dynamic figure in education, public health, and motivation. With a rich background as an educator, researcher, public health consultant, and change agent, she has spent the past decade empowering students and educators to advocate for themselves on their educational journeys. Dr. Kassimu's diverse educational background, spanning Sociology, Public Health, Health Studies, and Educational Leadership, fuels her passion for education, improved quality of life, and enhanced health equity. Her platform, Dr. K.'s Health Minute, delivers courses, academic writing coaching, and accessible health and wellness information, driven by her commitment to reduce health disparities, promote health equity, enhance health literacy, and expand academic opportunities. Her publications include recommendations and best practices in mental health, Black maternal health, and health inequities.

Elizabeth Wachira is an Associate Professor at East Texas A&M Commerce and Public Health program director. Her research aims to understand the often-covert pathways of oppression and injustices that marginalized populations face. She aims to inform and expand authentic, lived-experienced knowledge on health vulnerabilities as determinants of health among marginalized individuals. As an educator, through service-learning, her students do a community needs assessment to implement initiatives that have community impact, such as a peer led mental health promotion program for campus students.

***

Amutah-Onukagha is the Julia A. Okoro Professor of Black Maternal Health in the Department of Public Health and Community Medicine at Tufts University School of Medicine. Her current research interests include maternal health disparities, reproductive health and social justice, infant mortality, and HIV/

AIDS in Black women. Dr. Amutah-Onukagha also serves as the inaugural Assistant Dean of Diversity, Equity, and Inclusion for Public Health and Professional Degree Programs. In 2022 Dr. Amutah-Onukagha founded the Center for Black Maternal Health and Reproductive Justice (CBMHRJ) at Tufts University School of Medicine and is one of the first centers dedicated nationwide to addressing maternal health inequities. Ndidiamaka is the Principal Investigator of two multi-year studies on maternal mortality and morbidity, an R01 funded by the National Institutes of Health and an interdisciplinary grant on health equity funded by the Robert Wood Johnson Foundation. Additionally, she is a member of the MA-COVID 19 Maternal Equity Coalition and was honored with the American Public Health Association's Maternal and Child Health Section's Young Professional of the Year Award in 2019. She is in the 2020-2021 class of the top 40 under 40 Minority Leaders in Healthcare, an annual award given out by the National Minority Quality Forum. Ndidiamaka is a life-long member of the American Public Health Association and is currently the co-chair of the Perinatal and Women's Health committee in the Maternal and Child Health section. Dr. Amutah-Onukagha also serves on the editorial board for the Journal of Women's Health Issues, and as a board member for the Neighborhood Birth Center in Boston, and the National Women's Health Network. Dr. Amutah-Onukagha is the Founder and Director of the Maternal Outcomes for Translational Health Equity Research (MOTHER) Lab, a research lab with a keen interest in reducing maternal health disparities as experienced by Black women. A well-published author, Dr. Amutah-Onukagha has over 70 manuscripts, 6 book chapters, a best-selling book on Amazon, and a textbook on culturally responsive evaluation. Her research has also been featured across a series of platforms, including, The Lancet, TedX, USA Today, and MSNBC. She also serves on the editorial board for the Journal of Women's Health Issues.She lives in MA with her husband and two sons.

Vickie Dugat is a Maternal and Child Health Postdoctoral Fellow at the Center of Excellence in Maternal and Child Health. She earned her Ph.D. in Health Education from the University of Toledo with a concentration in Maternal and Child Health and Diversity. She earned her Bachelor of Science degree from the University of Florida in Family, Youth, and Community Sciences and her Master's in Public Health from Morehouse School of Medicine. Her research interests include exclusive breastfeeding, racial and ethnic health disparities, and stressful life events during pregnancy. She has also taught undergraduate public health courses and served as a certified Diversity Ambassador for the School of Population Health at the University of Toledo. As a first- generation Haitian American and college graduate, she aims to aid in reducing breastfeeding disparities in underrepresented populations and advance the overall health of mothers.

Jennifer Edwards has a passion for service and energizing organizations. She has expert-level capability in actionable strategy, optimizing programs, and convenings. Throughout her career, Jennifer has had an opportunity to lead US Centers for Disease Control, US Department of Labor, and Health Resources and Services Administration federally funded grant programs. She has also managed Susan G. Komen, American Psychological Association, and Robert Wood Johnson Foundation-funded national nonprofit projects. She received National Institutes of Health-funded training, and wrote U.S. presidential appointee testimony submitted to the Congressional Record, and has served as a committee co-chair for a World Health Organization (WHO) non-state actor. Jennifer served on undergraduate public health and graduate health administration faculty for 10 years. She also designed and curated the Maternal & Mental Community Health Worker Training Program™ hosted by Renewell Foundation. The Amazon best-selling author has served as a reviewer for five national journals including Public Health Reports, the peer-reviewed journal of the U.S. Surgeon General's Office. As a fourth generation entrepreneur, she's also a graduate of the Nasdaq Milestones Program and a member of the Forbes BLK Community. By invitation, the Grow with Google™ Co-Host and invited TEDx™ speaker activates audiences on resilience and strategy topics. Jennifer earned a Ph.D. from Howard University, an MBA from Walden University, and a B.S. from Florida A&M University. She lives in the Dallas area with her family and enjoys hiking, trails, gardening, and yoga.

Chinonye "Chi Chi" Egbulem, PMP, MSW/MPH, LCSWA is a Behavioral Health and Change Management Consultant with over 10 years of global experience as a public health social worker. Drawing from her deep roots in social justice, somatic healing, and systems transformation, Chi Chi empowers individuals and communities through trauma-informed care, inclusive policy design, and holistic wellness practices. She is the founder of BLOOMWELL HEALTH, where she integrates research, technology, and community-centered approaches to address youth development, mental wellness, and economic empowerment—particularly in low- and middle-income communities. A certified Full Spectrum Doula, she centers body-based healing in her advocacy for child and family wellbeing. Chi Chi currently serves as a Guest Researcher at the CDC, exploring the effectiveness of violence response programming for children. Her career spans roles with the CDC, NIH, UNC School of Medicine, and Baltimore VA, with a strong focus on reproductive health, injury prevention, and gender-based violence. She holds DEI certifications from Cornell University and the University of South Florida, and is a Project Management Professional (PMP) with dual master's degrees in Public Health and Social Work. A Nigerian-American and former Peace Corps volunteer, Chi Chi brings a global, embodied lens to mental health, organizational wellbeing, and community resilience.

Tyra Gravesande is a passionate Research Assistant at the MOTHER Lab, serving on the Research and Grants Committee. She earned her BA in Comparative Women's Studies from Spelman College and is pursuing an MS in Bioethics at Clarkson University. Tyra's focus on feminist theory, women's health inequities, and the intersections of gender, race, and health drive her commitment to examining healthcare policies through a social justice lens. As a board member of the National Women's Health Network, she has honed her leadership through programs at Harvard Business School and Management Leadership for Tomorrow.

Aliyu Tijani Jibril, As a PhD in Nutritional Sciences graduate, I am committed to delivering responsive, top-notch services. Throughout my academic journey, I have engaged in practical projects and teamwork activities that have highlighted my exceptional strengths in research, analysis, leadership, and troubleshooting complex problems. My ability to adapt quickly to changes, coupled with a strong passion for learning and expanding my capabilities, makes me an outstanding candidate. With my skills and experience, I am confident in my ability to contribute significantly to any organization.

Solimar Santiago-Warner, DSW, LCSW, PMH-C, is a perinatal mental health therapist, grief educator, and founder of Solmaterna Psychotherapy & Consulting. She specializes in supporting BIPOC birthing people through perinatal loss, reproductive trauma, and identity transitions, offering trauma-informed, culturally responsive, and justice-centered care. With clinical roots in the NICU, PICU, obstetrics, and perinatal palliative care, her work focuses on the intersection of perinatal mental health and grief. Dr. Santiago-Warner teaches at NYU, Manhattan University, and with the Zelda Foster Studies in Palliative and End-of-Life Care, where she mentors social workers and advises doctoral students. Her scholarship centers on perinatal palliative care, embodied grief, reproductive justice, and the neurobiology of trauma. She has published on perinatal palliative social work and culturally grounded grief practices, and co-led the needs assessment group for the National Coalition for Hospice and Palliative Care's Pediatric Palliative Care Task Force..

Lena Sharara was born in Egypt and spent her early childhood in Khartoum, Sudan before moving to Pittsburgh, Pennsylvania. She now resides in Boston, where she's pursuing a Master's of Public Health at Tufts University School of Medicine. Driven by a passion for addressing maternal health disparities, Lena aims to become an OB/GYN, integrating cultural competence into her practice. She is an EMT, student leader, and researcher at the MOTHER Lab (Maternal Outcomes for Translational Health Equity Research Lab), committed to improving healthcare access in underrepresented communities. At the MOTHER Lab, Lena serves as Co-chair of the Community Engagement, Advocacy, and Policy Committee and produces The MOTHER Lab podcast.

Arika Wiggins, PhD, LMSW, is an assistant professor at Southeast Missouri State University. She teaches in the Department of Criminal Justice, Social Work, and Sociology. Prior to joining the CJSWS department at Southeast, Dr. Wiggins practiced social work for 11 years, starting as a Licensed Bachelor Social Worker (LBSW), and with most of her practice experience as a Licensed Master Social Worker (LMSW). Dr. Wiggins worked with children, youth, and families in the child protective services domain, older adults and adults with disabilities in nursing homes and assisted living facilities, and hospice care. Dr. Wiggins' research interests are qualitative methods focusing on various traumas, the social determinants of health and mental health disparities and service provision for underserved populations.

Farida N. YADA, MPH, is an international scholar from Burkina Faso (West Africa). She obtained her doctorate in Health Services Research and Master of Public Health at the University of North Carolina at Charlotte. Her research interests include disparities in Maternal and Child Health outcomes and Global Health. More specifically, her research focuses on the reproductive health disparities experienced by Black/African American women, sub-Saharan African immigrant women living outside of Africa, and the reproductive health outcomes of sub-Saharan African women living in Africa.

Index

A

B

C

D

P

R

www.ingramcontent.com/pod-product-compliance
Lightning Source LLC
LaVergne TN
LVHW081338300926
849161LV00008B/2008

* 9 7 9 8 3 6 9 3 4 2 7 2 5 *